The Parent's Guide
Natural Health Care for
CHILDREN

1.50

The Parent's Guide to Natural Health Care for

CHILDREN

How to raise happy, healthy children from birth to 15

KAREN SULLIVAN

Foreword by

Dr. Paula Elbirt, M.D.

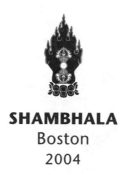

SHAMBHALA
Boston
2004

This book is dedicated to the people who matter most: my grandfather, Grant Brown; my parents, Paul and Judy Hurrell; and my reason for doing it all—my children, Cole and Luke.

Shambhala Publications, Inc.
Horticultural Hall
300 Massachusetts Avenue
Boston, Massachusetts 02115
www.shambhala.com

Copyright © 2002, 2004 by Karen Sullivan
First Published in the United Kingdom by Piatkus Books 2000
First published in Canada by Key Porter Books Limited, Toronto, Canada 2002
First published in the United States by Shambhala Publications, 2004

9 8 7 6 5 4 3 2 1

First Shambhala Edition

Printed in the United States of America

❂ This edition is printed on acid-free paper that meets the American National Standards Institute Z39.48 Standard.
Distributed in the United States by Random House, Inc.

Library of Congress-in-Publication Data
Sullivan, Karen.
The parent's guide to natural health care for children: how to raise happy, healthy children from birth to 15/Karen Sullivan; foreword by Paula Elbirt.—1st Shambhala ed.
p. cm.
Earier British ed. published as: Natural healthcare for children. London: Piatkus, 2000.
Earlier Canadian ed. published as: Complete guide to natural health care for children. Toronto: Sarasota Press, c2002.
Includes index.
ISBN 1-59030-107-2 (pbk.: alk. paper)
1. Pediatrics. 2. Naturopathy. 3. Children—Diseases—Alternative treatment I. Sullivan, Karen. Natural healthcare for children. II. Sullivan, Karen. Complete guide to natural health care for children. III. Title.
RJ47.S84 2004
618.92—dc22
2003059111

Contents

Foreword vii

Acknowledgments ix

Part One: Holistic Health for Body, Mind, and Spirit

1 Natural Nutrition 3

2 The Modern Child's Diet 44

3 When Food Becomes a Problem 59

4 Healthy Eating from Day One 76

5 Fit for Life 97

6 And So to Bed 114

7 A Natural Environment 140

8 The Key to Happiness: Emotional Health 168

Part Two: Illness and Natural Health

9 Understanding Illness 201

10 Natural Therapies for Children 232

Part Three: Natural Treatments for Common Ailments

Treating Common Health Issues 297

Appendix 1: Keeping Your Child Safe 399

Appendix 2: Vitamins and Minerals 434

Resources 438

Notes 450

Index 456

Foreword

··

The march of time never seems faster than when we examine it in the moment. This observation seems most true whenever the subject of child care and parenting philosophies are examined. Indeed, we live in speedy times and our concerns for the impact this pace is having on the development of our precious children is both warranted and real.

We live in a time of paradox. Never before has the disparity between what we know and what we can apply been so great. Technology has driven forward while our wisdom may not have had the chance to get its arms around this progress in time to sanely direct it. Into this broad chasm between reason and progress has fallen one of the most basic of man's tasks. It is widely believed that there has never been a better or worse time for raising children. Detractors grimly point at the myriad risks of toxic exposures, actual and metaphorical, that bombard our offspring via computer electronics, a diverse range of media, and through the chemically and genetically modified foods we feed them. They rightfully direct our attention to the apparent increase in diagnoses of neurologic malfunction such as learning disabilities, pervasive developmental disorders and the patently terrifying implications of a downwards shift in the average age of pubertal onset making itself apparent in female children in developing nations.

The optimists point instead to the decreasing health risks from common infectious diseases as the result of better medical diagnosis and the pharmaceuticals and vaccines that are so accessible to all of us, even to those living at or below the poverty level. They direct our attention at the advances in early childhood education and the research that has uncovered for us what we may have once known but since forgotten: that native intelligence can be nurtured from the earliest hours of life with substantial differences in outcome depending on what we put into the process.

The debate between champions of today's parenting styles and detractors who fear the outcomes of our errors in this arena is also fast and furious, and often so torched by passion the ordinary parent is inclined to shut it out all together. We all too often hold our collective breaths as our children move on, often mostly unguided.

What is needed are fair and balanced guides. Works that cut through bias and supposition to provide us with solid information that we can use to make the individual choices we are ultimately left to make on our own. Karen Sullivan's comprehensive work *The Complete Guide to Natural Health Care for Children* provides just that opportunity. Culling through the vast plains of information to present only what is substantiable and of reasonable source, Karen Sullivan allows us to face the difficult choices we parents have to make with regards to our children's welfare in an orderly, and intellectually sane manner. Often not taking a specific stance, this work leaves us better prepared to understand the potential ramifications of both sides of health related choices for our precious charges. Unintimidated by unconventional approaches to health care, yet fully respectful of the advantages borne by some of technology's medical marvels, this work presents what is so vitally needed—choice in daylight, rather than the murky darkness of ignorance when information is blighted by bias and paranoia.

For the past twenty years in pediatric practice and medical teaching I have watched as parents from all walks of life sincerely struggle towards a better future for their children. As the medical director for the Children's Aid Society I have learned that neither economic class nor level of education can divert parents from their determined efforts to seek the best for their children. It would be a precious and much needed gift for all parents and practitioners of child health care to take the messages within this volume to heart and mind. To treasure the vastness of our accumulated knowledge over the ages and pay due honor to the awesome wonder of tomorrow's children is our most glorious duty. With the wisdoms shared within these pages parents can begin to move through this with comfort and clarity, both so desperately needed.

—Dr. Paula M. Elbirt, M.D.

Paula M. Elbirt has spent the majority of her career in private practice and in medical school teaching positions. Trained in Philadelphia and New York City she is a certified pediatrician who appears regularly on talk shows, news reports, and in magazine articles. She is the author of *Dr. Paula's Good Nutrition Guide for Babies, Toddlers, and Preschoolers: Answers to Parents' Most Common Questions Plus Help for Coping with Fussy Eaters* as well as *Dr. Paula's House Calls to Your Newborn*.

Dr. Elbirt's work with the American Academy of Pediatrics helped establish their Steering Committee on Media and Children and the AAP's Media Resources Team in New York City. Elbirt also runs *www.myfavoritepediatrician.com*, a pediatric advice website that helps parents learn more and deal better with the vital job of raising our children.

Acknowledgments

A great deal of research has gone into the making of this book, and I have called upon the expertise and resources of more people than I could possibly mention here. Special thanks are due, however, to Melanie Woollcombe, homeopath and friend, who acted as a sounding board for many of my ideas, a library for my constant need for material, and a fact-checker when I needed it most. Thanks also to Giles Davies, Tricia Allen, Dr. Charles Fairhurst, Chuck Spezzano, Dr. Hilary Jones, Paul Shattock of the Autism Research Unit at the University of Sunderland, Ann Coote and Jackie Fletcher of JABS, Simply Organic, Child Nutrition Research Center in the U.S., Institute of Food Research, Flower Essence Society, The Pesticides Trust, Health Canada, Food Allergy Network, Homeopathic Educational Service, Feng Shui Association, American Music Therapy Association, Royal Society for the Prevention of Accidents and RoSPA Road Safety, National Society for the Prevention of Cruelty to Children, Institute of Complementary Medicine in the U.K., NAPS, Association of Reflexologists, the Health Development Agency (formerly the HEA), Massage for Therapy Council and the Soil Association. Thank you to Dr. Michael Apple and Dr. Margaret DeJong for checking this book thoroughly for possible errors or misinterpretation!

Big thanks go to Piatkus Books, for their (instant) belief in this project and their determination to make it the best book possible. Thanks to Gill Bailey, Rachel Winning and Judy Piatkus in London for showing faith. And thanks are also due to Clare McKeon and Linda Pruessen at Key Porter in Toronto, who embraced this project with such insight and enthusiasm.

On a personal level, I would like to thank everyone who put up with my enthusiasm (obsession) with the subject for seven long months (and a lot longer before that), as well as my inability to focus on anything other than the book for just as long! Thanks, then, to Mel, Gill Paul, Katja Moegel, Debbie and Malcolm Gill, Tracey

Lawrie (who let me try out my ideas on her brand-new baby), Lisa McGown, Elaine Gawin, Phyll, Chris and Mrs. T. Final thanks to the kids who put up with my experiments: Ralph, Rowan, Fergus, Eleanor Daisy, Kyla, Tristyn and, of course, my own two extremely patient children, Cole and Luke, who gave up an awful lot of holidays and Pokémon trading sessions to allow me to finish this on time.

Part One
Holistic Health for Body, Mind, and Spirit

chapter one

Natural Nutrition

···

What our children eat will affect the rest of their lives. If it sounds like an exaggeration, consider this: almost all cancers are linked in some way to nutrition. So are fertility, heart disease, immune function, mental prowess, weight, the health of our bones and teeth, allergies and, of course, well-being.

As parents we spend a great deal of time and energy choosing schools for our children. We take them to swimming lessons or other activities, and we worry about their illnesses, any problems they might be having with friends, and their future. It's natural to want the very best for our children, but many of us neglect one of the areas that can affect our children's future the very most—what they eat.

All of us know children who seem to live on canned spaghetti and air. Others have a diet that seems to consist of nothing more than milk and toast with jam. They look healthy enough, and seem to be thriving. So what's in this nutrition business? It's difficult to be concerned about diet when a child is growing well, is happy at school and seems content.

Why is nutrition important?

There are many reasons why nutrition is important, and they fall into three obvious categories: the present, the future and then beyond. Let's look at them in detail.

There's no question that many children are picky, picky eaters, and mealtimes can be a nightmare. It's also fairly obvious that, in a busy day, battling with a stubborn child about food is a stress that most of us can do without. The result? Children often win, and with the advertising to which they come into contact, and peer pressure, it's not surprising that what they want is not always what they should be having.

Think of it this way: we are responsible for growing our children. We must ensure that they get everything they need in order to grow up strong and healthy. At no other time in their lives do humans grow and develop more quickly than they do as children. Everything children eat contributes to that growth and development, and lays the foundation for their future, and for their own children's future. It affects their emotions, their ability to concentrate, to ward off illness, to play sports, to grow and to develop into happy, healthy adults.

Giving in to junk food and fads might seem like a short-term solution, and we can argue that they will eat well when they are old enough to understand why nutrition is important. After all, we were picky eaters and we are perfectly healthy, right?

Wrong. Chances are that our diet was much better than that of our children. Most of us were exposed to only a small percentage of the chemicals that now make up the vast majority of the foods we buy and eat. Processed and fast-food sales have increased by over 100 percent over the past two decades, which means that they are forming an ever-increasing proportion of our diet. So our children are at a disadvantage to begin with. We've adopted a peculiar diet where children's food has become an entity of its own. In many cases, we don't eat children's food, and they don't eat ours. Any niggling worries we might have about our children's diet is silenced by the fact that the freezer sections of every supermarket are filled with animal-shaped, cartoon-colored kiddy offerings that everyone buys. Everyone buys it, everyone eats it, so it's easy to turn a blind eye. There is some comfort in numbers.

But bad diets don't just change overnight. There is overwhelming evidence that people who develop poor eating habits as children will continue to eat inadequately later in life, so we are doing our children no favors if we serve them unhealthy food. The majority of foods aimed at children are high in sugar and fat. Younger children tend to burn off the excess calories, but when they become less active as young adults, such a diet will lead to the children's being overweight and the health problems that go with it. There are also a host of diseases linked with the Western diet, and they can affect our children now and later.

Most of us remember the overcooked meat, potatoes and two soggy vegetables that formed the basis of our diets as children. In contrast, our own children's food looks magnificently more edible—pizzas, burgers, chips with a brightly colored splash of ketchup, chicken nuggets (shaped as dinosaurs and cartoon characters no less), 30 different flavors of chips, cakes and cookies of every variety and neat little pots of yogurt with candies to put on top. But despite the appeal of this food, the problem is pretty clear—the manufacturers invested a great deal of money into making it all attractive. That's what we are paying for. In reality, the food our children eat has little nutritional value and, even worse, it takes the place of food that would actually do their bodies and minds some good.

The wide variety of foods now available has broadened our diets enormously, but has the way we eat changed for the better? Not according to recent research. According to the USDA, 50 percent of us don't eat a single piece of fruit a day, and only 23 percent of Americans manage to eat the daily recommendation of five portions of fruit and vegetables. Some eat none at all. If we're not eating well, it's unlikely that our children are faring any better. In fact, only 9 percent of American children aged six to eleven eat the recommended five-a-day of fruits and vegetables. Pop, cakes, cookies, candies and popsicles edge out fruit and vegetable consumption by a wide margin.

The point that needs to be made to all parents is that poor nutrition has a dramatic effect. Let's look at the short-term effects first.

The short-term effects of poor nutrition

- The incidence of overweight among children in all age categories has more than doubled since the 1970s, with the greatest increase in the past decade. Over the past 30 years, obesity in children has more than doubled. In the U.S., 21 percent of children are considered obese, and in the U.K. a recent study suggests that 14 percent of primary school children are overweight. That number increases dramatically as children hit their teens. By adolescence, overweight kids have a 70 to 80 percent chance of carrying extra weight into their adult years. Quite apart from the serious health risks, obese children face social discrimination in a (wrongly) thin-oriented culture.

- One in six teenagers shows significant early signs of heart disease, with plaque growing on at least one artery wall. In other words, they have heart disease to such an extent that there is a real threat of heart attack—before the age of 20.

- Learning difficulties? Diet may be the cause. A 1995 study showed that pupils showed a rise of between 1 and 15 IQ points after beginning a program that eliminated sugar and refined foods.

- Behavior, learning and health problems were compared between boys with high and low intakes of essential fatty acids (see page 12). More behavioral problems were found in those with low omega-3 intakes, and more learning and health problems were found in those with lower omega-6 intakes.

- It is estimated that 3–4 percent of children in primary school have severe iron-deficiency anemia. In the 18-month to 2½ year bracket, the number increases to 1 in 8 toddlers. A far greater number of children most likely have mild forms of iron deficiency. Low blood iron levels translate to poor school performance for many of these children. Studies link low iron levels to decreased attention and concentration, irritability, low IQ tests (especially in vocabulary), perceptual difficulties and low achievement.

- There is compelling evidence that undernutrition during any period of childhood can have detrimental effects on the cognitive development of children and their later productivity as adults. When children eat poorly, they do not develop at normal rates, and some fail to develop normally at all.

- Children who are deficient in just one or two key nutrients can show symptoms that will affect their development and their school work. For example, a shortage of B vitamins can translate as fatigue, listlessness, moodiness and even attention problems. The B vitamins are crucial to the development of a healthy nervous system, and long-term deficiency (even mild deficiency) can lead to depression and neurological problems, among other things. A shortage of vitamin C can result in an impaired immune system, constipation and bleeding gums. A low calcium intake will affect bones and teeth, and cause muscle cramping and poor growth. Most of the "children's food" is deficient in these nutrients.

The longer-term effects of poor nutrition

- A joint report by the World Cancer Research Fund (WCRF) and the American Institute for Cancer Research (AICR) claims that 30–40 percent of cancers may be caused by dietary factors. For example, breast cancer, the number-one killer among women aged 35–54, could be triggered early in life from an unhealthy diet, and 30 percent of tumors in the prostate and colon are associated with nutrition.

- According to a study published in *The Lancet*, average sperm count in Britain fell from a high of 113 million per milliliter in 1940 to 66 million in 1990. In the U.S., the National Institutes of Health confirmed that sperm count is dropping by an average of 1.5 percent every year. If this trend continues, we can expect infertility to become a mass epidemic by the middle of the 21st century. A huge number of studies show that nutrition is the main cause, with estrogens in the water, our food and the environment playing havoc with male fertility. Men with low vitamin C also have a markedly increased likelihood of genetic damage to their sperm. It may sound ludicrous to be concerned about the future fertility of a toddler, but it is an issue that could dramatically affect the later lives of our children.

- Heart disease is the number-one killer in the Western world. Apart from smoking and lack of exercise, the main cause is diet. More than 20 percent of children already show some signs of heart disease, which means that the problems are beginning long before they make their own choices about food.

- Osteoporosis (thinning of the bones) is a condition that normally affects the elderly, but studies show that low bone mass (bones that are not strong enough) may be caused by a high intake of carbonated soft drinks, which rob the body of the minerals necessary for bone health, and seem to have taken the place of milk in many diets. And not just in the future—experts suggest that not only will the incidence of osteoporosis increase in our children, but they will and do suffer more bone fractures now as a result of their diet. If you want your children's bones to last their lifetime, their diet—in particular, their calcium intake—must be changed.

■ Apart from the fact that processed foods have little nutritional value, they also contain a huge number of chemicals, the effects of which are only just beginning to be made clear. Many additives have now been banned, but some—particularly tartrazine or E102—have been linked to hyperactivity in children, allergies, asthma, migraines and even cancer. Scientists are also investigating a possible link between aspartame (found in low-calorie drinks) and changes in brain function. Caffeine is linked to peptic ulcers, insomnia, nervousness and birth defects. Although all additives go through rigorous testing, in combination they may prove to be a deadly cocktail (see page 73). Most of the chemicals in our foods are "anti-nutrients" in that they stop nutrients from being absorbed and used. These crucial nutrients are the same ones that keep our children healthy, encourage healthy development and growth, and prevent illnesses such as cancer and heart disease, among other things.

And the future?

Chemicals in our food and environment generate "free radicals," which are capable of causing cancer and many other diseases. The only known natural defenses against free radicals are the antioxidant nutrients (see page 284), vitamins A, C and E and beta-carotene, and the mineral selenium, now dangerously deficient in the Western diet. Unless we eat sufficient quantities of fresh fruit, vegetables and whole, unrefined foods we will, unquestionably, not get enough to prevent cancer and other diseases. Even more worrying, perhaps, is the fact that free radicals can cause cell mutation (changes in our cells) that can be passed on to our children and our children's children. What does that mean in the long term? If our genes, which carry the information that determines how our cells are formed, become damaged, our children's own children could be born with birth defects and have a higher chance of getting cancer and other conditions that are now being linked to genes.

What's going wrong?

We've never had it so good. We have choice and variety and dozens of different means by which to cook our food. Supermarkets are big business and consumers have more power than ever before. Look at the organic revolution—according to Minnesota-based Organic Consumers Association, 10 million families in the United States are buying organic food each week, and that number has increased by 25 percent every year in the last decade. This year, grocery stores across the U.S. will sell $10 billion in organic food, about 2 percent of all food sales. Change is afoot because consumers are becoming educated about nutrition and taking a stand on the issues. We are literally voting with our feet, and we have the power to see that our demands are met.

That's all good news. So what's the problem?

Lack of time

Our eating habits have changed dramatically over the past decades. We might be demanding organic produce and GM-free food (food free of genetically modified ingredients), but we are also insisting upon ready-prepared meals and a wide variety of processed goodies that look delicious and will appeal to picky eaters. If you've got two kids hanging on the cart at the supermarket and you have to collect a third from hockey practice in 20 minutes, you are unlikely to find the time to read the labels or to plan family meals. You choose the quick-fix solution that you know the kids will eat, and you buy a selection of different meals to prepare for yourself. Everyone needs a break in our overscheduled lives, and one of the easiest ways to save time is to cut corners on the food front. But it's a false economy and, in the long run, everyone suffers.

Kids' food

We no longer eat with our children on a regular basis. Obviously one or more parents returning home late from work precludes the idea of a 5 o'clock sit-down family dinner, but we've taken it one step further. In the majority of families, children eat on their own. Because we believe that they are unlikely to want to eat what Daddy and/or Mommy are eating later, they are given kids' food—in other words, food that they will eat, even if it is much the same fare every single day. It's an impossible pressure on most parents to produce two wholesome, separate meals every day, and rather than even try, we choose the easy option and give the kids something quick and, very often, canned or frozen.

There should be no such thing as "kids' food." Children won't grow up to enjoy a wide variety of foods or have a clue about nutrition if they are fed the same, unhealthy foods every day.

Children learn what they live

Once upon a time, children were given the best bits of meat or vegetables or, if food was scarce, some of their parents' portions. Growing children do, after all, need good food in their bellies, was the reasoning. That "once upon a time" wasn't so very long ago either. Most of our parents will remember being the priority at the dinner table. Things are quite different now. We seem to believe that feeding children good food is a waste of money, and that it is unappreciated. What's the point of preparing nutritious stews, soups and fish dishes if they pick at them and squeal that their best friends have chicken nuggets *whenever* they want them? It's a curious state of affairs. You've seen it before—a summer barbecue with hot dogs and potato chips for the kids and steaks and salad for the adults. All of us need good food, but none more than children, who are growing and developing so dramatically. As for appreciation, children learn what they live. If they are given bland, boring food every day, that's what they'll come to expect. Children don't appreciate food the way adults do. They eat to live and they eat because they are hungry. They'll never feel privileged or grateful if they are given an expensive piece of fish, and nor should they. Good eating should become a way of life for children just as it is for any adult.

Peer pressure

Pop culture has taken over. Rather than be seen as parents who stick out their necks, we feed the kids what their friends are eating because they don't want to be different. The average child watches somewhere in the region of 20,000 television commercials each year, many of which are for food products. They know what they want, and so do their friends, because they've seen it on TV. The target foods call out from the supermarket shelves with their special offers and familiar cartoon characters, and it takes a strong parent indeed to resist them. The fact is that advertising works. It convinces us that sugary, completely nutrient-free drinks are healthy, and we have come to believe that a few added vitamins and minerals make a chocolate breakfast cereal acceptable. If we have nagging doubts about the food our children are eating, they are swiftly assuaged by the fact that everyone else is feeding their children the same thing. Listen to your doubts. Children will not have a healthy present or future if they are fed what the advertisers say they should eat.

The "treat" cycle

We've developed a "treat" mentality. A glass of wine for Mom; a chocolate for good behavior; a bag of potato chips for finishing homework; a ready-made meal to take the pressure off a busy day. Better still, lunch at a fast-food restaurant complete with a toy from the newest Disney release. Treats are important, but we've got the emphasis all wrong. There's no harm in the odd unhealthy treat, but when it becomes a way of life, it's difficult to go back. The packet of candies for finishing dinner becomes a regular "dessert" and new treats have to be dreamed up to take their place. It's an unhealthy cycle, and it tends to get worse.

Setting a bad example

We are failing to set a good example ourselves. If we fill the house with junk food we don't want our children to eat, we are sending the wrong message. And if we eat poorly, our children will learn that it's acceptable and even appropriate to do so themselves. If your own dinner comes in a microwavable tray every night, it's time to think again.

There are many, many more reasons why our diets have become so poor, and we'll examine some of them in more detail later in this chapter. If it seems a mammoth task to change a routine or to set up a new system, don't despair. Eating well doesn't have to involve reading every label, baking your own bread and serving tofu stir-fries every night. It's easy to make little adjustments, and the road to recovery starts with an understanding of what children really need.

What children really need

This is the nuts-and-bolts section of the chapter, but it's essential reading for every parent, whether you are working on your first child, or trying to make some changes further down the line. A good understanding of the elements of different foods and what they do in our bodies also provides a basis for discussion with your child or children. If children grow up knowing that food can make a difference in their lives, they will learn to make choices based on that knowledge. That doesn't mean explaining essential fatty acids to a toddler. It simply means putting nutrition in children's terms, in a way that they will relate to it.

First and foremost, children need variety and they need balance. Too much of the same foods can trigger allergies (see page 301) and cause nutritional deficiencies. On the other hand, a diet that is weighted too far in the "food is not fun; eat your greens" direction can create an obsession for just the sorts of foods you want to avoid.

The essentials

There are seven principal elements that make up a healthy diet, and they are all essential for our children's growth and overall health. When there is a shortfall in any of these areas, health will suffer in the short and long term. The main nutrients are fats, carbohydrates and protein (called macronutrients, which basically means "big"), and then vitamins and minerals and other trace elements (called micronutrients because they are literally microscopic). Two other important elements are water and fiber. A balance of all of these nutrients ensures that our children heal, grow and develop, and that their bodies can carry out all of the processes that are necessary for life itself.

What we really need to know is why they are essential for children, how much they need, and what happens when they don't get enough. We also need to know the good from the bad, in order to make informed choices when we are planning our family menus.

Chewing the fat

Fat has become the scourge of the past decade and, if you believe everything you read, you'd think that it is entirely surplus to our requirements. We have no-fat, low-fat, half-fat, reduced-fat and chemically produced fatless fat foods, and they are widely available. Interesting, isn't it, that obesity is increasing almost as quickly as the number of fat-free offerings?

The fact is that we need fat. Too much fat is unhealthy, but rather than adjust our diets to ensure that we get less, we are determined to eat exactly the same foods we have always eaten, in exactly the same quantities, by choosing reduced-fat products instead.

There are two main issues with fat:

1. Saturated (mainly animal) fats clog up our arteries and cause heart disease. Obviously eating lower-fat food will reduce the risk of heart disease, BUT

2. Fats make us fat, which is one of the main causes of heart disease, blood pressure problems, illness, fatigue and all sorts of health problems. Half-fat products haven't changed our eating habits. We are eating more of them because we feel that the risks are minimized. The problem is not so much the fat, but the diet itself, and that's where we need to make changes.

We need fat for energy. It is necessary for the smooth functioning of our bodies—in particular, our nervous systems. Fats contain the vitamins A, D and E, which are essential to many of our bodies' processes. For children fat is even more important. When babies are breastfed, over 50 percent of calories come from fat. When babies are weaned on to table foods, they still need more fats than adults to ensure that they grow and develop properly. Fat provides the calories necessary for growth and essential nutrients required for brain function. Cut down on fat too soon, and your child could suffer.

What we do need to consider, however, is the type of fats our children are eating. Deep-fried fish and chips are a very good source of fat, but unfortunately, it's the wrong kind. Although children need more fat than adults, the balance between healthy and unhealthy fats must be right.

Bad fats

- These are the saturated fats, found in butter, lard, meat, hard cheeses and eggs, and they are the scourge of our modern diet. Fried foods, mayonnaise, pizza, burgers, many baked goods such as cakes and cookies, and cooked meats, such as salami, are all high in saturated fats. These types of foods need to be kept to the bare minimum.

- Too much saturated fat is linked with all sorts of diseases, including heart disease, asthma and eczema, stroke, obesity and cancer.

- Saturated fat clogs our arteries and prevents beneficial nutrients being absorbed by our bodies.

- We know that even young children are showing signs of heart disease, so it's clear that we need to remove this type of fat from our diets as much as possible.

Another type of bad fats are the "trans-fats," which are produced when oils are hydrogenated—even healthy oils. Hydrogenation is the process used to turn liquid fats into hard fats. Margarine is a good example of this process. A perfectly good oil is heated to give it a firmer consistency; in other words to make it more solid. We've been convinced that margarine is better for us because it uses "healthy fats." However, the hydrogenation process changes the nature of the fat so that our bodies cannot make use of it. Worse, it blocks the body's ability to use healthy oils (see below). Trans-fats are used in all kinds of processed and baked food, including cookies, pies, potato chips and cakes.

Avoid:
- foods that contain hydrogenated oils

- saturated fat products wherever possible. Trim the fat from your meat, and try not to offer red meats more than once or twice a week.

Good fats

Both children and adults should aim to get more of the good fats and less of the bad fats, while cutting back on fat overall. There are several types of good fats.

Unsaturated fats are broken down into two groups: polyunsaturates and mono-unsaturates. The polys include vegetable oils, nuts, seeds and oily fish. The monos include olive oil, avocados, nuts and seeds, and rapeseed oil. The polys do not seem to cause damage in our bodies, unless they are heated, at which point they become unstable and fairly dangerous. The monos appear to do some actual good, by protecting against heart disease.

Then we have the fatty acids, which are essential, and these fall into two categories: omega-3 and omega-6 oils.

- Omega-3 oils are found in leafy green vegetables, pumpkin seeds, flaxseed oil, walnuts, oily fish (including salmon, herring, sardines, mackerel and fresh tuna).

- Omega-6 oils are found in vegetable oils and seed oils (including corn, soy, sesame, sunflower and safflower oils), and in peanuts, peanut oils and olive oils.

Essential fatty acids are converted into substances that keep our blood thin, lower blood pressure, decrease inflammation, improve the function of our nervous and immune systems, help insulin to work, affect our vision, coordination and mood, encourage healthy metabolism and maintain the balance of water in our bodies. There's also exciting new research showing that fatty acids can affect our children's behavior and ability to learn. Children with a low fatty acid intake seem to be more at risk of attention deficit disorders.

▶ Top hints for increasing your children's intake of good fats

- Use cold-pressed olive oil for cooking, which does not become unstable when heated.

- Add flaxseed oil (available as capsules or as an oil on its own), which has the highest concentration of omega-3 oils, to your child's diet. It shouldn't be heated, but you can drizzle a little in salads, or add it to yogurts, or warm foods just before serving. A tablespoon a day is adequate for most children.

- Remember the daily spoonful of cod liver oil? Our parents and grandparents were not far off the mark. Cod liver oil contains substances that can help to prevent arthritis and other inflammatory conditions. Cod liver oil is a rich source of vitamin D, and therefore important for the development of healthy teeth and bones. Cod liver oil is also unlikely to contain mercury, which can contaminate other fish oils. Use a teaspoon a day for a young child (under age five), and a tablespoon a day for older children (age six and older).

- Children are unlikely to think that these oils are a delicious addition to their diets, so you might need to be sneaky. Blend it into favorite foods, or try whizzing it in the blender with some fresh orange juice at breakfast time.

- Offer lots of nuts and seeds, to ensure plenty of fatty acids.

Fatty acid deficiency?

There are some obvious symptoms of fatty acid deficiency. If your child suffers from any of the following, the symptoms could be reduced or improved by ensuring that fatty acids are adequately represented in her diet. Is your child:

- Particularly prone to infections (see page 207)?

- Overweight, but not responding to a healthy diet?

- Small for her age or growing slowly?

- Suffering from mood swings?

- Excessively thirsty (see also page 55)?

- Suffering from MS (multiple sclerosis) or diabetes?

- Prone to eczema or dry, itching skin?

IN SUMMARY:

- No more than a third of our total fat intake should be in the form of saturated fats.

- The remainder should be unsaturated, focusing on the foods that contain essential fatty acids.

- Overall, fat should not form more than about 20 to 30 percent of our children's diets. At present, many children's diets are more than 60 and even 70 percent fat, much of it the wrong kind.

Protein power

Protein is important, but the average Western diet contains much more than we really need.

- About 17 percent of the body is made of protein, including muscles, bones, skin, nails and hair.

- Proteins are made up of different combinations of 22 separate amino acids, which our bodies need to function and, of course, to carry on living!

- A lack of protein in the diet retards growth in children and causes a decrease in energy.

- Excess protein puts a strain on the liver and the kidneys, and leads to an increased risk of certain cancers and heart disease.

- Almost all unrefined foods contain proteins—some of them are surprising! In oranges and rice, for example, 8 percent of the calories are protein. Ten percent of the calories in potatoes are protein, and in most beans around 26 percent of the calories are protein. Wheat and oatmeal come in at a whopping 16 percent.[1]

What is healthy protein?

Traditionally we believed that protein had to come from meat and other animal products. In fact, experts now say that the healthiest proteins (because they are lower in fat and normally contain many other nutrients) are those found in vegetable products.

- Animal proteins include beef, pork, lamb, bacon, ham, sausages, chicken, turkey, game, fish and seafood, milk, butter, cheese and eggs.

- Vegetable proteins include meat substitutes, tofu, some pastas, potatoes, corn, black beans, legumes and brown rice. Even fruits and vegetables such as string beans, broccoli, seedless raisins, sweet cherries, oranges and bananas contain more protein per calorie than you'd imagine.[2]

IN SUMMARY:

- Meats with all visible fat cut off are much leaner, and much healthier sources of proteins than, say, marbled meat.

- The best proteins are those found in vegetable sources.

- Children need between three and five *small* servings of protein a day—no more.

- Protein is essential, but we normally get far more than we need. Breastmilk, for example, contains less than 2 percent protein, but babies can double their birthweight within six months on this exclusive diet.

- Choose vegetable proteins over animal proteins wherever possible. Go for animal proteins that are lower in saturated fats.

Get those carbs!

Carbohydrates are as wildly different as fats. What's good is crucial for our children's health. The bad carbohydrates form a great deal of our "junk food" intake, and they tend to act as "anti-nutrients," which means that they undo all the good effects of the healthy foods we are eating.

Carbohydrates are energy food, and they are the body's main source of fuel. There are two main kinds: refined and complex (unrefined). You can guess which are the good carbs, and which are the ones we need to avoid.

Good carbohydrates

Complex carbohydrates include:

- fruit and vegetables (and their juices)
- whole wheat unrefined flour
- whole wheat pasta
- brown rice
- whole wheat bread
- whole-grain breakfast cereals
- rolled oats
- legumes
- barley

The message is to eat *unrefined*. Complex carbohydrates supply a sustained source of energy, which means that the food takes longer to digest and assimilate. Unrefined foods contain vitamins and minerals, and proteins as well, making them excellent forms of balanced nutrition. If it's white, it's not likely to do you any good at all.

What about bad carbohydrates?

Refined carbohydrates supply energy, but they are quickly assimilated, causing a sudden energy boost, and a subsequent fall. You've seen the effects of refined carbohydrates after a birthday party—children eat cakes, cookies and lots of candies and become manically energetic. A short time later, it all falls apart as their blood sugar levels slump. This crazy rise and fall can cause mood swings, irritability, temper tantrums, lethargy and tears.

After school, children are often tearful and tired. This is caused by low blood sugar. In other words, they are hungry and need more fuel to raise blood sugar levels. Children whose lunches have been based around refined carbohydrates (including white bread, cookies, candies, tinned pasta, jams and soft drinks) will have a noticeably worse postschool slump than those children whose lunches included fruit, whole grain breads or fresh pastas, vegetables and fresh juices. Don't be tempted to offer a quick pick-me-up in the form of a candy or a chocolate. The symptoms will improve instantly, but you'll have a showdown well before dinner, as the levels slump again.

Quite apart from the blood sugar issue, refined carbohydrates have had the majority of their nutrients stripped from them in the refining process. Almost all chromium, for example, is lost when flour is refined. Why do I mention chromium in particular? It's the mineral that governs our glucose tolerance levels—in other words, blood sugar. Other big losses are calcium, B vitamins, iron, zinc and potassium.

Refined carbohydrates include:

- white sugar (and everything that contains it, including candy, carbonated drinks, fruit "juice" drinks, jams and jellies, cakes, cookies, chocolate, breakfast bars, breakfast cereals, pies, tarts and most baked goods—the majority of some children's diets)

- white flour (and everything that contains it, including bread, pasta, breakfast cereals, crackers, cookies, cakes and pies)

- white rice

What about fortified breakfast cereals?

Manufacturers would have us believe that adding a few token vitamins and minerals to children's breakfasts cereals, breads and even cookies or crackers balances the refining process (and of course the addition of an awful lot of sugar). It doesn't. Adding 2 or 3 nutrients to something that has been stripped of at least 15 other nutrients does not make it a healthy alternative.

Granola-belt kids

There have been scare stories about children eating too many of their carbohydrates in complex or unrefined form. The result was that children were getting too much fiber, causing diarrhea and inadequate absorption of nutrients, among other things. Some doctors then recommended that children should be given white breads, pastas and rice in favor of the unrefined versions, until the age of five.

That's nonsense. What happened was that some children were given diets that were inappropriate for children. They were eating high-fiber cereals containing too much bran, no fats, an overabundance of fruits and vegetables (some stories claimed that children as young as 3 were having 12 to 15 portions) and high-fiber products aimed at constipated adults. There can be too much of a good thing, and once again it's a question of balance. Swapping nutrition for stodge is not the answer. As long as your child's intake falls within, or even just slightly above, the recommended number of servings, there should be no problem.

What's the ideal balance?

60 per cent carbohydrates
20–30 per cent fats
10–20 per cent protein

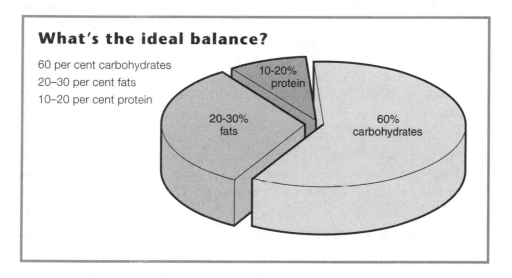

10-20% protein

20-30% fats

60% carbohydrates

IN SUMMARY:

- Children need between four and nine servings of healthy carbohydrates every day.

- About 60 percent of a child's diet should be made of up of these healthy carbohydrates.

- Choose a variety of unrefined carbohydrates. White, refined carbohydrates have virtually nothing to offer.

What about fiber?

Fiber is a relative newcomer to the key nutrient list, and its importance in our diets, and those of our children, is often underestimated. Paradoxically, fiber does not actually provide any nutrients. Instead, it has a host of roles in our bodies that encourage them to function properly.

- Anything that contains fiber requires considerable chewing. This stimulates the flow of saliva, which protects our teeth and encourages healthy digestion.

- Fiber literally acts as a broom in our bodies, clearing away debris from the digestive tract and keeping it healthy.

- It also adds bulk to our diet, which helps nutrients be absorbed more efficiently.

- Pectin, a soluble fiber found in apples and carrots, is particularly important. It absorbs heavy metals, such as lead, and stops them from being absorbed. Pectin also helps our bodies to eliminate waste products, and prevents the reabsorption of toxins in the bowel.

- The two main types of fiber are soluble (found in fruits, vegetables and grains such as oats and barley) and insoluble (found in wheat and wheat bran). The best fiber for children is soluble fiber, which is easier on the digestive tract and less likely to cause irritation. Don't be tempted to give young children foods that are high in insoluble fiber (including cereals like All Bran, and even Bran Flakes), which can cause diarrhea and inadequate absorption of nutrients (see page 326).

- Fiber is an excellent way to prevent constipation, and most experts believe that it can substantially reduce the risk of bowel cancer. Fiber has also been positively linked with the prevention of such health conditions as heart disease, diabetes, hemorrhoids, IBS (irritable bowel syndrome) and appendicitis.

How much do children need?

There's an easy way to calculate your child's minimum fiber needs: age plus five. So a seven-year-old would need about 0.4 oz(12g), a two year old 0.25 oz(7g), and so on. If your child's diet is healthy and varied, and she eats the recommended five-plus servings of fruits and vegetables, she will be getting all the fiber she needs.

For example, an orange at breakfast, a sandwich made with two slices of whole-wheat bread for lunch, a banana at recess, and a serving of peas and potatoes at dinner will provide adequate fiber.

▶ Top tips for increasing fiber the easy way

- Peels, such as those found on apples, potatoes, pears and plums, are the most fiber-rich part of the food. Leave them on whenever possible to boost intake. However, experts recommend we peel non-organic fruits and vegetables because of the number of toxins concentrated in the skin. Scrubbing is always better than peeling, but, wherever you can, choose organic and wash carefully.

- Whole fruits are richer in fiber than juice, so although a glass of fruit juice will count as a fruit serving, a child should consume at least two or three whole fruits a day to ensure that fiber needs are met.

- Raw fruits and vegetables have more fiber than cooked (see page 95), so try to encourage your children to eat some foods raw. Obvious choices are broccoli, carrots, celery, peppers, cucumbers and even corn canned in water. Keep them in a place where children can help themselves.

- Sprinkle beans or lentils into soups and onto salads. Children seem to like chickpeas, although they rank in the top ten of adult dislikes. Add them to casseroles, soups, stews and even pasta sauces or salads if your child is chickpea-friendly. Humus is popular as a dip for raw veggies.

- Rice crackers are a great source of fiber, and kids love them. Make them a regular treat.

- Healthy breakfast cereals are also a great source of fiber. Try to encourage oatmeal for breakfast to kick-start the day. Breakfast cereals don't always have to be for breakfast, either. Try porridge for supper or even a late-night snack, if your child has had a nutritious meal at other times in the day.

- Make an oatmeal buffet, with raisins, sesame seeds, sunflower seeds, and dried fruits, such as apricots, bananas and cranberries in small dishes. Each child can create his own extravaganza.

Water

About 65 percent of the human body is made up of water, so it's not surprising that water is the most essential element of our diets. Without food, we can last for several weeks. Without water, we'd be dead within a few days.

What does it do?

- Water is essential to the digestive process. If we don't drink enough between meals, the saliva flow slows down and digestion is less efficient.

- Almost 0.5 gallons (2 liters) of water is excreted from our bodies every day through our skin, urine, lungs and gut, and many toxins are removed from our bodies this way. If we are losing this much water, we need to replace it. The more water we drink, the greater the number of toxins eliminated.

- Without water, our cells cannot build new tissue efficiently, toxic products build up in our bloodstream, and blood volume decreases so that we have less oxygen and nutrients transported to our cells, all of which can leave us weak, tired and at risk of illness.

How much do children need?

According to their age and size, children will drink correspondingly less water. It's virtually impossible to drink too much (or, more to the point, for children to drink too much)—so as long as they are getting a minimum of 17.5 oz (500ml) to 70 oz (2000ml) a day, you can rest assured that they are getting enough.

What source of water?

About half our children's water intake will come in the form of fruits and vegetables, if they are eating properly. The other half should come from—you guessed it—water. Obviously, powdered drink mixes and juices contain water, as do carbonated drinks, but our bodies have to work harder to extract the water. Furthermore, adding toxins in the form of food additives, chemicals and sugars to water simply increases the toxic load, and more water will be required to clear it.

- Bottled natural mineral water is the best bet, although some experts have expressed reservations about the high levels of sodium (salt) it contains. If you drink bottled water, look for one with low sodium (lower than 20 mg of sodium per liter) and the weakest mineral concentration, to be on the safe side. Bottled natural mineral water is guaranteed to be free of all traces of pollution, and it is naturally free of bacteria.

- Bottled spring water is a waste of money. There are fewer regulations governing these types of waters, and there have even been reports of tap water being bottled and sold as spring water.

- The downside to bottled water is the fact that you have to pay for it. If your budget doesn't stretch, or you find the transportation of bottles from the grocery store too cumbersome, the next best option is filtered water. There are various types of filters, and you'll have to shop carefully to ensure that you are getting what you want. Unfortunately, this is one case where you get what you pay for. A plumbed-in filtering system is ultimately much more effective in removing unwanted pollutants and other chemicals from our tap water, but again, it might be unaffordable. Most "jug" filters remove only chlorine and floating particles, although there are some new ones on the market that claim to remove bacteria, pesticides, industrial chemicals and heavy metals. Always change your filter regularly, as they become useless, and a breeding ground for bacteria, over time.

Encouraging children to drink water

With the unbelievable range of brightly colored, highly flavored children's drinks available, it's not surprising that water ranks a poor second (or third, or fourth) with kids. There are, however, ways to introduce it fairly painlessly:

- If you have a baby, you can start with a clean slate. Offer only water to drink as food begins to replace milk in her diet. Very diluted fruit juices can be offered with food, but water should take precedence.

- Keep a jug of chilled filtered or bottled water within reach in the fridge. If it's the easiest drink to hand, they'll be more likely to drink it.

- Don't buy anything you don't want them to drink. In the end, if they are thirsty, they'll drink what's offered.

- For soft drink consumers, gradually dilute the amount of powder or syrup until they are drinking mostly water. They might complain, but they'll get used to it, and the transition to plain water will be easier. Eventually stop buying it. If they want an alternative, offer pure fruit juice diluted with water with meals only.

- If you have older children who drink too many carbonated drinks, explain the reasons why you are concerned (see page 55). Buy sparkling natural mineral water if they want something with a little fizz, and a variety of pure fruit juices to mix. For active kids, or aspiring sportsmen and-women, explain that water is the best rehydrator there is—all the top athletes drink it.

- Buy a plastic sports water bottle for each child, and keep it filled in the refrigerator. It will need to be washed and refilled daily to prevent a buildup of bacteria, but it can be theirs for the day—in the house, in the car or on the playing fields.

- Set a good example. If they see you drinking diet sodas with your lunch, they'll want some too. The whole family needs to convert if you are to succeed.

Vitamins, minerals and other important nutrients

So many claims have been made by neutraceutical (healthfood manufacturing) companies over the past decade, that most of us have become wary of and even bored by these nutrients. Interestingly, if you ask a child what a vitamin is, the usual reply is something along the lines of "a pill you eat with your breakfast." We've been rather beguiled into thinking that popping pills is the perfect antidote to an unhealthy diet, and happily consume billions of dollars worth every year.

The fact is that vitamins, minerals and a host of other substances are absolutely crucial to every single body process. Without them, we are seriously compromised. An average Western diet, based on commercially produced and processed foods, and low on the fresh, natural stuff, falls shockingly short of even the most basic recommended levels of vitamins and minerals. Many experts believe that this shortfall is a major contributory factor to many 20th-century diseases.

It's not surprising, therefore, that a lucrative and important industry has built up around vitamins, minerals and other supplements. See the Appendix (page 434) for details of what's required, and how to get it.

How it all fits together

The most up-to-date research suggests that the pyramid structure works best to analyze and graphically show how our diets should be set up. Pin the pyramid on your refrigerator so that the whole family can see how a good diet should be balanced. The diagram opposite shows what it looks like.

What's a serving?

Don't worry too much about serving sizes. The main thing is to get the balance right. In other words, if your child is eating a variety of different foods, weighted in importance according to the food pyramid, there should be no problem. However, don't put too much store in weights and measures. A child who eats three or four different vegetables and two or three different fruits in a day, along with some whole grain cereal, some rice, some potatoes and bread, some lean meat, fish and cheese, will be fine, even if the quantities seem inordinately small or large.

▶ Helpful hints on servings

- From the time an infant starts solids (four to six months of age) until the age of about six, the recommended serving size for fruits and vegetables is one tablespoon per year of their age. So, for example, four tablespoons of corn would constitute a

Ideal food pyramid

Other
To be eaten as an occasional treat
Candies, cookies, fast foods, cake

Fats and Oils
Use sparingly
Butter, olive oil, seed and nut oils, unhydrogenated magarines

Proteins
3 to 5 servings a day
Very lean meat, fish, poultry, cheese, yogurt, nuts, soy products (including tofu), legumes such as lentils, seeds

Fruit and Vegetables
5 to 7 servings a day
Any fruit or vegetables and their juices. Remember that the more colorful the vegetable, the more nutritious it tends to be

Carbohydrates
4 to 9 servings a day
Anything whole-grain and unrefined, including pasta, bread, brown rice, grains (such as rye, barley, corn, buckwheat), pulses, potatoes, sugar-free cereals

Fluids
A minimum of 500 to 2,000 ml a day
Water is the most important

serving for a four-year-old. After age six, serving sizes for fruits and veggies are roughly the same as those for adults—about half a cup. Remember that fruit and vegetable juices also count as servings. For children above the age of two, about 2 oz.(60 ml) would be an appropriate serving. A few sips is enough for a toddler.

- For other foods, the same rules apply. The younger the child, the smaller the portions.

- An adult serving of bread would be one slice, half a bagel or muffin, 25 g ready-to-eat cereal, half a mug of porridge, rice or pasta, or five to six crackers or oatcakes. A child above the age of six would need roughly the same-sized portions. A quarter of a piece of toast would represent a serving for a two-year-old, and so on.

- Protein portions for children above the age of six would be about 1.75 oz (50g)–2.5 oz (75 g) (about the size of a deck of cards). The younger the child, the smaller the portions.

Pyramids for kids

Encourage your children to work out whether their diets actually form a pyramid shape! You may find that they create a lovely hourglass or even an inverted pyramid when they break down what they are eating. The pyramid is an excellent tool for teaching about nutrition. Draw some blank pyramid shapes and see if your children can plan a healthy diet for a day (with help, depending on their ages). The good news is that if they've planned it, they are more likely to eat it!

Why fruits and vegetables?

According to the Child Nutrition Research Center at the Baylor College of Medicine in Houston, Texas, fruits and vegetables are beginning to achieve some recognition in a meat-oriented Western diet. The Center reports that the vitamins, minerals, fiber and protective substances called phytochemicals found in fruits and vegetables help kids grow and develop properly. Other advantages:

- They keep body weight under control. Snacking on low-calorie, fiber-rich fruits and vegetables helps keep both calories and hunger in check.

- They maintain cardiovascular health and prevent birth defects. Fruits and vegetables are naturally low in sodium, potassium rich and virtually fat free.

- Many also provide a healthy dose of folate, a vitamin found in asparagus, spinach, broccoli and citrus fruits that is important for preventing neural tube birth defects and keeping levels of homocysteine under control. Homocysteine is being investigated as a possible independent risk factor for cardiovascular disease.

- Research also suggests that the fiber and antioxidant phytochemicals found in fruits and vegetables also help prevent blood vessel damage.

- They reduce cancer risk. Folate (see above for sources) helps prevent cancer damage at the molecular level. Selenium, vitamin C and other antioxidant phytochemicals, such as the dark green and orange pigments called carotenoids, help prevent cancer by neutralizing harmful by-products of metabolism inside cells, while other phytochemicals appear to help detoxify carcinogens and block cancer growth.

- They help you live a longer and healthier life. A diet rich in fruits and vegetables is associated with a lower risk of stroke, cataracts and diverticulosis, as well as improved blood lipid levels.

Food Scares and Concerns

Absolutely safe food is impossible. Even natural, whole foods contain chemicals and toxins (albeit naturally occurring) that need to be broken down by the body. Our bodies are equipped to deal with these types of chemicals. The trouble starts when we begin to add extra work to the body's natural detoxification process, and the modern diet contains a minefield of chemicals and other substances that can play havoc.

Above and beyond this, food has been the subject of literally dozens of scare stories over the past decade, and wary consumers are beginning to believe that nothing is safe to eat. Let's look at the issues.

Mad cows and meat

While most readers will associate this problem with the U.K., it's worth knowing the facts. BSE (bovine spongiform encephalopathy) came about because of intensive farming practices that relied upon cheap animal feed in order to meet a demand for ever-cheaper meat. Those same issues are present in almost every Western country, so take note. BSE is a degenerative brain disease in cattle. CJD stands for Creitzfeldt-Jakob disease, named after the two men who discovered it. This condition is a degenerative brain disease, and until the link with BSE was made, it normally affected elderly people. In 1996, scientists confirmed a strain of the disease among younger people now known as vCJD (v for variant). There is no cure for vCJD, which causes holes in the brain and a host of physical and mental symptoms, eventually leading to loss of control over the entire body.

The 1980s saw the biggest-ever epidemic of BSE in cattle, and vCJD emerged shortly thereafter in humans. The link was made when it was discovered that most vCJD victims lived in the U.K. where the cattle epidemic took place. Scientists believe that the most likely cause of vCJD in humans was the consumption of BSE-infected beef between the years of 1986 to 1989. The origins of BSE are not entirely clear, but it is believed that its spread coincided with new feeding practices, where the remains of other cattle and perhaps even sheep and other animals, were processed and fed to cattle.

There are doubts about whether or not there will be a mass epidemic of vCJD. At least 80 people have died in the U.K. since 1995. But because the disease can incubate for 10 to 15 years, it's difficult to know how many will be affected. The result? Beef was off the shopping list for some time, British beef on the bone was banned, and only recently has it been declared completely safe to eat.

So is it safe?

The U.K. government (and others in Europe) arranged for the mass slaughter of millions of cattle at risk of infection, and only young cattle were allowed into the food chain. All young cattle are traced from birth to death to prove they are free of the disease, and they are issued with "passports," and tagged in the ear. Scientists now believe that any future cases will be in those who are already incubating the disease. The chances of acquiring the disease now are officially very remote, but there have recently been signs that the situation has not been controlled as well as hoped.

What about TSE?

In the U.S., BSE has not been an issue (although critics claim that the Department of Agriculture is inadequate, and may not present the real picture), but there is concern about other transmissible spongiform encephalopathies (known as TSEs). Although considerably less common at the moment, they are nonetheless a focus for concern: chronic wasting disease, a TSE found in deer and elk, may pose a threat to those who eat infected animals.

No one is sure to what extent the public is at risk from TSEs, which are caused by little-understood proteins called prions. The prevalence of the disease in livestock populations is still unknown. How humans are infected with a TSE from other species is undetermined. And the disease in humans is difficult to track, since it may take decades from the time of initial infection to show any symptoms.

A TSE specific to deer and elk, chronic wasting disease, is endemic in parts of Colorado and Wyoming and has been found on game ranches in Montana and Oklahoma. Chronic wasting disease was first observed in 1967 in captive mule deer, which were subsequently released into the wild. One theory has it that the captive deer were exposed to sheep that carry an ovine form of TSE known as scrapie, which is relatively commonplace. Another is that the deer contracted the disease by eating feed that contained rendered protein from an infected animal. In parts of Colorado and Wyoming chronic wasting disease affects as many as 8 percent of the deer and 1 percent of the elk.

At least two young hunters, who ate and dressed deer, have come down with CJD. And a third, a young woman who had eaten venison from a deer shot in Maine, also contracted the disease.

It doesn't sound that threatening, but given that we now know that BSE-and TSE-type infections can incubate for long periods, and that there is no available scientific research into the problem, this may be a disaster waiting to happen.

BSE-type infections have also been linked with lamb in the U.K., throwing up a huge warning for the meat industry worldwide. The main problem is that we don't know how and why BSE has arisen, other than the fact that it has something to do with feed. There is another theory that the immune systems of cows may have become weakened by the use of organophosphates, a pesticide used against the warble fly.

Whether or not BSE or TSE is anything but an irksome PR problem for the meat industry in the U.S. at the moment, it has caused consumers to question animal feed and pesticide use, and the possible implications of a CJD-type epidemic. Vigorous preventive measures to stop the spread of TSEs could threaten the bottom line of many industries (meat and human blood products, for example), and, as in many cases, big business has tended to win out over public health.

Interestingly, anyone who contracted a TSE from exposure to either deer with chronic wasting disease or cattle infected with an American strain of BSE would not test positive for nvCJD. Experts claim that this focus on nvCJD means that other chronic wasting disease in humans found in the U.S. are being ignored. They also say that there are TSE diseases in sheep, mink, deer, elk, humans and possibly in cattle and pigs. Feeding practices, such as weaning calves on cattle blood protein, could lead to exactly the same problems that exist in the U.K. The USDA has failed to institute a complete ban on the practice of feeding rendered animal protein to other animals (rather than the current partial ban on feeding rendered ruminants to other ruminants).

The verdict

According to the majority of research, theoretically we have nothing to worry about on the BSE front in the U.S. and the U.K., although experts are now beginning to question whether controls have been sufficiently stringent. New cases have cropped up in the U.K. and in Europe, and with the potential risk of other wasting illnesses on the horizon, for the time being, it's probably sensible to stick to organic beef and other meat products.

Hormones in meat

EU farmers are banned from giving hormones to cattle because of health fears, but in the U.S., natural and synthetic hormones are routinely given to cattle to boost the amount of quality meat they produce, without having to feed them more. The female sex hormones estrogen and progesterone stimulate extra muscle and fat, while the male sex hormone testosterone increases muscle growth and decreases fat production. Estrogen has been linked to breast cancer in women, and to infertility in men. Progesterone may increase the development of several "female" cancers, including ovarian, breast and uterine, while testosterone is linked to prostate cancer in men.

In the U.S., cattle are routinely injected with growth hormones to encourage weight gain. At least one in six farmers injects his cows with genetically engineered growth hormone. Around 90 percent of the 29 billion pounds of beef consumed by Americans each year comes from cattle that have been fattened by hormone implants.

For pork, the figure is almost 100 percent. The EU has, for this reason, banned American beef from the shelves.

There are also issues involving human hormone activity. In the U.S., six "natural" sex hormones are given to animals to increase their weight by as much as 50 pounds. These hormones are obviously contained in the meat itself. According to some estimates, an eight-year-old boy who ate two hamburgers made from this meat would, following the meal, have increased his levels of female sex hormones by 10 percent. According to a number of studies, lifelong exposure to high residues of natural and synthetic sex hormones in meat poses serious risk of breast and reproductive cancers, which have increased sharply since 1950, while sperm count has decreased. Hormone residues are also suspected to be causal factors in premature sexual development in young girls.

Is it safe?

Because there are concerns and associated risks, it is not safe to eat meat that has been injected with hormones.

The verdict

Organic meat is guaranteed to be free of hormones and other chemicals (see page 73), so meat doesn't need to be ruled out of a healthy diet. To be on the safe side, avoid giving children any U.S. meat products (including stock cubes and gelatin) until studies can show that it is completely safe.

Antibiotics

Intensive farming methods have ensured that most animals are raised in small spaces, under stressful conditions. The increased stress and close confines do two main things: they decrease the animals' natural resistance to disease, and they are an obvious breeding ground for disease itself. In fact, these conditions may have contributed to the recent increase in salmonella and E-coli infections in humans. An estimated 60 percent of chicken sold in the U.S. is infected with salmonella, and that figure may be as high as 75 percent in the EU.

For this reason, antibiotics are routinely given to pigs and poultry. They protect the animals against disease, and also encourage them to grow faster.

Is it safe?

The answer is no. When we eat foods containing high levels of antibiotics, we run the risk of developing a resistance to them. For more about the dangers of antibiotics, see page 211.

The verdict

Once again, organic meat and poultry is guaranteed to be free of antibiotics and hormones. To be on the safe side, children should not, as much as possible, be given anything but. The immune systems of children are immature, and their growing bodies are much more susceptible to both antibiotics and disease. Because we do not know the long-term effects of our new ways of producing foods, it is much safer to take no risks. Children don't need a lot of meat, so although organic products are still more expensive, the investment could save your child's life.

BST

One of the reasons dairy cows produce milk is a hormone called BST (bovine somatotropin), which is naturally produced by their bodies. Typically, when something works, we want more of it, whether it's natural or not. Genetic engineers are now able to program parts of genes so that cattle will churn out more of the hormone (lots more). This is injected into cows to encourage them to produce more milk—up to 20 percent in fact.

In the U.S., this hormone has been legally used since 1994, but it was banned in the EU and in Canada, following some disturbing tests and studies. The ban is up for review, and it's beginning to look like this is one battle that the EU may lose.

Is it safe?

Obviously not. Some farmers using the drug are finding that the levels of disease are rising in their herds. Long-term effects are as yet unknown. Veterinary experts claim that the hormone exhausts the cows to such an extent that they become more susceptible to infection, which means more antibiotics. Children drink a great deal more milk than adults, and the risks are, therefore, increased.

The verdict

Organic milk is the only answer. Not just because of the as-yet unknown long-term effects of BST on humans, but because of the higher use of antibiotics.

Do children need milk?

For many children, milk is a godsend. It's rich in vitamins, minerals, protein and fat, and for some picky eaters, it might be the only form of calcium they get. But many parents become too reliant on milk, and some children drink many glasses a day, which is not healthy. There is an abounding myth that children must have milk—and lots of it—to grow. I always point to my youngest son when this argument is raised. He has never had a glass of milk in his life, and won't even eat it on his cereal. He eats a little cheese and some yogurt, but his dairy intake is very low. He's the tallest child in his class, and he's strong and healthy. He gets all the nutrients he needs from a balanced diet that does not include milk, and there is no doubt that it hasn't affected his growth! See the Appendix for some of the best forms of calcium, vitamin A and vitamin B2.

Milk in moderation is a healthy drink. After the age of four or five, switch children to partly skimmed milk to ensure that their intake of saturated fats stays within healthy limits. Weaned children need no more than 21 oz (600 ml) of milk a day; many children need far less.

There's some evidence that adolescent girls should be drinking more milk than their male counterparts. A study published in the *British Medical Journal* suggests adolescent girls who increase their milk intake could help prevent the onset of osteoporosis. Adolescence is the crucial period to achieve a healthy skeleton, but calcium intake among teenage girls is below recommended levels. Researchers gave 40 girls aged 12 an extra 10 oz of milk each day for 18 months. At the end of that period their bone mineral density and content was significantly higher than that of another group of girls who did not receive extra milk.

But too much milk can have the following drawbacks:

- Milk is filling, and although it is nutritious, it does not contain anywhere near the number of nutrients required by growing children. When children drink too much, they fill up more easily and have no room for the foods that contain all the nutrients they need.

- Cows' milk is a common allergen, and some experts believe that we start our children on the slippery slope of allergies by feeding them baby formulas based on cows' milk. Cows' milk is vastly different from human milk and is not as easily digested or tolerated.

- Milk also increases the production of mucus. A healthy, well child can cope with the extra mucus, but if your child is tired or ill, it can lead to an increased susceptibility to disease. Chinese medical practitioners, for example, believe that milk might be at the root of many health conditions, including asthma, chronic colds and coughs, glue ear (see page 353) and digestive problems.

- A recent report indicates that a naturally occurring chemical that occurs in pasteurized milk may cause Crohn's disease (inflammation of the intestine) in susceptible children. While your child may not be in the risk category, there's no sense in giving him too much of something that may hold potential risks.

- Anything apart from organic milk will contain whatever chemicals were fed to the dairy cows that produced it. Whether it's antibiotics, pesticides, hormones or BST, they'll make their way into your child's body. Too much of any type of food increases the risk of toxic overload (see page 141), which can lead to allergies and ill health.

Barbecues

Another scare story to hit the headlines, and this one is worth noting. When we barbecue food, fat drips on to the coals. Some of this is not completely combusted, and it forms a smoke that contains carcinogens (benzopyrene), which is then deposited on the food. Furthermore, charring protein-rich foods (such as meat) may result in the production of mutagenic (which changes the structure of our cells) and carcinogenic substances.

Is it safe?

Sadly, no. Several studies show that the risk of cancer is greatly increased in people who eat a lot of charred or fried foods.

The verdict

If a barbecue is an odd treat, don't worry too much, but if it is the mainstay of your summer diet, think again. Children are particularly susceptible to carcinogenic and mutagenic substances. Burnt sausages, chicken, hot dogs, burgers or any other sources of protein, whether they are grilled, fried, broiled or barbecued hold some potential risks, so avoid them where possible.

Nitrates

These are chemicals that are widely used as preservatives for meat and meat products, such as bacon, ham and salami (and almost every smoked meat). Even larger amounts of nitrates are found in vegetables grown with nitrate fertilizers—for example, spinach and beets—and in drinking water in areas where these fertilizers are heavily used.

Are they safe?

Absolutely not. In food, nitrates appear in fairly minimal quantities, and most healthy children will be able to "detoxify" fairly easily. However, a child who eats lots of meat, salami, hot dogs, bacon and even smoked chicken, fish or beef, will be at higher risk. What are the risks? First and foremost, nitrates convert to substances that are known to be carcinogenic. Nitrates are also implicated in stomach cancer and "blue baby" syndrome in newborn infants. In rural areas where nitrate levels in water are up to four times higher than national averages, childhood diabetes appears to be 25 percent more common. In Yorkshire, England, alone, some 2,000 children have been diagnosed with diabetes since 1978, yet only one in ten has a relative with the disease, which was largely believed to be hereditary.

The verdict

We know that high levels of nitrates in food can cause cancer. Higher environmental levels can cause even greater problems. If you live in an area with high nitrate levels in the water—your local water company can test your water or you can buy a testing kit at your local hardware store—consider getting a filter that removes it. Avoid any nitrate-containing foods, to ensure that you aren't increasing the risks. For the average child, the odd piece of bacon at breakfast or in pasta or the occasional ham sandwich should not cause undue problems. If nitrate-rich foods are the mainstay of her diet, it's time to make changes.

GM foods

This is a tricky one. GM (genetically modified) foods have not been conclusively proved to cause damage to health, but the public is concerned enough to have demanded that they are adequately labeled and, in many cases, withdrawn.

Genetic modification involves isolating and identifying a gene that produces a desired characteristic. This gene is copied and then inserted into another species. The idea is that the very best aspects of plants (or even animals and humans!) can be fitted together like a jigsaw to produce the ideal product. For example, scientists have produced tomatoes that don't rot, insect-proof corn and potatoes and a host of other goodies, the best known of which is the soy bean. Soy plants are particularly susceptible to herbicides, so the plan was to engineer the plants to resist just one herbicide: then spray only that one product, leaving weeds dead but soy bean plants unharmed.

Soy beans are processed into oil and flour—and then used in 60 percent of processed foods, including cooking oils, margarines, salad dressings, sauces, bread, cookies, cakes, pizzas, noodles, ice creams and alternatives to dairy products, such as tofu, tempeh and miso.

Are they safe?

The answer is that we don't know for sure, but here are the main points:

- The average consumer is fed up with food issues. In the U.K., we weren't warned about beef and BSE until it was too late, and it's become pretty clear that the government was in cahoots with industry. In the U.S., consumer wariness has created an incredibly strong and growing organic food market. GM foods were yet another case of the government saying "We are sure it's safe," but this time the public didn't let them get away with it. In the EU, GM foods should now be labeled, and we can choose not to buy them, but in the U.S., there are as yet no rulings concerning GM ingredients. This should, in the future, change. Consumer polls show that

80 to 95 percent of Americans want genetically engineered foods to be labeled in order to avoid buying them.

- An increasing number of us suffer from allergies, and that number is growing all the time. Allergies are often caused by proteins, and genetic engineering results in new proteins in food products. Gene foods could trigger allergic reactions (some serious enough to cause death), or they could encourage susceptibility to more allergens. Again, we don't know for sure; the argument is not simple.

- GM foods don't focus on nutrition, and there is a real worry that we may end up with beautiful, quick-growing plants that have no nutritional value.

- An early GM amino acid is believed to have produced a powerful toxin that reportedly killed at least 37 people in the U.S. and permanently disabled up to 1,500 others.

- All plants contain their own natural toxins, which our bodies deal with adequately. We don't know what genetic modification will do to toxins in plants, and there is a very real concern that they could raise them to unacceptable levels, or alter them so that they become much more dangerous.

- The British Medical Association has called for a global ban on GM foods, while the *New England Journal of Medicine* has warned that "the allergenic potential of these newly introduced microbial proteins is uncertain, unpredictable, and untestable." Scientists warn that GM foods may set off allergies, increase cancer risks, produce antibiotic-resistant pathogens, damage food quality, and produce dangerous toxins.

- No one can yet say with certainty that GM foods are safe to grow or eat. The reason: these products have not been thoroughly tested for their long-term effects. Worryingly, too, many safety assessments are carried out on a case-by-case basis, rather than considering the likely overall impact of a series of new developments.

- We don't benefit from GM foods; the manufacturers and producers do. It's always necessary to be concerned about issues where there is big money at stake for the manufacturers.

- GM foods could destroy our natural environment, and once we've gone down this route, it's impossible to go back. Any mistakes are out there, transferred by pollen, animals, birds, water and the like, and we can't reverse the damage. We could be breeding super-pests, by creating plants that are pest-resistant or antibiotic-resistant; we are altering the very structure of plants at top speed, and without anywhere near adequate testing. Even organic foods can be affected, if they are, for example, downwind from GM crops. The ramifications of that could be massive.

Foods likely to contain GM ingredients

Always read the label. Many manufacturers are taking great pains to remove GM ingredients from their products. If it says GM-free, it is. The following may not be:

- reduced-fat and "light" foods

- processed foods from the U.S. (where genetic modification is worth billions of dollars every year, and where no restraints or labeling practices are in place)

- ready-prepared sandwiches and meals

- anything containing soy or soy milk (including tofu)

- prepared pasta and noodles

- burgers, meatloaf, sausages, sausage rolls, pies, hot dogs, pastries and quiche

- cooked sliced meats

- cooking oils, margarines and spreads

- frozen yogurts, ice cream and other desserts

- cookies, cakes, chocolate, candy

- flavored yogurts

- processed meat, fish, poultry or vegetarian foods, such as fish sticks, veggie burgers and chicken nuggets

- store-bought (and usually takeout) pizzas

- cheese—hard, soft and processed

- mayonnaise, sauces and dips

- dried fruits

- potato chips, tortilla chips and popcorn

- canned and dried soups

- soft drinks, hot chocolate and some coffees

Does that cover a good portion of your weekly shopping list? You can see why there is concern.

The verdict

Too much is unknown. GM foods are not natural and they have the potential to cause harm. Don't take a risk. Avoid GM products wherever possible. Organic food is GM-free (and will hopefully stay that way). Eat organic whenever possible, or look for labels that state "GM-free." GM-free products are increasing all the time.

Food irradiation

Irradiation is a fairly new technology, which involves exposing food to high doses of radiation in order to kill insects and pests that infest food; reduce levels of bacteria like salmonella and listeria; delay ripening and rotting, so that foods can be kept for longer; and completely sterilize foods, which is a bonus for anyone with a weakened or immature immune system, such as the chronically or terminally ill, babies and the elderly.

Is it safe?

Because it is a relatively new science, the dangers are as yet unknown. We do know that irradiation can substantially reduce the nutritional content of foods—up to 90 percent of the vitamins found in untreated foods are potentially lost. So the food may look better, taste better and last longer, but it will have very little nutritional value—the main reason for eating it. Studies show that irradiation may also leave some active bacteria, while killing off "healthy" bacteria that may have controlled whatever bacteria existed.

The verdict

Irradiated foods are not labeled at present, so it's virtually impossible to distinguish them from the natural thing.

In Europe, consumer resistance has slowed down the introduction of irradiation. When it does appear, foods should be labeled as "irradiated" or "treated with ionizing radiation." But this labeling requirement does not apply to ingredients that make up less than 25 percent of a labeled product. The situation is, however, different in the U.S., where irradiation is widely used, and there have been appeals for more extensive use.

Why say no?

- Irradiation damages food by breaking up molecules and releasing pieces of the molecules, known as free radicals. These damage vitamins and enzymes, and combine with existing chemicals (such as pesticides) in the food to form new chemicals, called unique radiolytic products (URPs). Some of these URPs are known toxins (benzene, formaldehyde, lipid peroxides) and some are unique to irradiated foods.

- Scientists have not studied the long-term effect of these new chemicals in our diet. Therefore, they cannot guarantee that irradiated foods are safe to eat.

- When the U.S. FDA approved irradiation for fruits and vegetables in 1997, it used a theoretical calculation of the number of URPs in one 7.5 oz serving (found in a large apple or pear, for example). It did not consider the fact that people may eat several times that amount of irradiated food over the course of a day.

- Irradiated foods can lose between 5 and 80 percent of many vitamins (A, C, E, K and B complex). The amount of loss depends on the dose of irradiation and the length of storage time.

- Irradiation weakens or destroys the natural digestive enzymes found in raw foods. This means the human body has to work harder to digest them. Furthermore, the liver is put under increased pressure to deal with the chemicals in the food.

- The FDA already allows irradiated fruits and vegetables to be labeled "fresh."

- Science has not proved that a long-term diet of irradiated foods is safe for human health.

- A CBS News poll says that 77 percent of Americans oppose irradiation.

Organic foods are not irradiated, so they are the safe option (see page 39) until we know more.

Pesticides

Pesticides are commonly sprayed to kill pests, but they play a dual role of contaminating the plants and the surrounding area, as well as the healthy animals and insects that would have eaten the pests in the natural order of things.

Are they safe?

Pesticides can damage our immune systems, making us more vulnerable to illness and disease. The immune systems of other animals are also affected. Both animals and humans suffer fertility problems. Much of the food that we eat contains measurable quantities of pesticide residues, even though the chemicals have been applied legally.

Some imported foods may even contain residues of pesticides banned in the West. Given that children are particularly vulnerable, and that we encourage them to eat lots of fruit and vegetables, their potential exposure is a matter of real concern. Among the most controversial pesticides in recent years have been organophosphates. Some of their effects are believed to attack the nervous system, with early symptoms including headaches, excessive sweating, breathing difficulty, vomiting, blurred vision, slurred speech, slow thinking and loss of memory. Later come convulsions, coma and even—in extreme circumstances—death. Organophosphates are commonly used on a variety of fruit and vegetables, including bananas and carrots.

▶ *7 points about pesticides*

1. The World Health Organization has estimated that between 3.5 and 5 million people globally suffer acute pesticide poisoning every year.

2. Forty percent of pesticides now in use have been proved to be cancer-promoting and linked to birth defects or decreased fertility in men and women.

3. Pesticide exposure is associated with depression, memory decline, destabilization of moods, Parkinson's disease, asthma, eczema, migraine, irritable bowel syndrome and rhinitis, not to mention more serious diseases like cancer.

4. Pesticides may pose a far more serious threat to public health than has previously been thought, and their use is on the increase.

5. It's ludicrous to think that a product designed to kill another living organism could have no effect whatsoever on our bodies.

6. A Danish study claims that some pesticides, found throughout the whole food chain, can lead to breast cancer.

7. The U.S. Consumers' Union found that many fruits and vegetables carry pesticide residues that exceed the limits that the Environmental Protection Agency (EPA) considers safe for children. According to the Consumers' Union report, even one serving of some fruit and vegetables can exceed the safe daily limit for young children. And it's worth noting that the EPA considers 60 percent of all herbicides, 90 percent of all fungicides and 30 percent of insecticides to be potentially carcinogenic.

The verdict

To be healthy, children need fruits and vegetables, carbohydrates, fats and proteins. We must encourage children to eat naturally, which involves unprocessed foods. The "natural foods," such as meat, fresh produce and even grains like wheat and oats, are either sprayed with pesticides or the animals involved are fed with substances that have been sprayed with pesticides. The answer is to eat organic wherever possible (see page 39).

Additives, preservatives and other chemicals

See page 74.

Sugar

Sugar has been viewed as evil for quite some time now. Not surprisingly, manufacturers have gotten smart and started calling sugar by its various generic names, including sucrose, glucose, fructose, lactose, galactose and others, in an attempt to ease the blow.

But why is sugar so bad?

- First and foremost, sugar has a strong depressive effect on the immune system. According to a 1997 study, as little as six teaspoons a day can reduce the immune response by 25 percent. Most common foods—particularly those geared toward children—contain a substantial amount of sugar, which can have a dramatic effect on our children's health.

- Sugar causes blood sugar to rise dramatically—causing the "hyperactive" symptoms witnessed following a birthday party or even just a bag of candy. Following the rise, there is a dramatic slump, which causes the other set of familiar symptoms—tearfulness, fatigue, temper tantrums, mood changes and lack of concentration.

- Sugars provide calories and no other nutrients, and they damage the enamel of the teeth, causing decay.

- Foods high in sugars (cookies, chocolate bars, cakes, pastries, for example), are also often high in saturated fats, which can lead to weight-excess heart disease and even diabetes.

- Most importantly, however, the extra calories of sugars often displace more nourishing food in the diet. Diets high in sugar are also often high in fat and low in fiber. If your children fill up on sugary foods, they are likely to be at risk of vitamin and mineral deficiencies.

We get far more sugar than we need in even the most healthy diet. The message is to cut out the extras. Don't, for example, be tempted to sweeten cereal or porridge with sugar. If sugar falls within the first three or four ingredients in a particular food, you can be certain that it's too much for children. Some foods are surprising; I found a granola bar containing eight different types of sugar. Beware of "healthy"-sounding foods!

The best advice is not to buy processed foods that contain sugar, and then to cut down on other sweet foods. Obviously a chocolate cookie needs to contain sugar, but look for brands of "treats" that have "reduced sugar" content, and look at the label to see how much it actually is reduced. See page 50 for tips on making changes to the family diet.

Sugar content of common foods

Food	tsp	sugar
1 plain cookie	½	(.07 oz)
1 fruit yogurt	4½	(.77 oz)
Smarties (1 box)	7½	(1.295 oz)
1 Mars bar	9½	(1.645 oz)
Canned corn (sugar added)	2½	(.42 oz)
Ketchup (2 tsp)	½	(.07 oz)
Ice cream (1 scoop)	2	(.35 oz)
1 bowl sugar-coated cereal	3	(.525 oz)
1 bowl cornflakes	trace	(.035 oz)
2 tsp jam, honey or marmalade	2	(.35 oz)
2 tsp sugar-reduced jam	1	(.175 oz)
1 small can fruit in syrup	10	(.07 oz)
1 small can fruit in juice	5	(.875 oz)
1330 ml can of cola	7	(1.255 oz)

▶ Top tips for natural sweeteners

- The most natural sweetener is fruit juice or fruit juice concentrates, which simply use naturally occurring sugars in fruit to add sweetness to other products. Fructose is simply fruit sugar that has been extracted, so it is much sweeter than fruit juices.

- Dried fruit purées are a healthy choice.

- Molasses and maple syrup are also natural products, and they are both highly nutritious.

- Cold-pressed organic honey is an excellent choice.

- Date syrup and rice malt syrup can be used as well.

An organic revolution

The mounting number of food scares has made most of us deeply suspicious about what we are eating. While labeling standards are undoubtedly improving, we still can't be certain that our carrots are, for example, free of pesticides and our meat does not come from cows fed hormones and antibiotics.

Most of us have busy lifestyles, and the prospect of investigating everything that we feed our children can be daunting. Yet, it's clear that we need to know what's in their food.

There is a solution: eat organic. Organic food is undoubtedly more expensive, but it is the only source of food that meets the guarantees we need. Fortunately, consumers are buying organic in increasing numbers, so the price is coming down. Product ranges have been dramatically expanded (see page 7), and this bodes well for the future.

Why organic?

- Organic food is more than just a new trend in eating—it is the food of the future, and one of the few ways to eat safely and to be certain that what you are eating is healthy. Organic food is grown or produced under strict regulations, and an organic food label (such as the new USDA National Organic Program approval stamp, COAB's Canada Organic Biologique mark or American Organic Growers & Consumers kitemark) is notoriously difficult to receive.

- Organic food is grown under natural conditions without the use of chemicals.

- Organic vegetables are grown without artificial fertilizers or pesticides in ground that has been tested and declared free of contamination. This prevents the practice of intensive farming, where land is artificially fertilized to produce the greatest number of crops.

- Nothing labeled organic is irradiated (see page 35), or contains any genetically modified organisms (see page 32).

- Choosing organic food means avoiding all of the hundreds of additives, preservatives, fillers and other chemicals added to food during its production, and regularly found in conventional foods. Many additives are known to cause cancer, hyperactivity, insomnia, birth defects, anxiety, asthma and allergies.

- Organically raised animals are given comfortable surroundings and fed food that has been organically produced. Land used for grazing must not have pesticides or any other chemicals sprayed on it.

- No antibiotics or other drugs are given to organically raised animals, unless they are genuinely ill. If drugs are required, the animal is not slaughtered for some time, to avoid any residue being left in the animal's system, which could eventually reach our plates.

- Organically raised animals are not fed anything containing animal products, if they are natural herbivores, and most of their food is found in their natural environment—the fields of the farm.

- Organically raised animals are "free-range," which means that they can wander outdoors instead of living their lives in a stable or cage.

- Organic food is higher in vitamins, minerals and other nutrients. This has been an area of some dispute over the past year, with some experts claiming that organic food is no better for us nutritionally, but consider the following: if foods are grown naturally, ripened naturally by the sun (which increases their nutritional content), not sprayed with preservatives that allow them to sit for months in the backs of trucks or on supermarket shelves, and grown in soil that cannot be treated with artificial fertilizers, we have a much better chance of getting the nutrition we need from our food. There's evidence to back that up (see Organic facts box).

- Intensive farming depletes the soil, creating a need for increasing amounts of fertilizer. This fertilizer eventually makes its way into our food through the plants we eat, and through the animals that ate the plants themselves. Fertilizers are dangerous for a number of reasons. The first worry was the run-off into rivers—where the extra nutrients caused algae to grow faster—and the stripping of oxygen out of the water, as they decompose, suffocating fish and other wildlife. Then the focus began to shift to the risk of nitrates from nitrogen fertilizers gradually working their way down into underground water, with the result that drinking-water supplies became contaminated. This is now a major problem in some arable farming regions (see page 31).

- The amounts of antibiotics required to treat farm animals, and to boost their growth rates, can enter our food chain and, through that, our bodies. More and more bacteria are becoming resistant to the antibiotics used, which means a race to find even more drugs to treat the new strains. The problem is that bacteria that are resistant to antibiotics can be passed on to humans, and become impossible to treat.

Organic facts and stats

- The Soil Association, the British organization that campaigns for organic farming, has provided evidence that organic crops contain more nutrients. Their research shows that organic foods contain more "secondary metabolites" than conventionally grown plants. Secondary metabolites are substances that form part of plants' immune systems, and help to fight cancer in humans. The group says that research from Denmark and Germany shows that organic crops also have a measurably higher level of vitamins, and that this can benefit people who eat them. By contrast, intensive farming is devitalizing our food.

- In 1995, the U.S. Environmental Working Group tested levels of pesticides in jars of baby food made by Heinz, Beech Nut and Gerber. Sixteen different pesticides were discovered, including eight linked with cancer, eight that were known to affect brain function, and five known to disrupt hormone activity. Children are even more vulnerable to toxins and carcinogenic substances than adults. No organic baby food contains any pesticides.

- Research carried out in 1994 by the Department of Occupational Medicine in Denmark found that men who regularly ate organic food had twice the sperm count of those on a conventional diet.

- Organic produce is believed to have higher vitamin C levels, and organic tomatoes have been found to contain 23 percent more vitamin A than conventional ones. Vitamin C and A are two of the antioxidants that can prevent cancer and heart disease, and, in some cases, reverse it.

What to do if you can't afford it

The cost of farming organically is higher than conventional farming because its producers do not receive the same subsidies that support intensive farming, and because it's cheaper to keep animals indoors in crowded conditions. Funding for organic farms is pitiful, and despite the real risks involved in eating foods that have been intensively farmed, very little money or land has been turned over to it so far. Thankfully many other countries have taken note, and we are able to import organic goods from around the world, although this isn't really the answer either, since food traveling long distances both increases pollution and is open to damage or infection en route.

Thankfully, the demand has increased dramatically and we have witnessed a significant reduction in price. The more we buy it, the lower the price will fall.

▶ Top tips for buying organic on a tight budget

- First and foremost, consider what your children eat the most of. If your baby or toddler has a particular preference for apples, buy organic apples. If your 12-year-old eats toast all day long, buy organic bread. This will reduce the chances of buildup of any one particular pesticide or group of pesticides.

- Similarly, many children seem to drink a great deal of milk, so it's sensible to reduce the risks by buying organic.

- Meat, eggs and root vegetables are most likely to contain dangerous chemicals that are the result of intensive farming. Children are most at risk of chemical residues and it's wise to play safe with these foods in particular. (Remember that children do not need a lot of meat and can get protein from other sources.)

- Soy products should be organic, if possible. With the problems associated with genetic modification, it's sensible to buy something that you know does not contain GM ingredients.

- The real answer is to buy as much as you can afford. If you eat too many fresh products to buy all organic, then wash everything very carefully and, in the extreme, peel it. There are now specially produced detergents that remove waxes, pesticides and any other substances sprayed on the skin of fruits and vegetables (see Resources, page 438), which can help to limit the damage.

- Consider buying organic produce from a local greengrocer. They tend to be cheaper, and the food is fresher, because it is generally collected from the market that same day. Another good option is the organic delivery services. These can be cheaper than supermarkets and very convenient.

- Above all, a healthy diet needs to contain plenty of fruits and vegetables, and increasing the number of servings your children eat, whether they are organic or not, will have health benefits over and above the risks of pesticide poisoning and other negative impacts.

- Cancer research organizations are frightened by the emphasis placed on organic food as they fear people will stop eating fruits, vegetables and whole-grains, because of the risks associated with conventional farming methods. They have a point. Organic is best, but fresh is next best, so don't be tempted to give up healthy foods. In the end, a processed food diet is far more likely to cause health problems than one with the recommended servings of good healthy foods. If your children have a varied diet, they will be getting a wide range of different nutritional elements, and the risk of taking in unacceptable levels of any one additive or pesticide will be greatly reduced.

chapter two

The Modern Child's Diet

....

The majority of our children eat too much junk. Even healthy diets are peppered with bags of the ubiquitous potato chips (see page 49), and tempting treats aimed specifically at children. It takes a determined parent to resist the pleas of a child faced with an array of chocolates or sugar-coated cereals (complete with free toys) at the supermarket. It's also considerably easier to give in to a package of candies than to spend an afternoon bickering about it. It's not lack of education or even apathy that steers most parents in the wrong direction—it's usually exhaustion. Anything for an easy life. And that's fair enough.

But what we are only just beginning to realize is that parents hold their children's future health in their hands. We need to find ways to resist the move toward over-processed, nutrient-free food in favor of a diet that will give our children the best possible health—both now and as adults. The fact is that we cannot change the world around us overnight, so we have to find ways of living with it. We cannot insist that our children avoid all the foods that their friends are eating because children hate to be different. There's nothing like being a 5-year-old social leper. Along the same lines, we cannot insist that they opt out from the real world. They need to learn to eat well in a society that does not eat well. They need to learn about balance—countering the odd bad with lots of good—and they need to learn to make choices.

As adults, we can do a lot to guide them in the right direction. We can educate them about food. This doesn't mean nutrition lessons every Friday evening. It simply means explaining what you are cooking or choosing at the supermarket and why. It means pointing out, whenever you get the opportunity, why some foods are healthier than others. Children love facts. They love to be able to show them off. Give them lots.

Most of all, we need to instill in our children a love of food—a variety of foods.

Children need to taste a variety of foods in order to appreciate them, and they need to experience different ways of cooking, flavors, textures and ingredients. If we feed our children chicken nuggets, hamburgers, potato chips, french fries, pizza and canned spaghetti over and over again, they become accustomed to those tastes. They will not develop a gourmet palate overnight. Unadventurous children do not become adventurous adults.

Eating well doesn't mean giving up what our friends are eating. It doesn't have to mean baking our own bread and serving up lentil soup. It doesn't mean ignoring the culture of food that has grown up around us. It means finding a balance that works for the whole family.

The following examples represent the daily diets of three real children.

Jenny

Jenny is six and has rather unusual tastes. She loves salty foods like olives, but also enjoys a wide range of fruits and vegetables. She's not so keen on meat, but her diet is otherwise varied. Jenny is small for her age and quite thin.

Breakfast
- Sugar puffs with milk
- Apple juice

Snack
- Cookie and water at school

Lunch (packed)
- Whole wheat bun with coleslaw and olives
- Pepperoni stick
- Canned pineapple in natural juice
- Graham cracker

After school
- Fruit juice

Dinner
- Spaghetti with meatballs, with organic beef and organic pasta. The tomato sauce also contained organic carrots, onions, leeks and turnips.
- Apple juice
- Ice cream cone
- Mango

Pre-bed snack
- Rice cakes and water

Assessment:

- Jenny has eaten more than the required servings of fruits and vegetables, which is good news. One (the mango) was raw, which also helps supply essential nutrients. Her protein intake is slightly low. There is protein in the ground beef, the cereal milk and in the pepperoni stick, and some in the pasta and whole wheat bread and bun, but probably not enough for a growing child. Carbohydrate levels are good, with some complex carbohydrates offered at every meal.

- The low points are the following: sugar puffs for breakfast are not the ideal start to a day. She will experience a blood sugar surge and then dip that could affect her concentration and mood.

- Olives are healthy, but they can be very salty. Too much salt is not recommended, as it places a strain on the kidneys, among other things.

- Pepperoni is also salty and contains nitrates (see page 31), which aren't recommended for children.

- Coleslaw is very high in saturated fats, but since Jenny ate very few other saturated fats throughout the day, it represents a small proportion of her diet and is acceptable.

- She had three "treats" in the day—two cookies and an ice cream cone. On balance, her diet is healthy enough to sustain that.

Possible changes:

- Jenny could add a banana to her breakfast, and switch to a sugar-free brand of cereal to provide the energy she needs (see page 52).

- Jenny's sandwich could include a source of protein, such as canned tuna, sliced meat or even cheese to be better balanced. Swapping the coleslaw for fresh lettuce, cucumber or sliced tomatoes is a healthier option.

- The pepperoni stick could be replaced with a healthier form of protein, such as a granola bar or a yogurt.

- For dessert, a yogurt or fromage frais would provide more nutrition than an ice cream cone, and probably make her more relaxed at bedtime.

Luke

Luke is also six, and attends school with Jenny. His diet is fairly varied, but he has constant cravings for sweet foods. He is a tall boy, with a big appetite, but he is not heavy for his height.

Breakfast
- Apple juice
- Whole wheat toast with peanut butter and whole fruit jam

Snack
- Cookie and water

Lunch
- Tuna in mayonnaise with peppers and green onions on two slices of whole grain bread
- Pineapple juice
- Fromage frais
- Fresh apricot
- Granola bar with raisins and nuts
- Canned peaches in natural juice

After school
- Granola bar
- Apple juice

Dinner
- White rice
- Stir-fried chicken with carrots, broccoli and corn in honey
- Raw cucumber slices
- Water
- A banana
- Yogurt
- Chocolate chip cookie

Snack
- Bread sticks

Assessment:

Luke has a good variety of protein (fish, nuts, whole grains and chicken) and lots of carbohydrates. He eats plenty of fruits and vegetables, some of which are raw. Substituting brown rice for white rice would be healthier, but everything else in his diet is whole-grain, so the odd refined food won't hurt. The granola bars are surprisingly sweet. One a day would be enough. The treat is at the end of a meal, which reduces the chance of tooth decay. Overall, a good, healthy diet.

Freddie

Freddie is nine, and slim for his age. He is a picky eater, which drives his mother to distraction. He is also pale, subject to mood swings, and often ill. He eats his lunch at school.

Breakfast
- Chocolate-covered cereal
- Milk

Break
- Milk
- Package of potato chips

Lunch
- Cold sliced ham
- White bread
- Cucumbers
- Milk

Snack
- Package of potato chips
- Water

Dinner
- Pasta with tomato sauce
- Chocolate-covered cookie bar
- Milk

Snack
- Package of potato chips

Assessment:

It's fairly clear that Freddie's diet is diabolical. First of all, he has only two servings of fruit and vegetables, which is not enough. His entire carbohydrate intake is in the form of sugars or refined foods (pasta, cereal and chips). He drinks too much milk (more than 8 servings a day). His only real protein source (ham) is high in nitrates, which are not a good idea for children. He eats far too many potato chips (see page 49), which will be affecting his overall health.

Possible changes:

- Freddie claims to not like fruit or vegetables, but he needs to learn to eat them. Offering fruit juice at breakfast with, perhaps a banana, or some dried fruit, will help him get a better start to the day.

- Switching to whole wheat pasta, cereal and bread will provide a better form of carbohydrates and some protein.

- Adding some grated vegetables to his pasta will help, as will serving a selection of raw vegetables, such as carrots or cucumbers alongside.

- Canned fruit in fruit juice (which many children do not seem to consider fruit) would be a healthy dessert, along with a little yogurt.

- The potato chips have to go. The odd package of potato chips is acceptable. His morning snack could be a "healthy" breakfast bar (see page 54). In the evenings, some sesame seed breadsticks would be a better choice.

- After school, some whole grain toast with peanut butter or even just a little butter would be healthier.

- Milk on his cereal and with his dinner is enough for a nine-year-old. Other times it should be replaced with water (between meals) and fruit or vegetable juice (at meals).

Potato Chips

There's a peculiar and pervading myth that potato chips are better for children than candy and chocolate. Indeed, I have heard countless proud parents proclaim that their children are not allowed sweet foods, and yet those same children are invariably seen clutching a package of potato chips or other salty processed snacks (cheesies, fried tortilla chips) after school. A 1998 British study showed that 20 percent of children buy potato chips or savory snacks on their way home from school, and 57 percent of children eat them in their lunchboxes. What are the issues?

- First and foremost, on the nutritional front, potato chips have no advantage over candy. Indeed, a chocolate bar, although high in sugar, has immeasurably more nutrition than a package of potato chips.

- Potato chips are not as likely to cause tooth decay, but they do often contain sugars (especially highly flavored brands) that can damage the enamel of children's teeth. Furthermore, many contain artificial sweeteners, which have been the subject of much controversy (see page 154).

- Even low-fat brands are high in fat and salt (see page 65), both of which are linked to long-term health problems.

- Many of these snacks contain additives and preservatives that can damage your child's health. For example, many contain MSG, which has been linked to all sorts of health problems in children and adults (see page 74). Additives and preservatives also increase your child's toxic levels, which can be at the root of many of our main health issues (see page 74).

- The high levels of salt, fat, sugars and flavors can play havoc with your child's palate. It's no wonder that children demand foods with such intense artificial flavors. A plate of broccoli, potatoes and fish, no matter how beautifully presented and cooked, will always come a poor second for children who are used to manufactured flavors and high levels of salt.

- Potatoes are obviously healthy, but in the process of becoming chips, they lose most of their nutritional value, and, even worse, they become a source of potentially dangerous toxins.

The odd package of potato chips is no cause for concern, but if your child is eating more than one package a week, it's time to consider other snack alternatives. Potato chips are not healthy, under any guise, and your child should be made aware of that. Certainly it takes more time to put together a snack pack (see page 88), or even to fill a whole wheat bun or wash a piece of fruit than it does to pop the packet into a bag, but your efforts will be more than worthwhile.

Alternatives to Kids' Food

Food	What's the problem?	Compromise	Best alternative
Chicken or turkey nuggets (or dinosaurs, or any other shape)	The meat contained in these products is low quality and will provide little or no nutritional value. They are also high in fats, fillers and additives.	If you don't have time to prepare you own, try chicken fillets made of 100 percent meat (not re-formed) in whole wheat flour. breadcrumbs. Look out for labels that say "no artificial ingredients." Still high in fat, but a better option.	Better still are whole strips of chicken, dipped in a beaten egg and then a little seasoned whole wheat Lightly fry in a tiny bit of olive oil, or grill.
Pizza	Frozen pizzas tend to have little or no nutrition, just a scraping of tomato sauce and a refined flour base loaded with additives. Takeout pizzas are often much higher in fat than the alternatives, and many contain GM ingredients.	Buy an organic or whole grain frozen pizza and add a little more sauce or chopped tomatoes (canned is fine, and it's also OK to put it on top of the cheese). Add your own fresh vegetables, meats, pineapple and cheese.	Buy whole wheat bases— or even whole wheat tortillas. Add fresh tomato sauce, cheese and fresh vegetables, meats and cheeses as above.
Hamburgers	Store-bought hamburgers use the lowest-quality meat, with a multitude of fillers and other unnecessary chemicals. They are high in fat and not nutritious. Takeout hamburgers are no better.	Frozen or fresh organic burgers aren't much more expensive, and they contain fewer of the problem additives. Serve grilled with a whole wheat bun.	Make your own. Use good-quality (organic if you can afford it) beef. Add an egg to bind and season. Grill or bake and serve on a whole wheat bun.

Food	What's the problem?	Compromise	Best alternative
French fries	Frozen french fries are high in fat and have little nutritional value. Deep-fried, they contain even more fat.	Oven fries are a slightly better option, but go for the low-fat variety, or those that use olive oil instead.	Make your own! It's easier than you think, and you can freeze them in batches. Slice a potato into strips. Blanch in a pot of boiling water for about 5 minutes. Toss them in olive oil and bake in the oven, turning frequently. Try the same with sweet potatoes.
Yogurt and fromage frais	Avoid the brands with sugar and flavors. These are high in sugar and other additives.	Yogurts and fromage frais sweetened with fresh fruit purées and no added sugar.	Greek or plain yogurt served with fresh fruit and a little organic honey to sweeten.
Sausages	The cheaper they are, the worse they are nutritionally. Frozen economy sausages are a false economy. They contain little meat—what's there is usually of the poorest quality—and many fillers and other additives. Fried, they are high in saturated fats.	Choose more expensive brands and look at the label to ensure that they are made up of good quality meat and the fewest number of extra ingredients. Bake or grill rather than frying.	Fresh organic sausages are your best bet, grilled or baked. Still, eat sparingly.
Canned spaghetti or other pasta (see also pasta below)	Canned pastas are much less healthy than you would imagine. Colors, flavors, sugar and salt are usually added. They have literally no nutritional value, as the pasta is made with refined flour, and the sauce is largely flavoring.	Cooked pasta with a canned tomato sauce. Choose brands that are low in sugar and salt, and that contain extra vegetables. If time is tight, make a large vat and freeze it in small containers to be heated up later.	Choose organic whole wheat pastas (or those made with other grains to add variety), and make your own sauce with chopped tomatoes, tomato purée, basil, pepper, fried onions and some grated or chopped vegetables, such as zucchini, peppers, mushrooms or even peas and corn. Purée it if your kids like it smooth.

Food	What's the problem?	Compromise	Best alternative
Fish sticks	Most fish sticks aimed at children contain chopped re-formed fish of various types. Chances are that there isn't much nutritious meat there, and you will be getting all kinds of fillers and additives to improve flavor and texture. The coating is high in saturated fat, and still more additives and refined products.	Whole fillet fingers with a whole wheat coating. Unevenly shaped fingers suggest that you are getting the real thing. Choose brands with the lowest number of ingredients on the label.	Make your own. Fresh or frozen cod or halibut fillets are much better value for money. Cut them into pieces, dip them in a little lemon juice and egg, then roll in seasoned flour and bake or grill. Alternatively, season some fresh whole wheat breadcrumbs and replace the flour. Best yet, serve grilled or foil-baked fish. It's quick and easy and the majority of children love it.
Cereal	Sugar-coated breakfast cereals are, obviously, high in sugar and very low in nutrients, even if they are fortified. They contain refined products and additives.	Choose whole wheat, oat or other grain cereals (organic cornflakes, for example), and sweeten with a little maple syrup if necessary.	Porridge or other home-made hot cereals are a good bet. Organic whole grain cereals are also good. Add fresh or dried fruits and sunflower seeds to increase the benefits.
Candies	Very few candies have any nutritional value, so they are empty calories. They can often take the place of healthy foods in a diet, and will rot teeth if eaten between meals.	Plain chocolate has a little more nutrition than sugary sweets, containing a little iron and magnesium (chocoholics would have you believe there's a lot more!), but it's higher in fat and has some caffeine. Still, a piece of good-quality chocolate is the best of the lot.	Dried fruits and dried fruit bars with no added sugar are a good compromise. For children over the age of about 4, chocolate-covered nuts are quite high in fat, but they offer substantially more nutrition. A chocolate covered brazil nut, for example, is high in selenium and iron.

Food	What's the problem?	Compromise	Best alternative
Cookies and Crackers	These range dramatically. Many cookies for children contain hydrogenated margarines and other fats, colorings, additives and preservatives, as well as a good helping of sugar and usually fat.	Look for labels that say "no artificial ingredients," and make sure that that list of ingredients is not too long. Avoid the hydrogenated fats, and make sure that sugar is well down the list. Go for those that contain whole grains, oats, nuts and seeds. Shortbread seems to be the best of the pre-packaged cookies with good-quality granola bars a close second.	Breadsticks are a good snack food. Choose ones with added sesame or poppy seeds. Rice crackers (brown are best) are also good. If a sweet cookies is called for, make them yourself (they freeze well) using as many unrefined ingredients as possible, and butter instead of margarine.
Pasta	White pasta is high in unrefined flour and often many other additives. The preservatives used in fresh pasta purchased in supermarkets often makes it an even less healthy option. Worst is dried, filled pastas, which have very little nutritional value. The sauce makes the difference. If you buy canned or bottled sauces, read the label and choose one with the least amount of sugar and other additives.	Whole wheat pasta is better nutritionally, but can be hard on the digestive system of young children. Choose fresh sauces with the fewest ingredients, and add your own vegetables.	Choose whole wheat pasta with home-made sauces. You can make big batches of sauces and freeze them, whether they contain meat or only vegetables. Add as many fresh vegetables to sauces as you can.
Ice cream	The ice cream normally marketed at children is full of all sorts of ingredients, few of which, if any, are natural. Expect milk powder, sugar, hardened vegetable fats, flavorings, emulsifiers, colorings and lots of pumped-in air. It's fatty and not nutritious.	Dairy ice creams are higher in fat and sugar, but they tend to be made with more natural ingredients and fewer additives. Choose brands with natural flavors and added fruit pieces, and, of course, the fewest extra ingredients.	Organic ice cream is the best bet, but frozen yogurt is less fatty and often less sweet than ice cream in any form. Once again, go for natural flavors, added fruit and a label that reads "no artificial ingredients."

Food	What's the problem?	Compromise	Best alternative
Breakfast bars	These have hit the headlines over the past months, when it was revealed that the average bar had more than 50 grams of sugar (that's nearly 2 ounces). Despite the fact that many are fortified with vitamins and minerals and may contain a few oats or whole wheat crumbs, these are not nutritious and they are not a good way to start the day.	A good whole-grain granola bar is good if your child is forced to eat on the run. Second best is a bag full of unsweetened, or very low-sugar cereal, eaten dry.	Breakfast at home is obviously the best choice, and one of the important aspects of a healthy diet is getting into the habit of sitting down to eat a proper meal. Grabbing snacks and eating on the run lead to unhealthy eating habits. If you really are running late, a whole wheat sandwich, with peanut butter and a banana, or even lean bacon, is healthier.
Toast and bread	A healthy option, depending on the type of bread and spread! White breads, even those that are enriched with nutrients, are not nutritious. Brown bread is usually just white bread flavored with something like caramel. Jam contains a great deal of sugar, as do many types of peanut butter. Avoid hydrogenated margarines, which contain trans fats.	Whole grain bread is the best option here. Peanut butter is high in fats, but fortunately not the worst kind. Look for a crunchy peanut butter with no added sugar or salt. The taste is not dramatically different and it's much healthier. If jam must be on the menu, choose one with only natural fruit sugars. It should be labeled a 100 percent fruit jam. Fruit compotes are another good choice, but choose one with as little sugar as possible. Cheese is good, but avoid anything processed.	Toast and bread should be organic (if you can afford it) if your child eats a great deal. Not only is it much more nutritious, but there will be no preservatives, additives or any other unnecessary chemicals. The best toppings are fresh fruits (mashed banana, for example), nut butters (but not for children under 3) or a scraping of fresh organic butter, which is much healthier than margarine.
Canned fruits and vegetables	Canned fruits containing sugar, and vegetables containing salt and sugar, are unnecessarily high in additives.	Choose canned fruits in natural fruit juice and vegetables in water.	Fresh fruit and vegetables are always best; frozen vegetables seem to have the next best nutrient total.

Healthy drinking

Water is always the best option when you are thirsty, but there are a variety of other options, some of which are positively bursting with nutrition. We'll look at the less healthy options first.

Carbonated drinks

The majority of carbonated drinks contain nothing but artificial sweeteners, flavors, sugar, caffeine and water. Some carbonated drinks contain a little fruit juice (watch for the percentage), but not enough to make these drinks worthwhile. Even carbonated mineral water, with a "hint" of a fruit juice tends to be artificially sweetened and flavored. The best advice is to avoid them.

Here's why:

- Most carbonated drinks do not add any nutrition to your children's diet, and are full of "anti-nutrients"—the types of chemicals that actually prevent the good elements from being absorbed. If meals are accompanied by carbonated drinks, many of the nutrients in the food will be negated, and still others will not be processed properly by the body.

- According to a recent report prepared by Cornell Medical College in the U.S., liquid intake has changed markedly among youth in the last several decades. For example, soft drink consumption has risen dramatically since 1978 with intake doubling in children ages 6 to 11 and tripling among teenage boys. In the U.K., the intake of carbonated drinks and sweetened non- or low-fruit juices has increased by more than 900 percent over the last 40 years.

- Soft drinks and sweetened beverages contribute extra calories to children's diets, compounding the problem of increasing fat stores among children and teens. The dramatic rise in soft drink consumption coincides almost exactly with the significant increase in childhood and adolescent obesity.

- Substituting soft drinks for milk is a particularly dangerous practice among pre-adolescent and teenage girls. Not only are girls missing out on the calcium needed to fully mineralize their growing bones but also there is some evidence that links the high phosphoric acid content of cola beverages and bone fractures in girls.

- One study of children ages 4 to 16 established a relationship between drinking carbonated soft drinks and fruit juice before bedtime and the severity of tooth erosion. The acids in soft drinks (regular as well as diet varieties) are responsible for breaking down tooth enamel while the sugars feed the acid-producing bacteria in the mouth.

- Substituting caffeine-containing soft drinks for water and other beverages may lead to dehydration because caffeine acts as a diuretic. This is particularly dangerous when youngsters rely on colas as fluid replacers during sports or active play.

- Sugar-free and artificially sweetened brands are not healthier. While they don't have the sugar and calories of regular soft drinks, they simply replace one bad thing (sugar), with another (artificial sugar). And as bad as sugar is, it is still better for you than artificial sweeteners, says the U.S. Center for Science in the Public Interest. At least two artificial sweeteners—acesulfame-K and saccharin—may promote cancer (see page 154).

High quantities of carbonated drinks can affect the health of your digestive system. In some parts of the U.S. and the U.K., children suffer from the oral equivalent of Crohn's disease, with mouth ulcers, bleeding and pain.

Powdered drinks

Powdered drinks have always been popular, because they are cheap and you can dilute them fairly heavily. They are, however, mainly sugar syrups and powdered sugar, and even reduced-sugar brands are high in calories and very bad for dental health. Highly sweetened drinks actually increase the body's need for water, so they are not the best option for quenching thirst. There are many varieties of fruit syrups and powdered drinks, and although some contain fruit or fruit extracts, they are not the real thing and add very little nutritional value.

- Fruit drinks are sold ready diluted or as concentrates. Concentrates contain at least 7% whole fruit and 10 to 15 percent sugar, plus some preservatives. Ready diluted fruit drinks sold in cartons have no restriction on fruit or sugar content.

- High-juice fruit syrups usually contain 35 to 50 percent fruit juice, but there is no legal limit, so check the carton.

- Powdered drinks normally contain no real fruit juice, merely chemical flavors, colors and sweeteners.

- Most importantly, however, watch out for "sugar-reduced" brands. These often contain artificial sweeteners, which can be dangerous for health (see page 154).

Are they healthy? The simple answer is no. Almost all of them contain additives, preservatives, flavorings and colorings, combined with an unhealthy dose of sugar or artificial sweetener. Even high-juice brands will provide very few nutrients, and what are contained will be counterbalanced by the additives.

Fruit and vegetable juice

Fresh fruit juice is the equivalent of a serving of fresh fruit, and will contain at least the recommended daily intake of vitamin C. In fact, fresh, fruit and vegetable juices are essential parts of anti-cancer diets. Raw juices do most of the things that solid raw foods do, but in a way that places minimum strain on the digestive system. The concentrated vitamins, minerals, trace elements, enzymes, sugars and proteins they contain are absorbed into the bloodstream almost as soon as they reach the stomach and small intestine.

If you are worried about the number of fresh vegetable and fruit servings your children are getting, consider purchasing a juicer and making your own fresh juices regularly. Carrot and orange is a particular favorite with children. Many children will happily drink a cup of bright orange juice but will balk at the sight of a steamed carrot. Mix them in any combination.

Are there drawbacks?

- Fruit juices are high in sugar (in some cases as much as there is in a can of cola), but the difference here is that it is a natural sugar (which puts less strain on the body), and it is counterbalanced by a wealth of nutrients. For example, a glass of orange juice contains folic acid, vitamin C, thiamin, vitamin A, niacin, vitamin B6, riboflavin, potassium, copper and zinc.

- Fruit juices can be as high in calories as regular colas, so take that into consideration when planning your children's meals. Fruit juices should be diluted with water, and most children do not need more than 300 ml/10 oz a day.

- Too much juice (or fruit) can cause diarrhea, particularly if your child is not used to it. Make sure you don't offer too much in any one sitting, and dilute with water.

Hot drinks

Tea and coffee are not suitable for children. They both contain caffeine, which is a nervous system stimulant and associated with various unhealthy symptoms. Tea is slightly healthier, in that it has some health-giving properties, but it shouldn't be considered before the age of about 12 or 13—later, if possible.

Hot chocolate is a favorite with kids, but it is high in saturated fats, sugars and caffeine, so it should be drunk sparingly. Don't go for the pre-packaged brands. If you want a hot, chocolatey treat, make your own cocoa, with a few squares of good-quality dark chocolate, a drop of pure vanilla essence and milk. Heat to the boil, and then allow it to simmer until all ingredients are dissolved in the milk. Add a little more sugar, if it needs it, but try to get your children used to the taste of pure cocoa or dark chocolate, which is much healthier than synthetic taste-alikes.

Most pre-packaged herbal teas are appropriate for children of any age. Even babies can drink very diluted, cooled teas. Watch out for herbal teas with added flavors. The natural ones are best. If your children find them a little bland, add a tiny bit of apple or other fruit juice, or, for children over one year old, a little good-quality pasteurized honey to sweeten. Here are some that can be served to children of any age:

- **Peppermint**—particularly good in the case of a tummy upset and even travel sickness. It's nice after dinner, and served cold in the summer with a splash of apple juice, a little lemon juice and honey and some ice.

- **Chamomile**—soothes the most fractious toddler or teenager. Make chamomile tea a bedtime treat if you've got an insomniac on your hands. Chamomile is also good for digestive upsets. If it was good enough for Peter Rabbit . . .

- **Rosehip**—is rich in vitamin C (choose freeze-dried brands) and considered to be an immune booster. Serve any time. It's nice chilled in the summer with lemon juice and a little fruit sugar or juice.

Never serve young children anything other than hand-hot tea. A huge number of children are burned each year by boiling water.

Milk

Milk is important for growing children, although not essential if your child is allergic or intolerant, or if it isn't part of your vegetarian diet (see page 91). If your child doesn't drink milk, make sure he is getting adequate calcium from other sources. Milk provides many needed nutrients and is also a source of fluid. Serve full-fat milk up to the age of four or five, switching to 2 percent thereafter, to reduce unnecessary fat in the diet.

Water

Water is best. See page 19.

Most importantly, make sure that your child has plenty to drink. Depending on their age, size and activity level, most children need at least a quart/liter of fluids a day.

chapter three

When Food Becomes a Problem

P icky eaters, excess weight, eating disorders ... the preponderance of conditions relating to what should be one of the most natural and enjoyable parts of living is alarming, and it reflects the unhealthy attitudes we now have toward food. Changing your attitude, and encouraging healthy attitudes in your children, can make a big difference to their future eating habits and their health. Let's look at some of the main issues.

Overweight Kids

In America, health authorities are calling the current levels of obesity in children an "epidemic," and have set up a wide variety of programs involving parents, schools and children to help counter this alarming trend. At present, obesity is the most prevalent nutritional disease of children and adolescents in the U.S. In the U.K., figures are slightly lower, but with a diet that has become more American in focus, they are not far behind.

What's the extent of the problem?

- According to the American Academy of Child and Adolescent Psychiatry, the problem of childhood obesity in the United States has grown considerably in recent years. Between 16 and 33 percent of children and adolescents are obese. The academy claims that weight gain due to poor diet and lack of exercise is responsible for over 300,000 deaths each year. The annual cost to society for obesity is estimated at nearly $100 billion.

Calculating your child's BMI

Obesity is calculated using a formula called body mass index (BMI). To calculate body mass index, multiply weight in pounds by 705. Then divide that result by inches squared.

For example, a child who is 40 in. tall and weighs 55 lbs. has a BMI of approximately 24 ((55 x 703) ÷ (40 x 40) = 24)).

A BMI of 24 or less is considered healthy, 25–29 overweight, and 30 or over, obese.

- In the U.K., Dr. John Reilly, head of Glasgow University's Childhood Obesity Group, found that the amount of obesity in children has risen from 5 percent in the late 1980s to as much as 17 percent in the 15-year-old age group in the late 1990s. Researchers in the Netherlands collected weight and height details for 14,500 children between 1996 and 1997 and found that 13 percent were overweight, mirroring similar studies in the U.K. and the U.S.

- The second National Children and Youth Fitness Study in the U.S. found 6–9 year olds to have thicker skinfolds than their counterparts in the 1960s (Ross & Pate, 1987). During the same period, others documented a 54 percent increase in the prevalence of obesity among 6–11 year olds (Gortmaker, Dietz, Sobol, & Wehler, 1987).

What to do if your child is overweight

Excess weight is only very rarely caused by another health condition. Most cases of overweight and obesity can be safely and successfully reduced at home.

The causes:

- The Dutch research team blamed the rise in obesity on not eating breakfast (see page 85), snacking and eating too many foods containing invisible fats.

- Experts speaking at a conference in the U.S. agreed that a lack of physical activity, increased time in front of television and a diet high in fat and calories are major factors contributing to this unsettling trend.

- Studies show today's youngsters are eating less than in the past, but are watching more television at an early age. Dr. Reilly said: "What we suspect is happening is that preschool children have been replacing natural active behavior with inactive behavior like watching TV. Children have been eating less, but are watching more TV—which includes watching videos, PlayStations or PC screens."

- Data from the Third National Health and Nutrition Examination Survey in the U.S. showed children who watched four or more hours of television per day were more overweight and had a significantly greater amount of body fat.

- A study showing the difference between a child's diet in the 1950s and our modern diet indicated that children are not eating any more calories than they used to, but that their activity levels have fallen substantially. Forty years ago children ate more fat and consumed more calories, but their sugar intake was substantially lower, and they ate more grains, fruits and vegetables, as well as drinking more milk. Some researchers have concluded that activity levels are only partly to blame—an unhealthy diet plays an equally important role.

The answers

- Don't be tempted to try to control your child's diet completely. According to American specialist Leann Birch, high levels of parental control are associated with poor self-regulation of energy intake. In other words, when parents attempt to control their child's food intake, the child loses the ability to respond to his other cues of hunger and fullness. Dr. Birch's research shows that children with the most controlling parents actually have a higher level of body fat. The most positive step that any parent can take is to promote a nutritious diet, acting as a role model rather than a disciplinarian.

- Focus on the food pyramid (see page 23). If your child is getting all of the recommended quantities of fruits, vegetables, unrefined carbohydrates and good-quality proteins, there is little room for fattening, unhealthy foods.

- Get children involved in the family diet. Let them choose some of their own meals (from a pre-arranged selection). If they feel empowered, they will feel better about themselves and learn that they can control some parts of their lives.

- Learn to use "non-food" treats and rewards. If a child grows up believing that food is associated with good behavior, good marks at school, and making her parents happy, she will associate it with satisfaction and happiness. When children are old enough to make their own food choices, children will, often instinctively, go for the foods that have these good associations. If chocolate, dessert, candy, ice cream or a meal at a fast-food restaurant are your family treats, make some changes. Try, for example, a star chart for good behavior, with a family outing, a small toy or an article of clothing as the reward.

- From early on, it's important for children to learn good eating habits. If you have a house full of fattening foods, you are sending the wrong messages. Buy only foods that you want the whole family to eat—in other words, foods that are delicious, fresh and, above all, healthy.

- Don't put your child on a diet. If he feels that he is "different," he'll lose self-esteem and it can create obsessions for foods that are not allowed. Instead, change the eating habits of the whole family. Weight stabilizes at healthy levels when we eat a good, balanced diet. It's also important to recognize that *all* children need adequate calories and nutritious foods in order to grow and develop normally. Restrictive diets rarely work and are not appropriate for children, even those deemed "overweight."

- Ensure that your child feels good about himself. If he grows up with a positive self-image, he'll be that much more likely to look after himself, eating well, taking care of his body and choosing healthy over unhealthy. Many obese children feel ugly and fat, a self-image that is compounded by playground taunts. Praise your child often, and help him to feel attractive and good about his body.

- Don't make food an issue. Educate your children about a healthy diet, but don't dwell on it too much. Serve good, healthy food and enjoy it around the family table. Don't withhold certain foods from an overweight child if everyone else is eating it. Once again, it can create an obsession.

- Don't let him feel that he is missing out. All children need to feel part of their culture, at home, in the playground or at school. If every other child has potato chips or chicken nuggets, it might be too much to expect your child to forego them completely. Strike a deal—a package of potato chips on Fridays, for example. Try some of the healthy alternatives to junk food. If they feel that they are the "same" as their peers, children are less likely to develop obsessive habits. Better to offer one small candy after the main meal, or a little piece of good-quality chocolate, than cut out something that plays such an important role in our children's environment. Children learn the art of balance and don't feel deprived.

- Encourage children to eat slowly and to chew their food properly. Try to avoid eating on the run or in front of the television. When we focus on what we are eating, we tend to feel full more quickly.

- Watch the snacks. Most snack foods are high in fats and sugars, and many other unhealthy ingredients. Put a "help yourself" policy in place: the fruit bowl, a kitchen drawer containing rice crackers, dried fruits and nuts, unsalted, unsweetened popcorn, oatcakes, even whole wheat bread, a shelf in the fridge with good-quality yogurt and raw vegetables. These can be "choose your own snack" centers, which children can raid when they are hungry. Children who learn to eat healthily when they are hungry (not when their parents say they are hungry) are more likely to learn good eating habits and self-control.

- Make sure your child isn't filling up on unnecessary calories in his liquid intake.

Offer only water between meals, with milk (2 percent after the age of about 4) and diluted fruit juices offered only with meals.

- Boost activity levels. All children can benefit from becoming more physically active on a daily basis. School-based physical education programs have been continually eroding over the past decade. There are often fewer classes available, and overcrowding of schools means that children often stand around waiting their turn rather than participating in a continuous aerobic activity. For ideas on improving fitness, see chapter 5.

- Reduce the amount of television your child watches. Physical activity should be the first choice for leisure. Not only do children who sit in front of the TV get less exercise, but they are the target of literally hundreds of advertisements, many of which are for the wrong types of foods. It's hard not to feel hungry when faced with hamburgers and fries, chocolatey breakfast cereals, potato chips and carbonated drinks for hours on end. Similarly, children will be seduced into thinking that these types of foods are acceptable—and even necessary to feel part of the crowd.

- Talk to people at your child's school. If children are offered lunch at school, make sure your child isn't getting second or third helpings. Ask them to reduce the number of fatty foods on the menu. No child benefits from high levels of saturated fats. Plan your child's diet with him in advance—fries only once a week, for example, and a star on a chart for every serving of fruits and vegetables that he eats.

- The entire family must make positive lifestyle changes in the area of activity, television viewing and nutrition for children to realize a more healthy body weight. By becoming involved in their children's health, it is likely that parents will achieve better health as well.

- Look at your own attitudes toward food. Not only is obesity on the increase, but eating disorders are too. If you are constantly on a diet, or complaining that you are fat, children will grow up believing that food is something to feel guilty about. This can work both ways—with young girls (in particular) putting themselves on diets, or hungry children "stealing" inappropriate snacks because they feel bad about eating them. More than 50 percent of Americans are on a weight-reducing diet at any one time, so there is a clear message to children.

John

John is an active child who has played competitive sports since he was old enough to take part, and his favorite activities involve a ball and lots of fresh air. John is popular, does well at school and eats a normal diet. But despite taking lots of exercise, John was significantly overweight and as other children have started to notice, and to call him names. John's mother became concerned. She'd always made an effort to serve him healthy foods, and to make him feel good about himself. In fact, John doesn't think he's fat. He considers himself to be big and strong, and is looking forward to a career in football.

Having ruled out any medical causes, John's mother eventually came to the conclusion that he was overeating on the sly. She asked around and discovered that John was rather obsessive about food at other people's houses—clearing away leftovers, complaining of being hungry, and eating much more than the other children. She also discovered he was having second and third helpings of everything at school. She was rather shocked, having controlled his intake carefully since he was an overweight toddler. Therein lay the problem. At home, John's food intake was so carefully regulated, he felt he had no control. He had to resort to hiding forbidden snacks in his room, and to eating as much as possible when he was out of the house. He had become a food junkie.

John's mother immediately set about making changes. She arranged a "healthy" snack cupboard and allowed John to eat anything he wanted when he was hungry. She also allowed him to choose his portion sizes and to stop eating when he was full. At the beginning of this new program, she was alarmed. The snack cupboard was emptied within a couple of days and he was eating far more than was healthy at mealtimes. But she stuck to her guns, and continued to allow him to choose. Over the next few months, food lost its overwhelming importance for John. He still ate a great deal, but the healthy options paid off and because he wasn't always hungry, he didn't overeat when he was out of the house. He also didn't need to resort to subterfuge. John lost all of his excess weight within six months of having been given some freedom and personal responsibility.

Is my child fat?

It's not difficult to spot an overweight child, and you will undoubtedly notice if your child has gained weight. If your child is much bigger than his peers, and has obvious rolls of fat, particularly on his abdomen, chances are he is overweight. Try the BMI formula if you are concerned (see page 60), or see your family doctor for an assessment. But bear in mind the following:

- Some children are naturally sturdier than others, and will weigh more without being fat.

- Children come in all shapes and sizes. Big does not mean fat.

- Many perfectly healthy children are extremely thin, and your also perfectly healthy sturdier child may look fat in comparison. Don't compare. Keep an eye out for excess fat, but remember that most healthy children have some visible fat on their bodies.

- Many children seem to put on extra weight just before a growth spurt. If your child has a good, nutritious diet and takes plenty of exercise, a sudden weight gain might just indicate fat stores being laid down for growth.

- Don't panic, and don't let your child believe he is "fat." Focus on the positive things the whole family is going to do to improve overall health.

- If your child's eating habits suddenly change, try to see if there is an emotional cause. Is he comfort eating for any reason?

Salt

Children need no more than .06 oz (1750 mg) of salt every day, and chances are that they are getting more than that in their diets at present. For example, bread contains a whopping .02 oz (500) mg per slice, cornflakes contains more than .03 oz (900) mg per bowl, and even cheddar cheese comes in at 12 oz (335 g) per 2 oz (50 g).

Why should we worry?

Too much salt puts a strain on the kidneys and can increase the rate at which calcium is excreted from the body (putting children, particularly girls, at risk of osteoporosis later in life). It has also been linked with high blood pressure, stroke, heart disease and cancer of the stomach.

Even supermarkets have begun to take note. Most stores in the U.S. and Canada now offer low- and no-salt alternatives to most foods. In the U.K., they've gone even further. On major chain has just pledged to reduce the salt content of their salt and vinegar potato chips by 12 percent, and to reduce the ingredient in a variety of products. At present, bread contributes up to 25 percent of an adults average daily intake—and almost 50 percent of that of children. As a result, supermarkets are now offering bread with a substantially reduced salt content. Look for these brands when purchasing from the supermarket.

The best way to avoid salt is to read the labels. Many foods, such as breakfast cereals, are surprisingly high in salt. Once you cotton on to the problem foods, you can avoid or limit them in your child's diet.

Finally, never be tempted to add salt to your child's food. If they like the idea of additional flavoring, offer a little fresh ground pepper, fresh cut herbs, a squeeze of fresh lemon or even a little ketchup (see page 94).

Underweight kids

Although overweight kids are becoming the norm in the Western world, there are children who are underweight—often worryingly so. Being underweight can be the result of illness, and I'll discuss various health conditions and their natural treatments in chapter 11. On page 334, eating disorders are examined. Here, however, we'll focus on underweight that is not the result of illness.

Is my child underweight?

- Where does your child fall on the growth charts? If he's substantially below the average, he may be underweight. Talk to your doctor and ask her advice.

- Some children are naturally skinny, despite a healthy diet. If your child seems to be thriving, has lots of energy, good concentration and eats well, don't worry.

- Any child who suddenly loses weight should be seen by a doctor. Obviously short-term illnesses can cause weight loss, but anything dramatic should be reported.

- All children, even the skinny ones, should have some visible fat on their bodies. If yours doesn't, take a good look at his diet. Often very thin children have an imbalance or shortage of essential fatty acids (see page 11) in their diet, and it can be quickly rectified by supplements and by introducing the appropriate foods to their diet.

What to do

- Carefully consider your child's diet. If he eats too much junk food, he is probably not getting the nutrients he needs to grow. Although many junk foods are fattening, they can upset the metabolism and normal functioning of the body, and some children actually lose weight because they are not able to absorb what they need from food.

- The best advice is to follow the food pyramid (see page 23). If your child is getting all the correct nutrients, in the right balance, his weight should balance out.

- Don't be tempted to add fatty foods to your child's diet. By all means offer more foods with fat, but choose carefully. Unsaturated fats are always best. Increase calories and quantity rather than fat. Your child may be one of those lucky individuals with a quick metabolism, and he may be able to eat much more than his peers or even siblings and not put on weight. This is, however, a double-edged sword. Even very thin children will not benefit from a diet that is high in unhealthy fats—heart disease affects thin people, too. If you set up bad eating habits now, they can be there for life. Secondly, metabolism can change, and it often slows down as we get older. If your child becomes used to eating lots of fatty foods, he'll find it hard to change his diet when it begins to matter most. Many skinny children become overweight adults for this reason.

- Offer more healthy snacks. Some thin children find a big meal too daunting, and prefer to eat smaller meals more often. Make sure they are healthy, and contribute to a good overall diet.

- Don't panic. If your child senses that you are anxious about his weight, he will become frightened and, probably, anxious himself. Leave him to it. Offer lots of healthy food as often as you can, and encourage good eating habits. If he doesn't eat, don't push it. He will eat when he is hungry. If he is alarmingly thin and doesn't seem to want to eat at all, investigate the possibility of ill health, or some sort of emotional upset that may be affecting him. See chapter 10 for some natural treatments.

- Offer a vitamin and mineral supplement every day. This can help to address any shortfall in your child's diet, and if there is an imbalance or mild deficiency at the root of the problem, this can come some way to rectifying it.

- Look at the tips for picky eaters (see page 69). Even if your child eats well, but not enough, he may benefit from a different approach. Eating together or with friends at a companionable dinner table may encourage a better appetite, for example.

- Look at the liquid intake. If your child is drinking too much juice, water or milk, he may not have room for adequate food. Cut it down, and serve drinks only when he is genuinely thirsty. Conversely, he may not be drinking enough. Offer milk, yogurt and fresh fruit shakes, almond or rice milk and fruit drinks, or just lots of fresh fruit juices with snacks to boost nutrient intake and provide a little more sustenance.

- Watch the fiber. A diet that is too high in fiber can mean that your child is not absorbing nutrients properly. Bran, for example, is not really appropriate for small children as it can irritate the gut. Fiber is important, but if it makes up a large proportion of your child's diet, it can be doing more harm than good. Cut down on the unrefined carbohydrates for a while, and see if that makes a difference.

- Make sure that he's getting enough protein. Protein is essential for healthy growth and development. If your child is a vegetarian (see page 91) or a picky eater, he may not be getting enough. Add nuts, seeds, cheese, eggs, lean meats and fish to his daily diet to increase calories and protein intake.

- Could an overactive lifestyle be the cause? If your child is very active every day his calorie needs will be greatly increased. Make sure he is getting enough to meet the demands placed on his body. Consider cutting down on some of his active leisure pursuits. Exercise is essential for many reasons, but like everything else, balance is the key.

Picky Eaters

Herein lies the root of the problem facing many parents. It's very, very difficult to plan healthy, balanced meals when you've got children who refuse to eat them. Early in life, most children cotton on to the fact that their parents are concerned about how much and what they are eating. Making a fuss about food guarantees instant attention, and many children slide into the habit of using food to wield power over their parents. Other children are simply not interested in food, and the concerted efforts of their parents to make them eat put them off even further. For parents of all picky eaters, the best advice is to remove the pressure. If children fail to get a response, they get bored. If they realize that they won't get attention for eating badly, they'll stop using food as a tool to do so. If the pressure is off at the dinner table, children will start developing a healthier attitude to food—it's there to eat. It's neither poison nor is it a miracle medicine. Food can be enjoyed when it is not associated with parental nagging.

How can I change my child's eating habits?

Let's start at the beginning. If you have a baby who is just beginning her first table foods, you have a blank canvas, and chances are you'll be successful if you bear the following in mind:

- Offer plenty of variety. If babies eat the same foods all the time, they'll become accustomed to them. Babies like routine and they like the familiar. If they eat only the same few foods, they'll be more likely to resist new additions to their diet. Start as you intend to continue—introducing different foods every few days.

- Even babies have likes and dislikes. Don't worry if your baby has an instant aversion to spinach or avocados, for example. It's natural for babies to have defined tastes. The secret is to persevere. Try them mixed with other vegetables or fruits, or serve just a little. If you get nowhere, take them off the menu for a couple of weeks and then try again.

- Don't rely on little jars of food. The odd organic meal from a jar won't affect her eating habits, but using them exclusively will. Some babies refuse to eat anything that doesn't come in a jar and I've seen parents forced to purée their own foods and "hide" them in empty baby food jars so that their babies will eat them.

- Always take the food out of the jar and serve it in a bowl or cup, with a spoon. Even the most canny baby won't be able to identify where it's come from! Children need to learn that all food does not come from a jar!

- Serve your children what you are eating. Even picky babies will want to be part of the action. If everyone else is eating it, they'll want some too. Obviously some adult foods are not appropriate for babies, but purée or chop the parts of the meal that are, before the sauces are added, for example, or before you add that glass of wine for flavor.

▶ Top tips for dealing with picky eaters

- Don't make a fuss at mealtimes. There will be times when your child is starving and will demolish anything in sight. At other times, she will pick and graze and seem to need nothing substantial. Go with the flow. Never force a child to clear her plate. She'll grow up associating food with stress and bad behavior. The clean plate brigade was disarmed a long time ago.

- Children need to learn to recognize when they are hungry and when they are full, and ultimately they will learn self-control and self-regulation. If you decide when they are full for them, they'll never learn when to stop. That doesn't mean giving children free rein. If your child genuinely doesn't like something—mushrooms, for example—don't force it. Suggest that she try one bite. Or if she's not very hungry, suggest three bites of everything on the plate. Children need to learn to try foods, and they need to eat a variety of good foods in order to stay healthy. Provide that variety on a daily basis. Variety is one of the keys to preventing food allergies and sensitivities (see page 344).

- Show some respect. We all have foods we don't like, and there are very healthy eaters who simply cannot abide a particular vegetable, meat or flavor. Don't force food that a child dislikes. The problem with picky eaters, of course, is that they claim not to like anything. That's a different scenario. If your child eats well, tries new things and eats a healthy, varied diet, then the odd "no-way" food can be dropped from the daily diet. But don't give up. Try new recipes. Introduce it again in a month's time. Children's tastes change, and what may have been considered revolting one week may be the new favorite later on. If your child rejects a food after trying it a number of times, and continues to dislike it despite your best efforts, leave it for a period of time. Some children instinctively dislike foods to which they are sensitive—a type of instinctive defense mechanism.

- Don't buy what you don't want your child to eat. If you have a cupboard full of potato chips and cookies, and a refrigerator full of processed foods, you are fighting a losing battle. If there are alternatives to hand, you are unlikely to convince a child that he should eat what's put in front of him—particularly if he knows that you will cave in later and allow an inappropriate snack. Make a concerted effort to change the eating habits of the whole family, and start by cutting down on the junk food. If your child will only eat chicken nuggets, don't buy them. If he fills up on potato chips, leave them on the supermarket shelves. If there is nothing else, children will eat what's put in front of them.

- Don't offer alternatives. Serve a healthy meal for the whole family and don't panic if your child doesn't eat much. If she is hungry, she will eat. Even the most resolute child will not starve herself to death.

- Invite a good eater around for dinner—often! My youngest son was converted to salad, avocados and olives by his adventurous friend. Children like to do what their peers are doing, and if that involves eating new foods, they'll do it.

- Educate your child. Explain what foods are healthy and what they do for our bodies. Children love information, and they'll feel important if you take the time to explain things. Don't assume that they won't be interested. That doesn't mean boring them with facts about vitamins and minerals. Make it relevant—if you have a sportsman, point out that unrefined carbohydrates will give him more energy for the big game. If he's got a cold, explain that fresh fruits and vegetables have lots of vitamin C which will help his cold to go away. Bring children to the supermarket and show them food labels. Compare good and bad labels and look appropriately shocked at the labels for junk food. Let them feel that they are part of your program. Enlist their help and ask their advice. Encourage them to choose fresh produce—teach them, for example, to look for firm cucumbers, and how to tell if a melon is fresh by its scent.

- Don't label your child. Parents often create self-fulfilling prophecies. If a child thinks he's picky, he will be. If you continually praise your child during meals for what she does eat, and insist to everyone around that your child is such a good eater, she'll take some pride in this achievement.

- Don't give up! Picky eaters are often picky because we allow them to be. If you give in and serve only what your child will eat, you will be setting up unhealthy eating patterns that can run through his whole life. Serve good healthy meals at every sitting. Offer the normal treats, and balance the good with the bad parts of his diet.

- Empower your child. If your child feels that he's lost control, he'll dig in his heels or revert to tears or tantrums. Make up a list of eight or nine good healthy meals, with a variety of different vegetables on the side. Let each child in the family choose a particular night's menu. You can suggest that there have to be at least four fruits or vegetables with every meal, and at least two have to be different from the meal chosen for the previous night. If you make it into a game, children will be more likely to become involved. They'll also feel that they have some control.

- Involve your children in preparing and cooking food. Even very young children can help in some way, even if it is just stirring, or adding ingredients. Ask a vegetable phobic to make the salad. Praise the result. If they made it, they'll feel proud of it, and they'll be more likely to eat it.

- Introduce new foods alongside the old favorites, and then slowly drop the parts of your child's diet that concern you most. Don't be tempted to launch a dramatically different eating program overnight. You'll incite mutiny! Instead, make small changes. Every new food that your child eats is a step in the right direction.

- Introduce a star chart or the equivalent. Children can be encouraged to put a star up for every healthy or new food they eat. When they reach an agreed total, you can offer a toy, or some extra allowance.

- Watch the snacks. If your child is filling up with food between meals, she's that much less likely to want to sit down and eat again. Offer small snacks when your child is genuinely hungry, but if dinner is nearly ready, encourage her to wait.

- Drinks are filling, too. If you child drinks a lot of milk, he's not likely to feel very hungry. Milk is a nutritious addition to a diet, but it is not a complete food. If your child seems to be living on milk alone, he won't be getting enough of the nutrients he needs from other foods. Serve milk with meals or midafternoon or morning snacks. Stick to water or diluted pure fruit juice the rest of the time.

- If you have a grazer on your hands, make sure that the snacks she eats are nutritious. Some children just can't seem to stomach a big meal, and prefer to eat little and often throughout the day. This style of eating is fine, as long as the foods eaten are nutritious and balanced. But whatever your child eats throughout the day, sit her down and make sure she eats it at the table. You don't want to encourage eating on the run, which can develop into a bad habit. If she's had plenty of small meals throughout the day, she won't want a big dinner, but serve smaller portions of whatever you are serving the rest of the family.

- Don't overfill plates. Even the best eaters are daunted by a pile of food placed in front of them. Offer small servings and encourage second helpings.

- Place the serving dishes on the table and encourage children to help themselves. They'll naturally choose more of the things they like, but as long as they are encouraged to eat a little of everything, they can be allowed to make choices about quantity.

- If your child refuses food or just picks at his food for a long time, don't push it. Don't make your child feel guilty if he's just not hungry, and don't ever make him eat to please you. This sort of emotional blackmail can lower your child's self-esteem and make him insecure.

- If your child hates meat, talk to your dentist. Many children have bite problems that make chewing a nightmare. My eldest son hated all types of meats until his bite was corrected by a brace. Literally overnight he developed an interest in meat, when the problem was resolved.

- Eat the same foods as your children. There should be no distinction between children's food and adult food. Good, healthy food is appropriate for the whole family. If children see their parents enjoying a broad range of foods, they'll be more likely to try some.

- Picky parents are more likely to produce picky kids. Try to expand your own diet to include foods that you don't normally eat. You might find that your tastes have changed, too. Don't serve only foods that you like. Try new recipes and be more adventurous. What you want to aim for is variety. If your child sees you eating something different, he'll naturally think he has the right to an alternative too.

- Eat with your children. If they see you eating the same things that they are eating, they will feel reassured. Like anyone else, children enjoy company. If they are faced with a solitary dinner, they'll probably not be very interested. Make mealtimes fun with lots of conversation or laughter. Children will eat more if there is no pressure to finish their plates and no intense focus on what they are eating. They will also learn to associate food with pleasure. It can be difficult to sit down together as a family, particularly if one or both parents work late. If you work, encourage your child's caregiver to sit down and eat with him. If you are at home with your kids, and want to eat with your partner much later, you can still sit down and have a little bit of what your children are eating. Sip a cup of soup or eat a salad later on. It's much healthier to eat earlier in the evening, to give your body a chance to digest the food before bed. Alternatively, give your children a nutritious English "tea," with fresh vegetables, fruit and maybe some toast after school. They can then last a little longer and eat a proper meal with you a little later.

- Studies show that many picky eaters have a zinc deficiency. Increase your child's intake of zinc-rich foods, and ask your pharmacist for a special prepared zinc supplement for children (usually sucked).

Food allergies and intolerance

This subject is covered in depth in chapter 11. See pages 344–349.

Eating disorders

Eating disorders, including anorexia and bulimia, are covered in depth in chapter 11. See pages 334–337.

Don't forget chemicals in food

Chemicals in food can be one of the most dramatic causes of toxic overload (see chapter 7) and a whole host of other conditions. In Chapter 1 we discussed the impact of pesticides, growth hormones and other nasties that are a common feature of our modern food supply. Here we'll look at one of the worst offenders: food additives.

Any parent who wants to ensure their child's health needs to be aware of the issues here. Not only are food additives a major cause of health problems but they also can play havoc with the immune system, affecting growth, mood, concentration, sleeping patterns and overall resistance to infection by overloading your child's system with toxins. Children's food is full of the worst additives, largely because manufacturers (rightly) believe that something brightly colored, oversweetened and refined and processed to look like your child's favorite cartoon character is more likely to appeal to a picky child. As boring as it may sound, learn to read the labels, and take some time to educate yourself about this problem.

Every food contains natural chemicals, and many other chemicals are added to foods to make them safer for us to eat. Some chemicals change the consistency of a product, others make it last longer, and still others give it flavor or color. Vitamins and minerals are often added to foods to make them more nutritious. How do we differentiate between the good and bad?

The good, the bad and the ugly

Additives in foods have been cleared for use in the U.S. and Canada, and, officially, foods contain too little of them to do any harm. Some, in fact, are healthy, such as vitamin C (also called ascorbic acid). Others are preservatives, which are necessary for a product to survive for any length of time.

Many manufacturers understand that people are wary of chemicals and have begun putting the full, scientific name of the chemical, which, in some cases, makes it sound more official and even healthier. Longer names are bound to confuse the consumer, so beware of long lists of unusual-sounding words, particularly in foods that are brightly colored, highly flavored or very sweet. Watch out for tartrazine, which is a yellow food coloring that is now believed to cause hyperactivity, particularly in children. Also on the danger list are amaranth and crythrosien (red colors), which are possible carcinogens.

What to look for

- The main additives that have been linked with health problems of various descriptions include Curcumin, Tartrazine, Quinoline Yellow, Yellow 2G, Sunset Yellow, Cochineal, Carmoisine/Azorubine, Amaranth, Ponceau, Erythrosine BS, Red 2G, Patent Blue V, Indigo Carmine, Brilliant Blue FCF, Green S/Lissamine Green/Acid Brilliant Green, Caramel, Black PN, Brilliant Black BN, Carbon Black, Vegetable Carbon, Brown FK, Brown HT/Chocolate Brown HT, Lithol Rubine BK/Pigment Rubine, Carageenan/Irish Moss, Benzoic acid, Sodium benzoate, Potassium benzoate, Sodium sulfite, Sodium hydrogen sulfite/Sodium bisulfite, Acid sodium sulfite, Sodium metabisulfite/Disodium prosulfite, Calcium hydrogen sulfite/Calcium bisulfite, Biphenyl/Diphenyl, 2-Hdroxy-biphenyl-2-yl-oxide/Sodium orthophenylphenate, Hexamine, Hexamthylenetetramine, Potassium nitrate, Sodium nitrate, MSG, Propyl gallate/Propyl 3,4,5 trihydroxybenzene, Octyl gallate, Dodecyl gallate, Dodecyl 3, 4, 5, trihydroxybenzene, Butylated hydroxyanisole BHA, Butylated hydroxytoluene BHT, Sodium hydrogen L-Glutamate, Dimethyl polysioxane, Simethicone, Dimethicone, Chlorine, Chlorine dioxide.
- Healthy antioxidants are vitamin C (ascorbic acid) and vitamin E (tocopherol).
- Antioxidants (Propyl gallate/Propyl 3, 4, 5, trihydroxybenzene, Octyl gallate, Dodecyl gallate, Dodecyl, 3, 4, 5, trihydroxybenzene, Butylated hydroxyanisole BHA and Butylated hydroxy-toluene BHT are dangerous to asthmatics and to people who are sensitive to aspirin. They are also among the additives that are forbidden in baby foods.
- Potassium nitrate and sodium nitrate are, as their name suggests, "nitrates," usually found in cured meats, such as bacon and ham. These additives do cause some untoward effects, in that they can cause illness in young babies and may also be precursors to some carcinogens. However, they do also protect against botulism, which is one of the most toxic poisons known. Some experts believe that the slight risk of cancer is outweighed by the fact that you would most certainly die of botulism. See also nitrates, page 31.
- MSG (monosodium glutamate) is used to enhance meaty or savory flavors. Some people are sensitive to large quantities. It can cause headaches, giddiness, nausea, muscle pains and heart palpitations.
- The sweeter, more brightly colored or flavored a food, the higher the number of additives. Avoid these foods as often as possible.
- Some scientists have linked additives, particularly tartrazine, to hyperactivity in children, allergies, asthma, migraines and even cancer.
- Sulfites are a class of chemicals that can keep cut fruits and vegetables looking fresh. They also prevent discoloration in apricots, raisins, and other dried fruits; control "black spot" in freshly caught shrimp; and prevent discoloration, bacterial growth, and fermentation in wine. Until the early 1980s they were considered safe,

but the Center for Science in the Public Interest (CSPI) found six scientific studies proving that sulfites could provoke sometimes-severe allergic reactions. CSPI and the Food and Drug Administration (FDA) identified at least a dozen fatalities linked to sulfites. All of the deaths occurred among asthmatics. In 1985 Congress finally forced FDA to ban sulfites from most fruits and vegetables. The ban does not cover fresh-cut potatoes, dried fruits, and wine.

- The British Nutrition Foundation believes that more research is necessary before we can establish that additives are safe, particularly in light of the number of allergic reactions. It claims that there have been no properly controlled trials or tests looking at the effects. This view is echoed in the U.S. by concerned consumers, scientists and nutritional experts.

Does it sound like healthy eating is more trouble than it's worth? Think again. Healthy eating can easily be incorporated into family life with a minimum of fuss. The next chapter shows you how.

chapter four

Healthy Eating from Day One

O n paper, a healthy diet is entirely achievable, and most of us will be inspired by the fairly alarming statistics to do something about the way our children eat. In reality, however, it might be slightly more problematic. Whether you are thinking about weaning your first child, or you have a houseful of junk-food addicts, it is possible to set up a diet that suits you, your children's likes and dislikes, your schedule, your budget and, ultimately, benefits the overall health of the whole family.

▶ *Tips for implementing a healthy eating plan*

- The keyword is balance. Food is there to be enjoyed, and eliminating every treat from the family home or lifestyle is certain to cause full-scale mutiny. You need to find a way to get the best possible diet you can, and then take steps to balance the parts that aren't so good. For example, if your child has eaten the required number of fruits and vegetables, has had some good sources of protein and carbohydrates, there is no reason why an after-dinner chocolate treat can't be considered. A trip to McDonald's or a takeout pizza won't kill anyone, either. Try for balance on these occasions. Give up the carbonated orange drink for water or fresh orange juice. Buy mangoes or a fresh pineapple on the way home for dessert. Order a side salad, or pineapple, onions, peppers and extra tomatoes on your pizza.

- There are always weeks where time is short, there are birthday parties, or things just slide out of control. Once again, try to find a way to balance the negative with the positive. Do you have a tearful, tired child on your hands after a typical junk-food party? Offer a fruit platter treat with a yogurt or fromage frais when she gets home. Or a bowl of porridge and a cup of chamomile tea—great for calming the nerves!

- Don't be alarmed if you have a bad day, or even week. It's the overall balance that counts, not the daily or even weekly load. As adults, too many of us are used to diets that we slip in and out of at random. You know the familiar scenario—you blow the diet by eating a chocolate donut and decide to start again tomorrow. Eating well is a way of life, not a diet, and it should be adopted permanently. The odd slip, treat, chicken nugget, chocolate bar or even package of cookies will not make a difference in the long term if you adopt an overall policy of healthy eating. The more good there is in your child's diet, the less these slips matter.

■ Eating well means changing our approach to food. As families, we need to learn about food and what it does in our bodies. A healthy attitude is as important as healthy food, and we need to want what is best for our minds and bodies now and in the future. It is never too late, nor is it too early, to start taking steps toward optimum health and well-being.

Breaking it down

Many of us believe we are eating well until we stop and look at our diets in detail. The same goes for our children. If they are older, they may well be eating at school, or out with friends. Younger children and babies may be fed by a baby-sitter or at a day care center, and we may not be aware of exactly what they are getting.

The best place to start is to analyze your child's diet for a week. Write down everything she eats in as much detail as you can. You might have to rely on your child's memory to some extent, or on the willingness of a day care center or caregiver to supply details, but it's important that you come up with as accurate a picture as possible.

For each day, check your child's diet, adding up the points for each answer:

■ For every serving of fresh fruit and vegetables (and their juices), add 2 points.

■ Add an extra point for any servings that were raw.

■ For every serving of whole grain breads, pasta, brown rice, oats, barley, rye, corn, legumes, unsweetened breakfast cereal or potatoes, add 2 points.

■ For every serving of good-quality protein (fish, lean meat, chicken, turkey, cheese, milk, yogurt, tofu, nuts, nut butters (sugar-free), seeds or legumes), add 2 points.

■ For every full glass of fresh water, add 1 point.

■ For every serving of white bread, pasta or rice, add 0 points.

■ For every serving of food that was processed (for example, processed meats, cheeses, store-bought baked goods, including cookies and crackers), subtract 2 points.

- For every serving of food that was fried, or purchased "ready to serve," subtract 2 points. □

- For every serving of french fries, potato chips or other salty snacks, chocolate-coated or sweetened cereals, chocolate, candies and non-dairy ice cream, subtract 2 points. □

- For every serving of sweetened jam, jelly, dried and canned soups, subtract 2 points. □

- For every serving of carbonated drinks, artificial fruit drinks and drink powders/syrups, subtract 2 points. □

Total: □

Analyzing the results

Over 40: A brilliant diet. Lots of balance and plenty of the most important foods.

30–40: A fairly good diet. Look at ways to improve it even further.

20–30: Needs help. Your child will be missing key nutrients. Look at the foods that offer the most points (the fruits, vegetables, proteins and unrefined carbohydrates). By bumping up those, you can balance an otherwise unhealthy diet.

10–20: Very poor. Major changes need to be made to ensure that your child is getting the nutrients necessary for growth and development.

Less than 10: Desperately unhealthy. Your child's health will be seriously affected unless you take steps to redress the imbalance.

If you have a bad day, make changes to improve the score for the next day. It isn't daily intake that's important—it's overall intake.

Using the examples of the three children in chapter 2, here's how it works in action.

Luke had:

13 servings of fruits and vegetables (some in the form of juices)	x 2 = 26
2 of those were raw	x 1 = 2
5 servings of protein	x 2 = 10
7 servings of unrefined carbohydrates	x 2 = 14
4 glasses of water	x 1 = 4
Total good:	**56**
Minus	
1 chocolate chip cookie	x 2 = 2
2 high-sugar granola bars	x 2 = 4
	Total: 56–6 = **50**

Jenny had:

10 servings of fruits and vegetables (some in the form of juices)	x 2 = 20
2 of those were raw	x 1 = 2
3 servings of protein	x 2 = 6
3 servings of unrefined carbohydrates	x 2 = 6
4 glasses of water	x 1 = 4
Total good:	**38**
Minus	
2 cookies	x 2 = 4
non-dairy ice cream cone	x 2 = 2
processed meat	x 2 = 2
	Total: 38–8 = 30

Where's the shortfall? Jenny could balance the treats by adding more good-quality proteins and carbohydrates to her diet.

Freddie had:

2 servings of fruits and vegetables	x 2 = 4
1 of those was raw	x 1 = 1
2 servings of protein	x 2 = 4
0 servings of unrefined carbohydrates	0
1 glass of water	x 1 = 1
Total good:	**10**
Minus	
chocolate cereal	x 2 = 2
3 package of potato chips	x 2 = 6
chocolate cookies	x 2 = 4
	Total: 10–12 = –2

Where's the shortfall? That's pretty obvious. Freddie does not have anywhere near enough servings of fruits and vegetables. Protein is low, and there are no unrefined carbohydrates whatsoever. If he bumped up those, and dropped the potato chips, his long-term health would improve, he'd put on some much-needed weight, and his concentration and mood would be enormously improved.

Once you have an overall picture of your child's diet, you can make the changes necessary to create a balance. The best place to start is at the beginning.

The best possible start

Every modern parent is aware of the importance of breastfeeding. Ultimately, it's a personal decision whether to breast- or bottle-feed, but it's important, in a book about natural health, to reiterate the reasons why breast is best. And, if you are uncertain, try breastfeeding first, because you can always stop and change to the bottle, but it is unusual to be able to do it the other way around.

You may wish to combine both methods to suit your lifestyle, or to involve your partner or other children in the care of your new baby. The best way to feed your baby is the way that is right for you.

Breastfeeding

Many women find breastfeeding a rewarding and nurturing experience, which establishes a physical bond between mother and baby, and helps to strengthen an emotional one. There are many advantages to breastfeeding, the first and foremost being nutritional. Breastmilk provides the ideal balance of nutrients for your baby, and can help protect him from infections to which you are already immune. The composition of breastmilk also seems to vary with your baby's needs, whereas the composition of formula stays constant. You can put your baby to your breast as often as he seems to want it, and the baby will not gain weight too quickly, but a baby may become overweight with too much bottle-feeding.

Breastmilk is designed to provide complete nourishment for a baby for several months after birth. Before milk is produced, the mother's breast produces colostrum, a deep-yellow liquid containing high levels of protein and antibodies. A newborn baby who feeds on colostrum in the first few days of life is better able to resist the bacteria and viruses that cause illness. The mother's milk, which begins to flow a few days after childbirth when her hormones change, is a blue-white color with a very thin consistency. If the mother eats healthily, the milk provides the baby with the proper nutritional balance.

▶ 8 good reasons to breastfeed your baby

1. The fat contained in human milk, compared with cow's milk, is more digestible for human babies and allows for greater absorption of fat-soluble vitamins into the bloodstream from the baby's intestine.

2. Calcium and other important nutrients in human milk are also better utilized by babies.

3. Antigens in cow's milk can cause allergic reactions in a newborn baby, whereas such reactions to human milk are rare.

4. Human milk also promotes growth, largely due to the presence of certain hormones and growth factors.

5. Breastfed babies have a very low risk of developing meningitis or severe blood infections, and have a 500 to 600 percent lower risk of getting childhood lymphoma. Breastfed babies also suffer 50 percent fewer middle ear infections.

6. Research also indicates that breastfed babies are less likely to become obese children. Bottle-fed children have far higher blood concentrations of insulin, the chemical that stimulates the laying down of fat cells. Obesity in childhood is known to be a risk factor for developing cardiovascular disease in later life.

7. Other research has shown that breastfeeding for the first 15 weeks protects against both diarrheal and respiratory diseases, ear and urinary tract infections, and reduces blood pressure.

8. Breastfeeding also has psychological benefits for mother and baby because it helps promote a warm, close relationship between them.

Toxic breastmilk?

There have been recent concerns about levels of contaminants and toxins in breastmilk. One report suggested up to 350 contaminants had been found in various samples, including 42 times the safe level of toxic dioxins. Other chemicals identified came from suntan lotion and pesticides. Should we be concerned? If our breastmilk is contaminated by our environments and diets, certainly the milk of cows will be equally tainted. What it does show, however, is that a good diet is essential for parents in the period leading up to conception, and during pregnancy. Many experts now recommend a full detox for people considering planning a family. Another point to note is that women should not consider dieting while breastfeeding. Toxins are stored in fat, and when we lose weight, those toxins are released into the bloodstream, which could affect the toxic levels of breastmilk. Overall, breastfeeding is still considered to be the safest, most natural way to feed your baby.

IF YOU HAVE ANY problems in the first few days of breastfeeding, do not be discouraged. Talk to your doctor for support and advice, or ask at your health care center for a local telephone number for La Leche League International, a group that offers practical advice and moral support for women who are breastfeeding.

Bottle-feeding

Feeding your baby from a bottle is a viable alternative to breastfeeding, and it may be the right choice for you. Infant formulas available today are very nearly equivalent in nourishment to breastmilk, and you will be able to bond well with your baby, for it is the care that counts, not the breast or the bottle.

Milk formulas

Many formulas come as a dried powder in a can, although some are available in a ready-to-drink form. Everything on the market will be safe, with balanced nutrients and added vitamins, although you may need to choose between brands according to your baby's age and special requirements. Most formulas are based on cow's milk, but there are soy-based formulas available for babies who have difficulty digesting cow's milk, or who have allergies or intolerance (beware, however, that soy can be an allergen and there is a risk of phytoestrogens, which can play havoc with hormones). You can also get a goat's milk preparation, although some babies do not like the pronounced taste. If you are unsure which to choose, ask for advice from your doctor or midwife, who will be able to recommend something suitable. Watch out for baby formulas with GM ingredients. If possible, go for an organic formula, which will hold far less risk in the long term.

▶ *Top tips for preventing infection*

- Keep everything you use to feed your baby and prepare his formula scrupulously clean. Newborn babies are very vulnerable to infection, particularly of the gastrointestinal tract, and you will need to sterilize anything that comes into contact with his mouth, including bottles, teething rings and pacifiers, and all the equipment used to prepare his feed, such as knives, spoons and jugs, until he is at least four months old. A dishwasher should do the trick in most cases.

- Always use cooled, boiled water for making feeds.

- Never store formula milk for more than 24 hours; try to make up formula when you need it, rather than making dozens of bottles in advance. Never reheat an existing bottle, even if he has had just a few sips.

When should I wean?

The best advice is to wait as long as possible before weaning. Some babies show real interest in food at around four to five months, so it may be appropriate to start them with some tastes then, but foods introduced too early can cause digestive problems, and even allergies and intolerance (see page 344). Six months is a good time to start with a little table food—some rice, a few fruits and vegetables, for example—but leave it longer if you can, particularly if there are allergies of any nature in your family. Don't be tempted to replace milk in a baby's diet. Until your baby is about a year old, she will get most of her nutrition from her milk. Other foods will add a little variety, and introduce her to new tastes, but they should not be relied upon as a source of a balanced diet.

There comes a time, however, around the six- to ten-month mark (later in some children), when she will need a little more. Weaning your baby from the breast or bottle can be a time-consuming and long-term project, and it is best to start gradually by introducing new tastes one at a time. Don't be surprised if your baby isn't interested, and rejects anything that doesn't come with a teat on the end of it. If that's the case with your baby, try a few new tastes, and if she still won't have it, give up and wait for a few weeks and then try again. Early foods merely supplement milk feeds, and there is no reason to worry if your baby has nothing but milk for even the first year of life.

You may be impatient to begin solids for various reasons—perhaps because you are returning to work, and you think your baby will be able to go a little longer between milk feeds, or perhaps you wish to stop breastfeeding altogether. But try not to rush it—your baby will let you know when she is ready, and if you force solid food on her earlier, you can be setting up all sorts of problems that can be manifested in later months and years.

Your baby may be ready when he shows signs of being interested in food—perhaps he has begun reaching out for food on your plate when you are eating, or seems determined to eat his toys. Some mothers decide that their baby needs "more" when they continue to wake repeatedly at night, but beware! Many babies wake in the night for periods during the first six months, and their waking may be unrelated to hunger. Toward the end of the first six months, this waking is more likely due to the need for comfort than for nutrition or food.

Some babies will thrive on milk for the first 12 months, so don't panic if you have a slow beginner. If you wish to stop breastfeeding, you can switch to the bottle long before you need to give solid foods. Similarly, it is not advised that you give solid foods to a baby who is younger than three months. It is now believed that babies' digestive systems are not mature enough to cope with solids before this time, and they will be more prone to food allergies, rashes, diarrhea and tummy ache if you do. Wait as long as you can, and you improve the chances that your baby will welcome those first tastes.

First foods

Your baby's first foods are intended to be tastes, rather than nutritional supplements, although it is important to choose foods that are nutritious, and that will not put any strain on her immature digestive system. In the beginning you will need to purée everything, making it as sloppy as possible, as she will suck it rather than eat it, until she becomes accustomed to the different consistencies.

▶ *The best first purées*

- Apple, pear, peach, apricot, banana

- Parsnip, turnip, green beans, squash, sweet potato, cauliflower, carrots, peas, broccoli

- Baby rice

From about six months, you can begin to introduce other cereals to add some variety. Whichever solids you decide to offer, remember to introduce one new food at a time, for three to four days, to give your baby a chance to grow to like it, before offering another food. It may take some time for her to become accustomed to a new taste, and it will also give you an opportunity to pinpoint any adverse reactions to certain foods.

These first tastes are not intended to be meals so don't panic if she gets very little. Let her enjoy the food and make a mess if she wants to. She will need to learn that food, and mealtimes, are a pleasant experience, and if she feels forced to eat, or picks up tension from you, she will begin to associate food with stress.

Foods to avoid for babies

We mention specific foods in the section on allergies and intolerance (see page 344), but there are foods that should be avoided for other reasons:

- Pork and lamb should wait until your baby is at least nine months old, because they are too fatty to digest easily.

- Avoid food with any salt, which can put unnecessary strain on her kidneys.

- Spices should be very gradually introduced only after about six or seven months.

- Sugary foods or drinks can encourage a sweet tooth, and promote tooth decay.

- Fried foods are not good for her. Lightly steam foods when you cook them, and avoid using butter or oil.

Once your child is eating a variety of different foods, she can join in with the family diet. On most days, that starts with breakfast.

The importance of breakfast

For most children, breakfast is the first meal they have in more than ten hours, and sometimes even longer. Not only is it necessary to balance out blood sugar levels, but it can have a dramatic effect on health and well-being. In fact, breakfast is the meal most directly connected to school achievement. Experts say that children do better in the morning hours following a good nutritious breakfast. Their speed, response time and problem-solving skills are improved, and they are better able to persevere throughout the morning. Children who skip breakfast have shorter attention spans, do poorly in tasks requiring concentration and even score lower on standard achievement tests. And, when researchers compared the diets of children who regularly eat breakfast with those who don't, they found that the breakfast skippers never made up for lost nutrients. Children who ate a morning meal took in far more nutrients over the course of the day.

Also, eating a balanced breakfast (with at least three of the five pyramid food groups) will result in an increased supply of glucose available to the brain and enhance children's ability to think, concentrate and learn.

▶ *Top tips if your child is not a natural breakfaster*

- Some children are simply not hungry in the morning. Similarly, many children are grumpy in the morning (due to low blood sugar, in fact) and may be pickier than usual. Early morning tears and tantrums over food are, paradoxically, normally the result of hunger. Don't be tempted to wage a war over the breakfast table. Once they are dressed and feeling a little more alert, most children are hungry enough for some breakfast.

- Ask your child to choose breakfast the night before, and have it set up at the table for her when she comes down.

- Breakfast doesn't have to mean traditional breakfast food. There's no reason why a slice of healthy pizza, a bowl of soup or a sandwich can't be offered instead. The most important thing is to focus on getting a good source of unrefined carbohydrates into the meal, to ensure that blood sugar levels stay stable throughout the morning, and to get some protein, vitamins and minerals and fats.

- If your child won't eat before school, then make a packed breakfast to eat on the way to school. Add a bit of cheese, an apple, a whole wheat bun and a yogurt. Juice in a box will balance it out. Alternatively, a hard-boiled egg with an orange and a whole wheat bun is a good, balanced breakfast. An individual box of a healthy cereal can be eaten without milk.

Sweetened cereals

Don't be tempted by highly processed, sweetened breakfast cereals. They will artificially raise blood sugar levels, which will plunge before the morning is even half over. Furthermore, they offer very little in the way of nutrition, and contribute to an overall toxic load (see page 141). If your children will eat nothing else, simply don't buy them. If you have a variety of other healthy cereals on offer, and they feel they have a choice, they will soon forget about the sweetened versions. If they want a little sweetener, choose from the healthier options on page 39. Alternatively, chop a banana or add a little fruity yogurt to the top for variety.

Lunch

When children eat their lunch in the school cafeteria, many parents worry that they have so little control over their child's diet during the day. But don't despair. Studies show that children, regardless of income, generally have higher intakes of key nutrients when they eat school lunch.

There has been a fairly major overhaul of school cafeterias over the past few years, in the U.S., Canada and the U.K., and most schools base their menus around government-recommended guidelines. There should be more choice, as well as a greater number of fresh, whole foods available. If your school is the exception, find out why.

Many children eat better than they do at home because they mimic their peers. If a friend orders a previously untasted meal, others will try it as well. And a hungry child is more likely to eat what's put in front of him, particularly if there are no alternatives available.

If your child eats at school, make sure he is aware of the basics of nutrition. Explain how a healthy meal will give him lots of energy for sports or tests in the afternoon, and how it will make him feel happier. Negotiate an eating plan that is acceptable to both of you—fries only once a week, for example, ham only once a week, at least two vegetables and one fruit (different every day, if possible). If he knows the parameters, and knows that he can make the choices based on your agreement, he'll be more likely to stick to a healthy diet. Let him feel empowered rather than ruled. Show an interest in what he's eaten. Most children love reciting what they've had for lunch, right down to the last soggy Brussels sprout. Work out where the strengths and weaknesses are, and base the rest of his daily diet on those. For example, if he's been short on fresh fruits and vegetables at lunchtime, serve a picnic dinner with lots of fresh vegetables and dips, a platter of fresh fruit, yogurt, cheese and whole wheat toast. Even a bowl of fresh vegetable soup can make up for a less nutritious lunch.

Packed lunches

Lunchboxes give you a little more control over what your child is eating, although it's difficult to know what has been eaten if the lunchbox comes back empty every day. Many children simply tip out the contents rather than face an irate parent. The main solution is to discuss lunch in advance. Work out what your child wants and will eat, and try to incorporate that to some extent. Give a list to choose from; for example, would you like egg salad, cheese and cucumber, tuna salad, tomato and salad or peanut butter and banana tomorrow? Once again you'll be empowering by offering choices, and children like to feel that they have some control over their lives (see page 182). Children are also much more likely to eat something they have chosen.

The premise for healthy lunches is the same as for other meals. You want balance, nutrition, and as many elements of the food pyramid (see page 23) as possible. You also want to provide something that will appeal to a child, so that she'll be encouraged to eat it.

▶ *Top tips for healthy lunchboxes*

- Fruit doesn't have to be fresh and raw to be nutritious. Little containers of canned fruits in juice are also healthy and much more appealing to children.

- Peel oranges and tangerines before serving to make the job easier. You can also cut up fruit, but dip it in a little lemon juice before wrapping to prevent discoloration.

- Cut sandwiches into small bite-sized pieces that your child can pick up and eat while chatting to schoolmates.

- Picnic-style lunches are always popular. Choose from a range of small pieces of cooked chicken, yogurt, yogurt-based dips, fruit (such as grapes or strawberries), cheese, whole wheat pita bread, humus, boiled eggs, raisins, dried fruits, raw vegetables (such as carrots, broccoli florets, olives, sliced cucumber, sliced peppers, celery or corn), rice crackers or cheese crackers.

- Some children prefer to make their own sandwiches—either at home before school, or at school, if you supply the ingredients.

- Hot lunches—for example, leftover soups, stews or pastas—can be kept hot in a thermos for older children. With a piece of fruit and a whole wheat roll, this is a completely balanced meal.

Ask at your child's school how the children are supervised at lunchtime. Ensure that the children are encouraged to eat the healthy bits of the lunch before the treats, particularly if your child is a slow eater and some of the meal invariably comes home. Ask that the lunchbox is sent home unemptied so that you can see what has been eaten.

Super snacks

Few children can get through a day without a snack or two, and most school-aged children are encouraged to bring one to school for recess. Snacks are important and should never be dismissed as "fillers" or inconsequential to the overall healthy eating plan. Nor should they be considered "treats," which fall outside your normal nutritional guidelines. Some children eat little at meals, and snacks provide a large proportion of their daily requirements. Furthermore, children who fill up on unhealthy snacks are hardly likely to sit down to a nutritious meal.

If children are hungry, then by all means offer snacks. In fact, take it one step further and encourage your child to choose her own snacks from a "snack drawer" or shelf in the fridge (see page 62). Do, however, set some rules in place: no snacks before meals, for example, and a maximum of three in an afternoon. If you offer only healthy snacks, your child will eat healthy snacks.

Encourage your child to consider whether or not she is really hungry. Some children eat because they are bored, or lonely, or even upset. Sometimes they cry "hunger" when they want a little attention, or a treat. If they learn that hunger is satisfied by healthy foods, they will learn to eat only when they are hungry. And if hunger is no longer the cause of their discontent, they are much more likely to address the real reason they wanted food in the first place.

▶ *Top snacks*

- fresh fruit

- dried, unsulfured fruit

- nuts (after the age of five, and if there are no allergies)

- toast with peanut butter, cheese or a mashed banana

- make fresh popcorn (you'll need to supervise this) without salt or sugar

- breadsticks (choose those with sesame seeds, if possible)

- brown rice cakes (spread them with any of the toast topping suggestions, or eat plain)

- yogurt

- good-quality cookies (see page 53), preferably homemade

- non-sugary breakfast cereal with organic milk

- humus and pita bread

- raw vegetables (cauliflower and broccoli florets, peppers, celery, carrots, cucumbers, snow peas, for example)

- "milkshakes" with fresh milk (better still, rice milk), a banana, some fresh fruit juice and a little yogurt. Freeze a couple of bananas to add to the blender to make the milkshakes creamy cold!

- homemade or good-quality cakes, such as carrot or banana

- raisins

- cheese

- cold, healthy pizza

Adolescents and food

When hormones start to rage and rebellion becomes your adolescent's middle name, you can expect some battles about food. The typical adolescent is struggling to find his own identity, and to assert some power over his world. Growing up is a bewildering time and it's not surprising that family, household rules and eating habits become the focus of teenage rebellion. This will be particularly relevant if you are concerned about diet. Like toddlers, teenagers often choose to fight against the issues that matter most. They are guaranteed to get some attention, and it's the ideal way to assert their own authority, and show some control within the home environment. It's also a pretty easy way to wind you up.

Quite apart from that, peer pressure weighs the scales heavily in favor of a junk-food diet. Adolescents usually have some money of their own, and you can bet that at least some of it will be spent unwisely in fast-food outlets.

▶ 7 top tips for dealing with adolescent food battles

1. The key to managing this situation is to back off. Continue to serve the same meals that you always have, and don't hesitate to discuss food issues with your child. He will feel much more grown up if you confess your concerns about, say, a particular food and its link to cancer, and ask his advice or opinion.

2. Continue with the praise. Once again, you can create a self-fulfilling prophecy. If you continue to show faith in your child and his choices, he will feel in control. He will also be more likely to make good judgments because of your belief in him.

3. As your child grows up, reiterate the concept of balance. If a diet is 80 percent good and 20 percent bad, he is doing well. If your child knows the figures, he can make choices that allow him to have some fun with his buddies, but he will also know what to do and when to redress the damage.

4. Offer some fun foods alongside the traditional family meals. Buy different types of fresh exotic fruit juices and some sparkling water and set up a help-yourself drinks bar when he has friends around. They'll have such fun experimenting with concoctions that they'll probably forget there isn't cola on the menu. Offer make-your-own pizzas for late-night meals with friends, or homemade burgers and fries. Your child doesn't have to be a social leper to eat well with friends.

5. Most teens want to know how nutrition can help them now. If you can convince teenagers, particularly those who are interested in sports, or taking exams, that food is fuel and that the proper fuel will make a difference in their life today, you will be more likely to succeed in interesting them. For teens who are inactive, the challenge is to convince them of the importance of both exercise and proper nutrition in developing a fit mind and body.

6. Active adolescents do best when they fuel their bodies with a high-energy diet based on the food pyramid. By emphasizing a diet full of carbohydrate-rich grains, fruits and vegetables with a balance of lean protein foods and low-fat dairy products, the body will be tuned for peak performance. The more active the teen, the more carbohydrates are needed. Is your child a budding athlete? Explain the concept of "burnout" and lack of stamina, which indicate that body carbohydrate stores are low. If you put healthy eating in their language, they'll be much more willing to listen. More often than not, they'll pass on the information to friends.

7. When it comes to brain power, remind your child to eat a balanced breakfast every day. Good-quality food translates into better concentration, grades and ability to learn. If your teen is struggling with exams, or feeling tired or stressed by the competition at school, offer some practical nutritional guidance. Dietary changes can be one of the greatest factors in overall success at school.

Special diets

Vegetarians

The number of vegetarians in the Western world is rising all the time, and recent estimates indicate that at least 16 percent of the population embrace some form of vegetarianism, even if it is part time. Health is one of the main reasons people change to a vegetable-based diet, and in recent years ecological and ethical considerations have become more important.

Types of vegetarians

There are many different eating habits involved in vegetarianism, and certainly some people call themselves vegetarian and still eat white meats, such as fish, shellfish and chicken. Vegans eat a range of plant foods, but no products of animal origin. Lactovegetarians eat dairy food such as cheese and yogurt, and drink milk. This diet, with the addition of eggs, is also eaten by ovo-lactovegetarians.

Is a vegetarian diet healthier?

If saturated fats, such as cheese and full-fat milk are kept to a minimum, most vegetarians do have a lower blood cholesterol level, and a higher intake of fiber (nearly 30 to 50 percent higher than the average meat-eater), which reduces the risk of cardiovascular and digestive disease, among other things. Vegetarians are also generally less obese than meat-eaters, and suffer from fewer vitamin and mineral deficiencies, provided they eat a varied diet. This may seem unimportant when considering the health of a child, but healthy eating involves looking at the long term, as well as the immediate, and you will do your child a great service if you adopt an eating plan that offers a healthy future.

As long as your child's diet is not restricted, it is fairly easy for vegetarians to eat healthily. The main stumbling block is protein intake. A vegetarian diet should contain a variety of foods, such as cereals, beans, nuts, legumes and vegetables, which ensures a good balance of proteins and other nutrients. Cereals, beans, legumes, seeds, tofu, TVP (textured vegetable protein) and nuts should predominate in the diet, particularly if fewer dairy products are consumed. These foods are rich in protein and will ensure that adequate quantities are available for the processes of the body, including the rebuilding of the body's tissues. Lack of iron can also be a problem, particularly for teenagers. Increased amounts of beans, legumes, nuts, dried fruit or whole grain cereals should help to right the imbalance, and fresh fruit and vegetables will provide the vitamin C necessary for the iron to be absorbed.

> ## Cheese for teeth
>
> Research shows that children who enjoy sugary foods could neutralize the effect on their teeth by eating a chunk of cheese straight afterward. Researchers at Newcastle University dental school in the U.K. discovered that the plaque-calcium concentration was much higher for volunteers who had eaten cheese after a sweet treat than those who had not. Calcium encourages hardening of the teeth, and discourages softening, which is the first stage in the process creating caries, or tooth decay. If you are concerned about the sugar levels in even healthy foods, such as raisins and fruit, offering a small piece of cheese afterward may help to reduce any damage to teeth.

Children and vegetarianism

Children can thrive on a properly balanced vegetarian diet, but it is important that they get a higher percentage of protein and calories relative to their body weight. A diet that includes legumes at least once a day, whole wheat bread or cereals two or three times a day and (20 oz) 75 ml of milk or its equivalent in dairy foods such as cheese, yogurt or soya milk, plus the necessary fruits and vegetables, will contain more than enough protein and vitamins and minerals. It is also important to ensure that they get enough calories, since vegetarian foods tend to be bulkier and to satisfy the appetite more readily. If your child eats lots of pasta, for instance, ensure that he gets plenty of a nutritious sauce alongside, both to bump up the calorie and nutrition intake, and to ensure that he isn't filling his tummy with one type of food only. If your child continues to gain weight and grow normally, you can be assured that his diet is satisfactory.

Children raised on strict vegetarian fare, excluding all milk and meat products, do tend to be smaller than the average Western child. But they also tend to be healthy, as long as they are receiving a well-planned diet with adequate nutrients.

Veganism

A vegan diet contains even more bulk than a vegetarian diet, and it is therefore more difficult to ensure that your child is getting the required nutritional elements, and calories. The most common nutrients lacking in a vegan diet are calcium, vitamin D and vitamin B12.

The vegan diet does not provide vitamin B12 in sufficient quantities. B12 is found mainly in animal products, with the exception of miso, tempeh, brewer's yeast and soy milks that have been fortified. The latter foods cannot be eaten in large enough quantities to provide the required daily intake, so it is recommended that all vegans take a vitamin B12 supplement. Some experts recommend that children be given fortified soy milk regularly (see page 350), as well as a supplement.

Calcium is found in a variety of non-dairy foods, but it is important to ensure that these foods are eaten regularly. High-calcium foods include broccoli, soya beans, almonds, tofu, soy milk (or soy yogurt and cheese), dried fruits and dark green vegetables. Try not to rely too heavily on soy (see page 350).

Vitamin D can be synthesized by the body when it receives adequate sunlight, and sunscreens do not hamper this action. Ensure that your children get plenty of sunshine, and in the winter months offer a good multivitamin and mineral supplement containing vitamin D.

Family meals

There are several important factors to consider when planning family meals, and I've avoided listing suggested menus for that reason. Every family is different and has to adopt a program to suit their budget, time, interest in cooking and family likes and dislikes.

Family meals also have several functions. Not only do they provide the main meal of the day for most family members (therefore being the most important nutritionally), but they also provide an opportunity for families to interact socially. Children learn good eating habits and table manners when they eat with their parents. They learn to try new things and feel involved in the family unit. Mealtimes should, therefore, never be a battleground. Food should be fun, varied and interesting, as well as nutritious, and everyone—yes, everyone—should eat the same things. Even if small helpings are served, or children are encouraged to help themselves from serving dishes, everything should be tasted and even discussed. But keep it on a positive note. If your child doesn't like the spinach, tell a funny story about how you hated spinach as a child. Think Popeye. Or ask how they think it would be more tasty—in a salad the following night, for example, or cooked with a little cheese?

As much as possible children should be involved in the shopping (if that's impractical, ask them to check off a list of foods on your shopping list, or to suggest some menus for the coming week), the choice of menus and the preparation. See page 69 for more ideas on getting children involved in the process. It really does help to include children in every aspect of food. They'll feel they have some power within their household and they'll be less horrified by whatever is put down in front of them if they've had some warning and involvement. They'll also learn how to choose food, how to prepare a balanced meal, and how to cook, which will set them in good stead for the future. Offer a variety of seasonings apart from the ubiquitous ketchup and encourage them to taste foods as they cook. You may have some unusual suggestions—my son, for example, felt that our spaghetti sauce needed raisins, which I duly added. To our surprise, they tasted delicious.

Praise your children's involvement, their ideas and their efforts. Praise them when they try foods, even if they don't like them. Praise makes them feel good, and they'll associate mealtimes with that good feeling.

What are the basics of a good family meal? Variety, and lots of it. Choose from as many different foods as you can accommodate, and integrate them into your diet in new ways. You don't have to be a gourmet chef to grate zucchini into pasta sauces, or to soak some red lentils overnight. Many delicious foods are simple to prepare and extremely healthy—roasted vegetables, for example, or marinated chicken pieces. Fish cooked with a little lemon and cilantro or honey in foil takes only about 15 minutes to prepare, and is normally popular with the whole family. Children in particular love to have their own "foil" packet. If time is tight, get a steamer to cook your vegetables and rice for you. Cut corners if you need to, but ensure that you choose the best quality ingredients and cook them in a variety of different ways.

Above all, take pleasure from mealtimes. If you have a picky eater on your hands, gently work it out (see page 68) and focus your attention on the children who are eating, and on conversation and positive contributions to the meal. If your child is not getting the attention she expected, she's more likely to eat to feel a part of the action, and to share the good atmosphere.

Eat desserts, if you like them (children certainly do!). There are dozens of healthy

Ketchup

It's got to be the all-time favorite condiment for children, and parents have been concerned about its overconsumption. Ketchup tends to be high in salt and sugar, although the newer organic brands are free of these additives and much tastier. If you have trouble weaning your child from the sugary version, try mixing both in a big bottle, gradually adding more of the organic ketchup until she doesn't notice the difference.

There is some good news, however. It transpires that ketchup is actually healthy. In one study, it was found that tomato supplements helped slow prostate cancer in men diagnosed with the disease. The supplements contained lycopene, the chemical that makes tomatoes red. Lycopene, which survives cooking and is especially concentrated in tomato sauce and tomato paste, is a known antioxidant and a member of the carotenoid family of nutrients that includes beta-carotene and vitamin A. It cancels out the effects of free radicals, charged particles that damage the body's genetic material and can lead to cancer.

What's the verdict?

Put ketchup back on the menu, but try to make sure it doesn't drown out the taste of natural foods. Children need to learn to eat different foods both for their nutritional value, their tastes and their textures.

dessert ideas that take little time, including baked apples with raisins and maple syrup, fruit crumbles, yogurt with fruit and honey, dark chocolate fondues with fresh fruits, home-baked cakes or cookies, or even just exotic fruits. Don't withhold dessert until plates are cleared, or there will be undue emphasis placed on that course. Children need to learn that all food is equally delicious and healthy, whether it comes as part of a meal or afterward.

Is fresh best?

Fresh foods are almost always best. I say almost, because they are, in some cases, nutritionally inferior to their frozen counterparts. If you buy your foods from a supermarket, make extra certain that they are fresh and ripe. Many foods have traveled long distances from other countries, or sat in the back of a truck for long periods of time. Fresh foods, such as fruits and vegetables, become less nutritious the further they are from the day they are picked. If your fruits or vegetables are unripe, let them ripen naturally in the sun on your kitchen windowsill. This will help to promote nutrient content and improve flavor.

A local greengrocer may be a better bet for fruit and vegetable supplies, and all the better if you can find one that sells organic. Supplies are usually fresh, as the turnover is high and the produce collected the same day from the farmers' markets. An organic food delivery service is another good bet, and it can be enormously convenient for busy parents.

▶ *Top tips for preserving nutrients*

- Frozen is good, mainly because food is normally frozen immediately after picking, which preserves the nutrient content. On the whole, frozen foods retain their nutrient content far longer than fresh foods, so unless you are planning to eat your food within a day or so of eating it, frozen might be best. Some of the textures of fruits and vegetables are altered by freezing, so don't expect the crunch of fresh. They are a great addition to stews, pastas, sauces, however, and are fine eaten on their own if you don't mind a slightly soggier texture.

- Canned fruits and vegetables are less nutritious, and many of the nutrients have soaked into the water, juice or syrup in which they are suspended. Look for brands packed in water and natural juices and make sure to drink the juice as well. Canned fish, such as salmon and tuna, may have also lost some of their key nutrients (in particular, essential fatty acids, which may be lost in the canning process), but they are still nutritious, provided they are tinned in water, not brine or oil.

- Eat the skins of organic fruits and vegetables whenever possible. Many key nutrients are concentrated in the skins. Non-organic foods should be washed carefully before eating the skins, although some experts recommend that you peel them before eating. Wash *all* fruits and vegetables, including oranges and other citrus fruits. Although the peels are not eaten, the toxins can be absorbed in the oils of the flesh and you can transfer them on to the peeled fruit. Wash the fruit, wash your hands and then peel the fruit.

- Don't cut, wash or soak fruits and vegetables until you are ready to eat them. Exposing their cut surfaces to air reduces many nutrients. This may mean that advanced preparation may be impossible, but your diet will benefit from the freshness of the food.

In summary

Don't be put off by the idea of making lifestyle changes. Every step you take toward a healthy diet will have an immeasurable impact on your child's health, both now and in the future. The keyword is balance. Raising children naturally involves choosing and eating fresh, healthy, natural, unrefined foods, but it also means helping your children to live in the modern world. Fast food, junk food and convenience foods were the culinary buzzwords of the 20th century, and although things are beginning to change, they still dominate our popular culture. A life of abstinence is not the answer. We need to find ways to make a healthy lifestyle work today. In the future things may become easier, but it is the present that holds the most challenges. If you can manage to do it right 80 percent of the time, the other 20 percent really doesn't matter. The more good food your child gets, the better his body will work, and the easier he will find it to process and eliminate the less healthy parts of his diet. He'll grow up strong and healthy, be able to concentrate better, achieve a sense of well-being, fight off illness and, most importantly, he'll have the best chance of a rosy future.

chapter five

Fit for Life

Children are naturally active. Give the average child some open space and he'll explore it enthusiastically. Let go of a toddler's hand and she'll be off at top speed. Have you ever witnessed the after-school dash? The doors open and children fly out, stopped only by a restraining hand or their own front doors. Children seem to have two natural speeds—sprint (a super-speed race to be there first) and snail (no less active, but taken at a meandering pace as they stop to investigate the minutiae of life, from worms to cracks in the sidewalk). Whatever the speed, children *move*.

The importance of exercise

Given their natural inclinations, it's difficult to understand why exercise has become a problem for many children. And believe me, it's a serious problem. Here's why:

- In chapter 3 we investigated the growing number of obese children and examined the health effects from a dietary point of view. Lack of exercise is another major cause of excess weight, and its effects can be dramatic. Children who do not get enough exercise tend to put on weight on their bellies and chests—in other words, they adopt the unhealthy "apple shape." A study from the University of Cincinnati College of Medicine found that children with apple-shaped bodies (fat collected on upper body and stomach) had higher blood pressure and lower levels of "good" cholesterol than those with "pear-shaped" bodies (fat collected on hips and thighs).

- A 1998 study in the U.K. showed that the majority of children considered themselves "fairly fit," although less than 25 percent exercised or were active for more than six hours a week. This indicates that our children are simply not aware of what fitness entails, nor have they been educated about its importance.

- Children walk 80 percent less than they did just 20 years ago. While the health implications are obvious, it's also important to note that children who are not regularly exposed to traffic and roads fail to develop "road sense," which needs to build up over the childhood years. Child pedestrian casualties have dropped, probably because children are no longer walking as often, and they are kept away from traffic and busy roads. But, alarmingly, the highest incidence of deaths in children from pedestrian accidents comes between the ages of 10 and 13, a time when most children are first given the freedom to travel on their own.

- Exercise strengthens the cardiovascular system and increases heart mass. This reduces the risk of heart disease, the number-one killer of both men and women in the Western world. Because heart disease is becoming much more prevalent in the under-tens, it's fairly clear that exercise can reduce damage and prevent heart problems before they set in.

- Exercise also helps to increase the metabolic rate—the rate at which our bodies burn calories. Exercise burns enough calories to reduce body fat, leading to weight loss in those who are overweight.

- Children participating in a two-year moderate aerobic exercise program (running 20 minutes per day) showed a 30–40 percent decrease in body fat, and a 33 percent increase in lean body mass.

- Exercise reduces stress. Children and young adults can be exposed to a variety of stresses, such as problems within the family, poverty and social hardship, and difficulties at school such as bullying, peer pressure, boredom and exams. A young person under stress may have difficulty sleeping or have nightmares, seek constant reassurance, appear nervous and unhappy, and suffer from frequent headaches or abdominal pains. If any of these symptoms seem familiar, you might want to take a look at your child's activity levels. Exercise works by using up the adrenaline that is created by stress and stressful situations. It also creates "endorphins," the feel-good hormones that improve mood, motivation and even tolerance to pain and other stimuli.

- A 1997 study showed that physical activity may play a role in deterring cancer, particularly colon cancer, probably by reducing the amount of time that potential cancer-causing agents take to move through the intestinal system.

- Aerobic exercise is effective in helping to maintain bone strength. Weight-bearing exercise places stress on the bone and that stress helps maintain or increase bone strength. This is particularly important, as recent research shows that many teenagers (particularly girls) have reduced bone mass that can lead to osteoporosis and stress fractures later in life.

- Exercise is good for the brain. Aerobic exercise helps to increase the number of brain chemicals called neurotransmitters, so that messages can be carried more quickly over brain cells. This increases mental flexibility and agility over longer periods of time. Furthermore, regular exercise increases the supply of oxygenated blood to the brain, which can improve concentration, alertness and intellectual capacity.

- Regular exercise can promote good, regular sleeping habits. Many children are simply not tired at the end of the day, which pushes bedtimes later and causes disrupted sleep (see page 133). Children who are overstimulated by television, video games or even too much homework may suffer a similar fate. Children need to experience physical exhaustion before they will settle down at an appropriate time and get a good night's sleep.

- Several studies show that children who exercise regularly are more apt to do so when they become adults.

- Long-term aerobic exercise programs result in improved maximal aerobic power and enhanced physical performance, leading to better exercise tolerance and less "non-specific" fatigue.

- Strength/resistance training helps reduce the risk of injury for young athletes.

- Regular stretching to increase range of motion has a positive effect on flexibility in children. Increased range of motion in a joint allows it to give somewhat under stress, thereby reducing the chances of injury.

- Regular exercise significantly enhances the body's ability to move air into and out of the lungs, increases blood volume, and helps blood become better equipped to transport oxygen.

- Regular exercise reduces caloric intake. In a study of 43 overweight eight- to ten-year-old boys who attended a four-month physical education program, daily caloric intake spontaneously decreased by 12 percent.

- Regular exercise reduces fat around the chest wall, which helps decrease breathing efforts.

- Exercise can affect growth in a number of ways. Children whose activity levels fall far beneath their biological requirements may not achieve optimum development and growth. Furthermore, studies show that physical activity naturally stimulates the release of growth hormones into the circulation, and that the healing process (of wounds and from health conditions) is significantly faster in children who exercise regularly.

- Preliminary evidence suggests that exercise helps to increase insulin sensitivity and resistance to diabetes.

- Exercise increases health on many levels, and one side effect is an improved resistance to disease. What's more, all the systems in our children's bodies work more effectively when they are the recipients of plenty of oxygenated blood.

■ Exercise is also linked with self-esteem and mental attitude. Regular exercise produces muscle strength, gains in aerobic fitness, feelings of control over the environment and positive feedback from friends, which can make children feel better about themselves.

Exercise stats and facts[1]

Current research points to the fact that we are getting fatter and it's making us ill. How can we redress the balance? Exercise is one of the best ways to make changes that will affect health both now and in the future. Here are some of the main reasons:

• Fewer than one in four children get 20 minutes of daily vigorous activity.

• Nearly half of young people ages 12 to 21, and more than one-third of high school students, don't participate in vigorous physical activity on a regular basis.

• Data from the National Federation of State High School Associations suggest that less than 21 percent of high school students are involved in even one school sport.

• One out of four children do not attend any school physical education classes, while one in three get physical activity every day.

• While 47 states have state mandates for physical education, only Illinois has a mandatory requirement for physical education for grades K–12.

• The percentage of overweight young Americans has more than doubled in the past 30 years.

Why aren't children exercising?

If being active is the natural response for children, we need to identify what is preventing them from meeting their biological needs. Some of the reasons may seem obvious, but others are less so. In a study published in 1999, children claimed that they did not exercise as often as they would like because they did not have enough time. They blamed parents, homework and not being given choices about how to spend what little free time they had. On the other hand, parents interviewed by the same researchers claimed that their kids aren't interested in activities available to them, and are too busy watching TV, spending time on the computer or playing video games.

This presents an interesting conundrum. Both parents and children claim that they understand the benefits of exercise, but cannot agree on the way it should be undertaken. Perhaps both are partly to blame. Let's look at the reasons children are not getting what they need.

The homework dilemma

Certainly there is some truth in children's complaints. Homework has increased for the majority of children over the past decades, and it is now considered normal for even primary schoolchildren to do something at home in the evenings. With the school day running until 3 or 4 o'clock, and many children traveling some distance to school, it may not be until after supper that children are given any free time. In the winter, that might be too late for an outdoor play session. How important is homework? Several studies have come to the same conclusion—in children under the age of 14, homework has no benefit. If you feel your child is expected to complete more than is necessary, talk to your child's teacher or principal.

Television

There's no doubt that television is an easy option, and more and more children are opting out of regular exercise in favor of slouching in front of the box. In the U.S., the average child watches more than 24 hours a week and over half of all children have a television in their bedrooms. The message is clear: if children are sitting in front of a television, they are not active.

Computer games and consoles

The same problem exists here. Although computers and video games have taken over from television to some degree, they still comprise inactivity. An American study found that children who spent (the average time) four hours a day on the computer or using consoles (for example, Sony PlayStation, Sega Dreamcast and Nintendo Game Boy) had a larger waist size and more body fat than children who reduced these activities by just over an hour a day.

Is it our fault?

Children blame the parents and parents blame the children. There is, however, some truth in the idea that parents do not encourage exercise. Busy lifestyles mean that many parents are often too exhausted themselves to take part in active family outings, and it can be very easy to use the television, games console or computer as a babysitter. Furthermore, many parents fail to set good examples themselves. According to a 1999 survey, eight out of ten of us get no regular exercise, so it's not surprising that our children are less active.

We also need to ensure that our children are exposed to a variety of different sports and activities, in order to find one or more that appeal to them. Setting them up in swimming lessons when they hate the water doesn't encourage fitness. Inline skating, skateboarding, skiing, water polo and football are equally good exercise and your child might enjoy these more. We also need to take the emphasis off schoolwork. This may sound ridiculous, particularly if you've got a reluctant learner on your hands, but schoolwork has its place and it shouldn't take up more than a tiny percentage of your child's free time. Every child needs time to play, explore, run and enjoy sports and other leisure activities. If your daily schedule doesn't allow for this, it might be time to figure out why.

Safety

There's no question that safety is a big issue. When most of us were growing up, we were able to play outdoors on our own, and walk to and from school. According to a new study, parents do not feel that it is safe to let their children play on their own, the major concerns being the threat of abduction, pedophiles and traffic. The experts agree with this (see page 415), and it is unfortunate that we cannot offer our children the same freedom that we had. What we do know, however, is that exercise needs have not changed, and we need to find ways to incorporate exercise into our daily lives, even if activities must be supervised.

School

As school funding drops, many gym-only teachers are forced to take on other portfolios and teaching projects to make their role affordable. The result? Many school sports programs are cut to a minimum. The average child gets one or two hours a week. Large class sizes also mean that children stand in lines for long periods—waiting for instruction or their turn on the apparatus or the team. Some schools offer videos or computer classes in breaks and at lunchtime, so the traditional "let-off-steam" period is curtailed or nonexistent. With many schools selling off playing fields, break times often take place on cement playground courts, with little room for running. Some schools have even banned balls and playground equipment because the number of children in close confines make these activities dangerous. All of these factors multiply the possibility that children will go for days without actually getting some exercise.

What's the cost of exercise?

After-school activities can be prohibitively expensive and time-consuming for many parents. A sports-crazy child could be involved in a variety of sports—for example, judo or karate, hockey, swimming and gymnastics. The cost of these extracurricular activities and the arrangements for getting them there and back can put many parents off.

How much exercise do children really need?

According to the first comprehensive set of exercise guidelines for kids, issued by the American National Association for Sport and Physical Education, children should be active for at least 60 minutes a day, and ideally for much more.

What type of exercise?

Children need the same types of exercise as adults—that is, exercise that promotes flexibility, builds muscle, gives the heart and lungs a good workout (aerobic) and makes them stronger. That doesn't mean heading down to the gym every night. The majority of these needs can be met by playing, which is how children have always stayed fit and healthy. What we need to do, however, is to ensure that children are given the time and space to play, and the room to run!

- Large-muscle groups are worked by a variety of fun activities, including walking, climbing, gymnastics, kicking (a ball, preferably!) and skipping. These activities are also aerobic, providing they are undertaken for long enough (about 15 minutes).

- Aerobic activities are the best for the cardiovascular system. The best aerobic activities for kids are swimming, skating, cycling, running, active team sports (basketball is an excellent example) and inline skating.

- Exercises that improve and increase flexibility include gymnastics, judo and karate, playground fun (hanging from climbing frames is ideal) and ballet. There are even yoga classes for kids, which can be great for stress reduction and grace.

- Children become stronger by taking part in any activity that uses their muscles—pushing and pulling on playground apparatus, swinging (which works the leg muscles), climbing and other activities such as running and skipping.

- Go for sports that involve hand-eye (or foot-eye) coordination, including throwing and catching, baseball, soccer, tennis or squash, which improve grace, skill and, naturally, coordination.

- Rest. For every 15 minutes of activity, children need to rest. You'll probably find that children tune out naturally. Watch a child in the park—he'll run and jump for about 10 to 15 minutes and then take a self-imposed break. If you have a driven child, you may need to impose rest time, even if it's just for a few minutes. Rest doesn't mean stopping activity altogether, and it's not a good idea to plop in front of the TV, which can lead to sore or stiff muscles. Offer plenty to drink during rest periods.

Making time for exercise

- First and foremost, you'll need to assess your schedule. If time is a problem, you may need to book "fun" appointments for your children, to ensure that they are getting playtime. Given some freedom and a little open space, most children will get plenty of exercise with little prompting from their parents.

- Make sure that your children get fun time every day. If it means turning them out into the backyard, or making a visit to the local park, playground or gymnasium every day after school, you'll have to allow time.

- Make sure that playtime takes place before homework. While it is tempting to "clear the decks" when children get home, they will be tired from a day at school and will perform more efficiently after they have had some energizing exercise and probably something light to eat. Let them run off the steam that has built up over the school day. It will reduce stress levels and ease any tension that has built up.

- Don't rely on structured activities too much. While these are undoubtedly good for fitness levels, they can mean a lot of waiting around and are less useful for releasing built-up energy. Sometimes children just need to run and play, left to their own devices (see page 194) and without strict supervision.

- But do try some organized sports as well. Children need to have a flavor of all types of activities before they can decide what they like best. Don't be concerned if your child is not a natural athlete, and never criticize or suggest quitting, particularly if your child enjoys a sport. Team sports teach many things above and beyond fitness, and your child will benefit from a group activity. Many children begin sports in childhood that become hobbies in later life, so it's important to find something that they enjoy and will want to practice regularly.

- If the weather precludes outdoor activity, arrange some indoor games—running up and down the stairs, playing tag in a suitable room or even helping with the housework are all better than sitting still. You can be certain, however, that most children are undaunted by wet or cold weather. If they are dressed properly, they'll have as much fun in inclement weather as they will when it's sunny.

- Try to plan some family activities that involve exercise. After dinner, suggest a family walk around the block or a bike ride in the park. On weekends, try to get out together with a visit to the park, woodland or zoo, the local swimm[...] or gym club, or even the country, where you can spend the day in f[...] Everyone in the family will benefit from regular exercise, and you'll teac[...] children how to be active in their daily lives. For example, if they are u[...] "burning off their dinner" after a heavy meal, they'll be more likely to ado[...] habit in later life.

- Limit television and computer games. If your children have extensive view[...] habits, this will not be popular, but it's worth persevering. No child will benefit from inactivity, no matter how stubborn or determined she is to resist your attempts to make changes. Set an allocated period of time for each day, and relax the rules on the weekends. For example, you could suggest 30 minutes' television viewing per day (they can choose their favorite program) and 30 minutes on the computer. They can swap between the two, if necessary. Don't worry about holidays and special occasions. If your child is getting lots of exercise and is outdoors for much of the time, a little longer in front of the television (watching a video, or a film, for example) won't do as much harm as it will spending that long in front of a screen after a day behind a desk.

- Make exercise fun (see page 107). If they think it's healthy, children will not likely be enthusiastic. They'd probably say no to a chocolate bar if you called it healthy, so be prepared for resistance to doing what's good for them. Find activities that everyone enjoys and make them a normal part of your routine. Dragging kids away from the PlayStation for a jaunt in the park is unlikely to excite the average child. However, if you always go to the park after school, or before Sunday lunch, they'll accept it as a natural part of life. Try a variety of different activities to keep up their interest, and, above all, make sure they enjoy it (see page 108 for some tips on nudging lazy children into action).

- Focus on the positive. If your child worships a particular athlete or basketball player, point out how he trains and becomes fit. You'll be much more likely to inspire a child into action if you can relate it to something with which he identifies.

- Join a gym with children's activities. Many clubs now have programs for children on the weekends, and you can go for a swim or take a class yourself. Many local community centers also offer the same facilities and are a good deal cheaper.

- Set a good example. If your leisure time involves a glass of wine and the newspaper, your children are unlikely to think that riding a bike is a normal weekend activity. Try not to groan and moan when they want to head to the park for a ball game, or suggest a swim. If you are enthusiastic about exercise, and become involved as much as possible, they will respond with equal fervor. Most of all, they'll enjoy your company, and feel reassured that you also follow their interests.

- If walking to school or day care is impossible, park farther away than usual and walk part of the way. Consider organizing a "walking bus," which involves children walking to school in a large group, accompanied by a "driver" (a parent volunteer at the front of the bus) and a "conductor" (at the back of the bus). The bus stops at pre-arranged points to collect other children, who join the bus. This scheme has met with a great deal of success in the U.K., where children involved are given advice and information on road safety, and neon tabards to wear.

Active babies and toddlers

Most young children will be naturally active and it is important to encourage this instinctive behavior from the very earliest days. Some children may need to be kept in a stroller or on reins near busy streets, but always offer them the opportunity to get out and walk or run. Similarly, babies should be encouraged to investigate and explore their surroundings, whether they crawl or simply roll. Keeping a child in one place for any length of time will curtail their natural enthusiasm and curiosity. It can be a trying task to keep a toddler safe in a busy city or even within a house, but it's fairly easy to childproof a house for the few years that it matters, and it's even easier to take your child out to the park, the local baby gym, adventure playground, swimming pool or even music and movement classes.

Here are some ideas to keep little ones active:

- Turn on the music and dance. Most children naturally respond to music and if you become involved, they'll think it's great fun.

- Set up a play gym in the sitting room, using cushions from chairs or a sofa.

- Invest in a baby bouncer, which will allow older babies to sit upright and use their legs to jump up and down.

- Fill a plastic pool or the bath with a little warm water and lots of toys. You'll create the ideal setting for "splashaerobics."

- If you've got a reluctant crawler or walker, set favorite toys just out of reach. She'll soon learn that they have to move to get what they want. Make it into a game and have your little one chase the toy around an appropriate room.

- Make sure your child has toys that encourage him to walk, push or pull. All of these activities invite action and improve coordination. He'll also learn a great deal about his world by experimenting.

- Invite over children of a similar age. Very few children will want to sit on their own if there is a group activity under way.

- Encourage older toddlers to help around the house—carrying laundry to the washing machine, pushing a broom around or even helping to carry the shopping in from the car.

- Blow up a balloon and play volleyball, or just try to keep it in the air!

- Quiet times are also important, but don't be tempted to use the video as a baby-sitter. Although all parents need some peace and time to themselves, too much time in front of a video or television at an early age can encourage inactivity and make your child less enthusiastic about active pursuits.

- If it's manageable, consider accompanying your children to school on bikes. It's a good idea to enroll your child in a cycling proficiency program first, which teaches the basics of road safety, signaling and skills. Invest in a good helmet and a neon tabard.

Whatever you choose, make a decision to commit to it. As adults we are often wary of the term "exercise" as it calls up visions of enforced routines at school, or hours on a treadmill trying to lose unwanted weight. Exercise holds no such associations for children, and we need to ensure that it never does. If they start off being active, they'll be more likely to continue that way. Early on we need to plant the idea that exercise is fun and sociable, it makes us feel better, and, above all, it's a natural, normal part of life.

▶ *Top tips for making exercise fun*

- Change the name. If the idea of a walk does not excite your children, call it something else. Turn it into a game: a treasure hunt, for example. Get a local street map and ask each child to plan a different route each day. Or flip a coin at the end of every street to decide whether you will turn left or right (it may turn out to be a very long walk indeed). Go on a spying mission, where children are encouraged to find 10 different objects (all red, for example) before you can return home. Do your shopping locally and give each child a list of things they need to remember to get. If they feel that they have a mission, they'll be much happier to be involved.

- Start a get-fit campaign and make it fun. Children are enormously motivated by a little competition and if they see results, they'll be keen on making more. My son's school set up a program to improve the fitness of the boys. The children were assessed for fitness levels, and underwent a fitness improvement program, with regular testing to assess the results. The vast majority of children were enormously motivated by this project—partly because of the competition element, but partly because they could see for themselves what exercise could do.

- This type of program can easily be undertaken at home. Invest in a stopwatch and time your children running in the park, or around the block, even up and down the stairs. Write down the times on a chart and encourage them to better their results. How many sit-ups can they do in a minute, for example, or how many times can they touch their toes? Set up an obstacle course in the backyard or a local park and time how long it takes to get around.

- Dance! Turn on the CD player and get the whole family involved. Dancing is great aerobic exercise and any musical activity can be uplifting (see page 248). Make up your own line dances, or show your children how to jitterbug or tango. You might learn some more modern dances yourself. Allow the children to choose the music.

- Create your own exercise video. If you have a video camera, it can be great fun to prepare a homemade exercise program to music. Not only will the children have a good time (and get lots of exercise) while putting it together, but they might be encouraged to use it themselves on a rainy day.

- Make up an active game. Ask your children to come up with ideas for ball games, hopping or skipping games. The idea is to keep moving, whatever inspires them.

- Walk the dog. Dog owners have much higher fitness levels than any other pet owner, and for good reason. All dogs need regular daily walks, and it can be the type of enforced exercise that becomes a healthy and enjoyable habit. If you don't have a dog, perhaps your children can offer to take a neighbor's dog for a daily walk in the park.

- Set up a water park in the backyard, with a slide, the sprinkler, some buckets, an inflatable pool and even the swing set. Ask your children to design the park so that there are lots of different activities and then invite some friends.

- Ask older children to wash the car. On a warm, sunny day, this is best done in bathing suits! Give liberal access to a hose and lots of soapy water, and you can be sure they'll get lots of exercise and you'll be the owner of a clean car!

- Buy a packet of balloons and use wooden spoons or tennis rackets to play games in the backyard. Set up a net with a piece of string or some garden furniture. (This game can also be played indoors, using kitchen chairs as a "net.") Fill the balloons up with water and try to throw and catch them without breaking them!

- Try to plan holidays with plenty of outdoor activities for kids—skiing, windsurfing, bike riding, hiking, climbing, skating or swimming. The more activities children try, the more encouraged they will be to expand their repertoire of skills. They'll also begin to view exercise as something associated with leisure and fun, rather than just boring gym at school.

Inspiring lazy children

Have you got a nonstarter on your hands? Some children seem to be much happier in front of a screen, or in a corner somewhere with a book. While these activities all have their place in normal family life, chances are your child will not be getting the exercise he needs. Consider some of the ideas for making exercise fun, and keep the whole family as active as possible. Plan family outings involving active pursuits or invite more active friends to inspire some movement.

- Put up a star chart for exercise. For every half-hour of activity, offer a star. A completed chart can be rewarded with anything your child fancies—a new basketball, a new tennis racket or running shoes, judo or skating lessons, a new book or video, or even just 30 minutes of playtime with you, doing whatever your child wants!

- Be sneaky. Park as far away as you can from the mall so that you'll have to walk further to get where you are going. Send your children on local errands, or up and down the stairs to fetch things. Encourage them to make their own beds and to carry the shopping. All of these activities add up in terms of fitness.

- Talk to your child and try to work out why he doesn't like getting involved in active pursuits. It may be that he's had a bad experience in the playground or at school, or he may feel that he's hopeless at sports. Try to assess how you can help. Offer special coaching in a sport that many of his friends play. Encourage him to choose two or three sports that he's always wanted to try. You may find that his passion will be something that is not always routinely offered.

- Praise, praise, praise. If you offer lots of encouragement, your child will feel good about himself and take some pride in his achievements. Never put your child down or suggest that he isn't any good at a sport or other activity. Children learn confidence when they are encouraged, and they learn to like themselves when they feel that you approve of them.

- Don't nag and don't focus too much on the "healthy" reasons for exercising. While all children need to be educated about their bodies and their health needs, they don't want to feel that they are being lectured, or that they are under pressure to please you.

- In a 1999 survey, more than 1,200 children in the U.K. aged between 11 and 16 were asked about their attitude toward health and fitness. The youngsters said they wanted more information on how to be healthy—but they did not want to be lectured by adults. Take this advice to heart and offer some choices. Present information in a casual way—sounding shocked, for example, about a recent report that adolescents could have a heart attack. You'll open the door for discussion and an exchange of facts. Assess your own lifestyle and point out that you are concerned about how inactive you are. Ask your child's advice about becoming fitter and ask for suggestions about how the whole family can get more exercise. Make the information relevant. If your child is an academician rather than sporty, point out that exercise can improve memory and concentration and reduce stress.

- Get involved. If you are out there kicking or batting a ball too, they'll be much more likely to want to take part. Make fitness a family goal, with everyone playing a role.

- Offer appropriate choices to empower your child. Ask, for example, what she would like to do: play baseball in the park, go for a walk in the country, visit the local pool or plan a trip to an adventure playground. Make sure all the options include some activity. Children like to feel that they are in control of their lives and will believe that they have some stake in things when they are given choices.

■ Assign your child some household chores that require moderate exertion—raking leaves, washing windows, shoveling snow or even vacuuming the stairs. Make him feel proud of his accomplishments and consider offering an allowance as a reward, or a star on a chart leading to the promise of something fun later. All children like to be given some responsibility (see page 196), and it can have the dual purpose of keeping them fit and raising their self-esteem.

Adolescent apathy

The teen years are notorious for languorous living. Teenagers require a lot of sleep, and they grow and develop a great deal during these years. Not surprisingly, many adolescents have little energy or inclination to become involved in sporting activities, particularly if they are now considered "uncool." Family outings may not hold the same appeal that they did when your adolescent was younger, and you'll need to find ways to keep her enthusiastic and, most importantly, fit.

It's crucially important to create and maintain relationships as your child grows up. If your child views you as the enemy, your advice is likely to be ignored to the point of rebellion. We talk about this in chapter 8. Obviously if sport or physical activity played a big part in her younger years, she's likely to continue to enjoy exercise. That's one of the reasons it is so important to create healthy habits. However, if you are concerned about activity levels now, having either neglected that side of family life to some extent, or been unable to persuade your child to become involved in any sports or activities, it's not too late to make some changes.

The advantage of dealing with older children is that they can understand and reason (well, perhaps only on a good day!). You can best make headway by making things relevant to their daily life. Once again, draw parallels between famous athletes or even scientists, if that's appropriate. Everyone, in every walk of life, can benefit from exercise and you need to find a way to get that message through. Whether it's reducing stress, enhancing brain power or endurance that your teenager will respond to, there will be a way to convince her that exercise can help her do better. Whatever you do, try not to lecture or nag. Offer positive choices and let your teenager make her own decisions. Just ensure that the choices you offer are realistic and active!

Adolescence is a stressful period, and many teenagers find the transition from childhood to young adulthood very difficult. You may lock horns on many occasions throughout these years but, just like small children, adolescents do need to be guided and they need praise and encouragement. If your child feels good about herself throughout these years, she is more likely to communicate with you, with her peers and with other adults. She'll also have more respect for herself and her body. If a teenager takes pride in her body and her achievements, she'll be more likely to make healthy decisions. Raising self-esteem can be crucial to your child's long-term success (see page 173) in any part of her life.

It's well known that children involved in sports have less free time to experiment with drugs and alcohol. Focus on keeping your teenager active from the earliest possible moment. Busy, motivated teenagers have little free time for leisure activities that can harm health.

▶ *Top tips for motivating your teenager*

- The star system may be a little out of date for a teenager, but the principle remains the same. Offer rewards—and plenty of them—for behavior that you want to encourage. For example, if your child agrees to attend a sport of his choice once or twice a week, you could offer a lift (and possibly a ticket) to the movies on the weekend, or a new CD.

- Dancing is a good aerobic sport. Many unathletic children are very keen on music. Indulge this passion and maybe club together with a few other parents to get a karaoke machine or a few CDs that you can swap. Make sure your child has a room where he can feel free to move about comfortably, away from the eyes of his siblings or parents. He'll be much more likely to move around if he's not being watched!

- Set a series of fitness assessments, and offer a reward if your teenager can produce some good results and improvement over a period of time. Ask him to set up the program (including sit-ups, running around the block or a track, running up stairs) and offer to time him.

- Keep up the family activities. Many older children find it embarrassing to be seen with their parents, but agree, as a family, to do at least one session together a week. Try to make sure these times involve some physical activity. Similarly, family holidays are still appropriate for teenagers, and you can choose one that will appeal to the whole family—with sports and games for all ages.

- Encourage your child to get a part-time job helping out at the local swimming pool, sports club, soccer club or gym. He will more likely be inspired if he's in an environment that encourages fitness. The long summer holidays can be spent helping out at local school or sports club activity weeks, where older children and teens are involved in teaching and training the younger children. The majority of teenagers will respond to some responsibility, and will probably want to impress the younger children with their knowledge and skill.

- Consider some of the summer camp or adventure holidays set up for teens. It may be beyond your budget, but many offer concessions, particularly if your child can be of some assistance. Similarly, a summer job acting as a supervisor will keep him active, and he'll probably learn new sports and skills that can become passions.

- Most teenagers will respond to some competition. Set up a regular game of tennis or squash together. It's one way to ensure that you stay fit, and you might find that you are soon out of your depth!

- Offer to arrange courses in some of the more varied sports—horseback riding, cycling, athletics, diving, archery, martial arts, climbing, hiking or skiing. Anything that moves muscles will, in the long run, work toward fitness goals.

Assess your child's fitness

It's very easy to check a child's fitness levels. If your child is regularly active, you have no reason to worry. However, if you have a computer addict or bookworm in the house, her fitness levels may be inadequate.

Watch your child for an average week and note down how long she spends being active. If your child is in good health and is not asthmatic, answer the following questions and add up the number of points:

▶ *Does my child:*

- Get some exercise (run, play actively, skip, jump or simply move around) for at least an hour a day? Add 2 points for every day (out of 7) that this occurs.

- Take part in school gym or other sports classes? Add 2 points for every session; subtract 1 point overall if classes are larger than 30 children.

- Take part in extracurricular sports activities (baby gym, swimming, gymnastics, soccer, baseball, basketball, ballet, dancing, etc.)? Add 2 points for every hour spent at the activity.

- Attend classes, courses or activities where there is some physical activity involved (Brownies, Cubs, music and movement, etc.)? Add 2 points for every session.

- Choose physical activity above other hobbies or leisure activities on a regular basis? Add 1 point.

- Breathe heavily upon running up more than two flights of stairs (for children under the age of three, one flight of stairs)? Subtract 2 points.

- Continue to breathe heavily after a ten-minute break from high-exertion activities (in other words, has breathing returned to normal after ten minutes)? Subtract 2 points.

- Touch her toes easily? Subtract 2 points if she cannot.

- Spend more than two hours a day watching television, playing video or computer games, or reading? Subtract 2 points for every hour spent, above two hours.

- Fall into the category of being obese (see page 60)? Subtract 2 points.

- Have less stamina than her peers (able to run for less time, find keeping up difficult, etc.)? Subtract 2 points.

Working out the results

Total your child's score.

- **Above 20:** Very high levels of fitness, and should be in excellent condition.

- **14–19:** Good exercise levels, and should be fit and able to keep up with or exceed the efforts of her peers.

- **7–13:** Moderately fit. Could do with more regular exercise to really feel the health benefits.

- **Less than 7:** Unfit. Try to find ways to increase exercise levels even slightly. Every ten minutes spent being active will work toward substantial health benefits. Remember that lack of exercise is one of the main risk factors for heart disease and other health conditions. It's worth every bit of effort you can make.

chapter six

And So to Bed

M ore parents complain about their children's sleeping habits than any other issue. Nighttime wakings, inability to get to sleep, regular trips from the bed, nightmares and even adolescent sleep-ins are the source of great parental frustration and debate. They are also the source of broken sleep, which seems to affect parents far more than it does the children themselves. The interesting question is whether sleeping patterns have changed over the years and, if they have, what effect that is having on our children and, of course, ourselves.

One of the reasons sleep seems to matter so much is the fact that we have, as a culture, become obsessed by it. The majority of adults feel that they get inadequate sleep, so it's not surprising that this preoccupation has spilled over to affect the way we perceive our children's sleeping habits, and the way we deal with them. We feel anxious about getting enough sleep, and children undoubtedly take on this anxiety. Before you know it, sleep has become a problem or an issue—it's either a tool that children can use to gain attention, or it is associated with negative emotions, neither of which is conducive to good, restful sleep and sleeping habits.

AMERICAN RESEARCHERS surveyed over 2,000 parents of 6- to 18-month-old children. Over 90 percent had been sufficiently concerned about sleeping habits (night wakings, inability to get to sleep, bedtime struggles) to ask for expert advice. Of those who sought advice, only 6 percent of the children were found to have serious sleep problems. The study concluded that parental anxiety, intervention and feeding habits were the root of the sleep problems—in both the seriously affected children and those with normal sleep habits.

When we are not getting enough sleep, we feel frustrated and unable to cope with any disruption to the little rest we get. A perfectly normal newborn or a naturally determined toddler can undoubtedly alter household routines. The answer, however, is not to panic and self-diagnose a sleep problem, but to understand the sleep needs of children at various stages and to find an acceptable way to meet them.

ACCORDING TO the U.K.'s National Commission on Sleep Disorders Research, adults today are getting 20 percent less sleep than they did 100 years ago.

Our lifestyles are dramatically different from those of our forebears. We get inadequate exercise, our lives are stressful and our 24-hour society means that we often undertake what were traditionally considered daytime tasks long into the night. When you can buy your groceries at 3 A.M., get a haircut at midnight, or clock on to the Internet or do laundry at any time of the day or night, there is a temptation to fill every working hour with activity. The result? We have forgotten the importance of winding down, and then we are puzzled about why we feel tired. More importantly, perhaps, we are setting a poor example for our children. In the past, work had to end with the sunset, or shortly thereafter. Sleep was rightfully considered an essential part of daily life and in the absence of much else to do in the late night, it took priority. While most of us would argue that it is still a priority, there are very few of us who manage to unwind successfully and get the required hours of sleep to meet our individual needs. Our children have been born into this all-night culture, and it's difficult to explain or to put into practice good sleeping habits when the Disney Channel runs child-friendly cartoons late into the night or when parents don't sit down to eat or to begin their social life until after 9 P.M.

Many of us work and have little time to fit in housework and other household responsibilities. Add to that the fact that working hours have increased dramatically, and we have a fairly disastrous situation. Relaxation involves quick fixes, such as alcohol or fast-food meals, and then the customary plop in front of the television. At an appointed time—usually later than anticipated—we take ourselves off to bed, where we often find it difficult to sleep. You may wonder what this has to do with children, but I can assure you that it is of central importance. Here's why:

- First and foremost, lack of sleep makes it more difficult to cope with our children calmly and rationally. Small things are blown out of proportion, and at the end of the day when children are at their most fractious, tearful or hyperactive, it's harder to carry out a routine that will soothe them off to sleep.

- Secondly, if we are pressed for time and energy ourselves, we opt for one of two things: we bundle kids off to bed before they are tired, without an appropriate period of winding down and then snap when they fail to settle immediately, or waken in the night. Alternatively, we give in and let them set their own schedules, falling asleep on the sofa, in front of the television, or wherever and whenever they please. These two common habits are equally harmful, and will not create the type of sleeping habits and routines that are necessary for life-long health and well-being.

- Children pick up our negative feelings about sleep; they begin to feel that sleep is something that they have to do rather than enjoy doing, which makes it less pleasurable and a point of contention between parent and child. They also learn to believe that they are the cause of parental lack of sleep, which makes them feel guilty. Any anxiety around sleep can be transmitted to children, causing just the sorts of problems that keep parents awake.

- Children also learn what they live. If there are no set routines in place and everyone in the household is rushing around trying to fit everything in, they'll begin to think that relaxation and sleep are not essential parts of life. It's hard to convince an excited eight-year-old that it's bedtime when the household is chaotically active. For good sleeping habits, called "sleep hygiene," to take place, everyone in the family plays a role in setting up healthy routines.

Why is sleep important?

It's actually more important than you might think. All of us need good, restful sleep, but for children it's absolutely essential.

- Inadequate sleep lowers our immune response. A recent study showed that missing even a few hours a night on a regular basis can decrease the number of "natural killer cells," which are responsible for fighting off invaders such as bacteria and viruses. This will come as no surprise to those of us who succumb to colds and other illnesses when we are run down—normally after periods of inadequate sleep. Children are no exception, and with their immature immune systems, they are at particular risk.

- Even occasional sleeping problems can make daily life feel more stressful or cause us to be less productive. A survey in the U.S. showed that children who get enough sleep report a better ability to concentrate, accomplish required tasks and handle minor irritations. In contrast, those with a higher "sleep deficit" showed impairment of the ability to perform tasks involving memory, learning, logical reasoning and mathematical calculation. They also found relationships at home and with friends more difficult.

- Growth hormones are released during sleep, and while it is unknown what effect they have on growth patterns in children, research has shown that children who are chronically sleep deprived—those with severe asthma or sleep disturbances such as apnea (see page 380), for example—have retarded growth. There is also a great deal of evidence that abused children do not grow well because they are too afraid to sleep or wake too frequently to have sufficient deep sleep. When the same children sleep well in a more secure environment, their growth and development improve.

- Professor Jim Horne, who runs the Sleep Research Laboratory at Loughborough University in the U.K., feels that the brain is most affected by sleep deprivation in children. He claims that the organ for which sleep does seem vital is the cerebrum and this is clearly demonstrated by sleep-loss studies. Whereas most of the body can physically relax and recover in wakefulness to levels similar to those of sleep, the cerebrum cannot do this. Even when the eyes are closed and the mind is blank, the waking brain remains in a state of high activity and quiet readiness. He says that the cerebral (brain) metabolic rate is particularly high in three- to eight-year-old children, which suggests that this organ may be in need of even greater recovery during sleep at this time.

- Adolescents may be particularly affected. A recent study showed that when we do not get enough sleep, even over one night, a "sleep debt" begins to build and increases, until enough sleep is obtained. Sleepiness occurs as the debt accumulates. If too much sleep has been lost, sleeping in on the weekend may not completely reverse the effects of not getting enough sleep during the week. In general, pre-adolescent children may be getting sufficient sleep, particularly if parents help to protect sleep times. Older adolescents, however, are staying up later, rising earlier and incurring sleep debts that may never be "repaid." What's the consequence of this? A U.S. study indicates that adolescents commonly experience "microsleeps, attention lapses, decreased reaction times, impaired divergent thinking skills, impaired mental functioning, low mood, and a higher rate of accidents and injuries."

How much sleep does my child need?

Sleep needs differ dramatically between children, just as they do between adults. However, there is no excuse for thinking that a child can get by on what an adult gets. Sleep is crucially important in childhood and adolescence, and there are very, very few children who do not need to get at least the average required hours. The table on pages 118–119 lists the average number of hours that each age group requires. Don't be surprised if your child doesn't fit the norm exactly. It's simply helpful to have an idea of what to expect—and what to aim for. If you find your child is getting dramatically less or more than required, you may need to assess why (see page 380).

Age	Number of hours	Number of sleep periods
		Special notes
Newborns	16 to 18	In periods throughout the day. About half will be in the night hours, and half during the day.
3 to 6 months	15	Sleep occurs in about four or five periods. About two-thirds will occur at night. Somewhere between three and six months a baby will normally begin to sleep for long stretches at night.
6 to 12 months	14 to 15	Daytime sleep during this period is normally reduced from about four to two-and-a-half hours, which means that night time sleeping is increased accordingly. Naps will probably be regular (two a day, for example).
1 to 2 years	14	Naps still make up between one and two-and-a-half hours of sleep, with the remainder taking place at night. Most children drop the morning nap by the age of about two. In good health, most two-year-olds are capable of sleeping for about 12 hours at night without waking.
3 to 6 years	10 to 12	The afternoon nap normally disappears around age three or four, although some sleepier children may benefit from a rest in the afternoons.
7 to 9 years	8 to 10	Children may take longer to fall asleep, and this figure does not take into consideration the time between lights out and falling asleep. These hours refer to good-quality sleep only.

Age	Number of hours	Number of sleep periods
10 to 11 years	8 to 9 ½	Children of this age often don't get what is required, and many parents are surprised by how much children do need in these prepubescent years.
11 to 18 years	9 plus	According to research, very few adolescents get more than about six hours a night. See page 137.

Establishing routines

The key to successful sleep habits for children of all ages is a sound presleep routine that is undertaken on a daily basis. Many parents adopt extremely good routines when their children are babies and have little trouble throughout childhood. Others are careful about routine in infancy, but let it slide when toddlers and older children begin to assert their own ideas about bedtime. It is, admittedly, much easier to impose a regime when children are younger than it is to introduce something new later on. However, the importance of routine cannot be overstated. Children feel secure when they know their boundaries and what to expect. If the rules and routines shift repeatedly, they'll feel unsettled and will be more likely to create a prebedtime fuss or waken in the night.

Setting up your life in a series of ordered, sequential events may seem tedious and you may feel tied down by the thought of monotonous regularity. However, as your child slips into a routine that you have designed to suit all family members, you will all benefit. Your child will sleep better, with less disruption. You can avoid the distressing and exhausting bedtime battles, and you will have time on your own and get a good night's sleep too. Children who have slept well are less irritable throughout the day and do better at school.

Setting up routines doesn't mean that you have to be entirely inflexible or give up spontaneity. Good routines make it easy to comfort and settle your child wherever you are, which can be a huge advantage and provide you with freedom to go a little further afield.

Babies

There is no point in trying to force a routine on a small baby, who will have his own agenda and timetable—unfortunately one that runs around the clock. You will need to set up a routine that fits into your baby's inborn schedule, and gently adapt it to suit your lifestyle. The bedtime routine is one of the most important you can establish—even from the first days of parenthood. When your baby begins to recognize his own routine, he will relax and feel secure, and he will know what to expect. That means that you will be able to set the routine in motion wherever you are—in the spare bedroom of a friend's house for dinner, or perhaps on vacation.

Choose nighttime rituals that you know your baby enjoys, or that comfort him. You may wish to begin after the evening feed or meal with a short play session, winding down to some cuddling on the bed, or perhaps a short massage session with some relaxing aromatherapy oils. A bath every day is not necessary, but many babies feel settled and calm after one. Take time to rub him dry and talk to him about what you are doing, and then settle down for a story together. Even a newborn baby will respond to colorful picture books, and the sound of your voice. You may wish to sing to your baby, or rock him for a while before you give him a final feed, or settle him down to sleep. Whatever you do, try to repeat the same order of events every night, and bedtime will soon be associated with pleasurable sensations, rather than the fear of being left alone.

Try to plan your day around a series of regular events. You may wish to dress him about the same time each day, and perhaps take him for a walk in the park, or to a friend's house in the mornings. If he is agreeable, you may begin to settle him down for naps around the same time each day. In the early days, most of your time will be spent feeding your baby, changing him, bathing him and getting him off to sleep, with very little time for yourself in between, but you will soon begin to discern a pattern in his activities, and that is the time to swoop down with a routine that both he and you can recognize and work with. Paradoxically, a routine will give you freedom, and will help your baby to be confident as he goes about his familiar activities.

Toddlers

If you haven't already got a routine in place, it's not too late to start one. You may find that an existing routine needs to be altered slightly to take into account a slightly later or earlier bedtime, or your later arrival home from work. One of the most important things to remember about a bedtime routine is that it needs to be calm. It can be difficult for parents who have been away from their children all day to avoid boisterous playtime, but the sheer excitement of having a parent return home, coupled with some rough and tumble, tickling or chasing, can make it impossible for a child to settle down to sleep.

Some of the bedtime routine may have to be undertaken before you get home— by a nanny or other caregiver—and you'll need to make sure that she is aware of the best sequence of events to settle your child. The beauty of a routine is that anyone should be able to put it in place, whether you are there or not. If all of the sleep associations are in place—a warm bath, some time spent talking, a story or a puzzle and maybe a warm drink—your child will be less likely to make a fuss, even if you are not there.

If you or your partner do return home later, keep things low-key. Settle down with a story and a drink, or even just a little chat. Play some soft music, and take time to relax yourself. As your child gets older, she'll learn to welcome this peaceful period and you'll be much more likely to build up a good rapport if she knows that she always has this time allotted to her. This can be quiet time—a time for praise, gentle activities and comfort. If you are stressed or tired after work, try not to let it show, and never use this time to air disagreements or inflict discipline. It's certainly acceptable to talk things through—perhaps your toddler had a bad day at nursery school, or wouldn't eat her dinner—but keep things calm. If you are too enthusiastic, excited or angry, she will react in kind. *No* child will sleep well if she is anxious or overexcited.

Try to make a daily evening bath part of your routine. Although your child might not be dirty enough to warrant one every night, baths often have the positive psychological effect of "washing away" the stresses and strains of the day. Younger children may splash and become excited, but they will feel warm and relaxed when you have dried them off and put on their pajamas. Use a drop or two of tea tree and lavender oil, to relax and boost immunity (see page 243). This combination also works wonders for fending off head lice when your child reaches school age. A bath as part of a daily routine is a good way to instill some hygiene habits in children, and you can teach them how to wash and dry themselves properly.

Older children

As children get older, there are more demands on their time and many more distractions in the form of television, computers, games consoles and other activities. Routines are important not only to ensure that they fit everything in easily and comfortably but also will help to ensure that your child gets the sleep he needs.

Even older children find comfort and security in routines, and when good routines are in place, they'll learn the valuable skill of planning their own time in order to fit in homework, extracurricular activities, exercise and play.

If you've had a routine in place since babyhood, keep it in place and adjust it according to your child's needs. Most children will benefit from some quiet playtime, a relaxing bath, a chat and a story. As your child gets older, he may like to choose the story and read to you. Some children enjoy listening to a story tape at night, and as long as it's not too long or exciting, this can be a good way of lulling them off to sleep. If you haven't set up a routine, try to do so now. Start with dinnertime and begin the wind-down from there. You may need to put some new rules in place, but try to make it look like a series of lifestyle changes for the whole family rather than a rigid new routine, which is sure to be greeted with horror.

It's a good idea to get homework and other necessaries out of the way before dinner, unless you eat very early. Like adults, children need time to unwind before bed and if they are struggling with or resisting homework, it's bound to have its effect on their sleep. After dinner, give them a period of time in which to choose a favorite activity, but set a time limit and if necessary set up a star chart to ensure that it is maintained. If your child is used to watching television for several hours every night and you suggest a one-hour slot instead, you'll have to use some positive encouragement to implement the changes successfully.

After "free" time, work your way toward the bathtub or shower, and then play a quiet game or work on a puzzle together. You can listen to music, perhaps, or just chat. As long as the activity is quiet, anything goes. This may sound idealistic in a family with more than one child, but if you ensure that everyone has free time at the same time, and each party knows what happens next, you'll find that things do slip into place. Reading together or letting your child read to you before bedtime is a good way to end the day, especially if you can arrange to do it in her bedroom. Older children can be given time to read alone or listen to a story tape before lights out.

Adolescents

The sleeping habits of adolescents have become a serious concern (see page 137), and it is important that your teenager is able to get enough restful sleep. Adolescents may have activities of their own that take them out of the house in the evenings, and routines may be a little harder to put into place and adhere to. They may also have a great deal of homework, which can push bedtime later and later.

If you do not already have a household bedtime routine in place, encourage your teenager to set her own. Suggest that every night she spend some time doing her own thing, and some time with you, or with the family, after dinner. If homework spills over into the evenings, make sure that she gets it done early to avoid winding herself up so that she finds it difficult to sleep. Suggest a bath and a short reading session before bed every night. It's usually possible to reason with an adolescent, and you can use the same ploys that you did with exercise or eating—that is, make it relevant to her life. If you point out that sleep deprivation will affect athletic or academic performance, or even make her irritable with family and friends the next day, she may take this into consideration. If your child is a good sleeper, and has no trouble getting into bed and falling asleep at a reasonable hour, you don't need to worry. If, however, your child gets a second wind around midnight and seems glued to the computer or television screen long after she should be in bed, it is in everyone's interests to get a routine in place.

No child benefits from being allowed free rein to set her own bedtimes. Every one of us needs good, nurturing sleep in order to perform well at whatever age. Putting a good routine in action can help everyone in the family unwind and fall asleep at an appropriate time.

Creating the optimum sleep environment

A child's bedroom is an important part of restful sleep, and he will need to feel comfortable and relaxed in order to get to sleep and to sleep through the night. Like adults, children need to sleep in an environment that is free of distractions. It's not surprising that children resist going to sleep and wake at ungodly hours to play when their room is full of tantalizing toys, a television or favorite playthings. The answer is to keep the bedroom as clutter-free as possible.

If you don't have a separate playroom, and your child spends much of his free time in his bedroom, invest in some good storage, and make clearing away the toys part of the nighttime routine. Many children like to fill their beds with books and toys, but it's not a good idea to encourage this. By all means suggest a comforting book at bedtime, but if it's something interactive or likely to keep them awake, keep it away from the bed. Many children have a blanket or a soft toy that they associate with sleep, and may have had from childhood. Many experts believe that this is a useful tool for encouraging sleep, particularly in young children, and if you can keep a familiar item in the bed, they'll learn to associate it with comfort and with sleep.

Make the bedroom a haven, with comfortable blankets and soothing colors (see page 160). While a bright red-white-and-blue bedroom may be attractive, it could be hampering your child's sleep by overstimulating him. It's better to stick to cool, calming colors, such as greens, blues and creams.

Many children like having a tape-player by the bed, and this can be useful if your child likes to fall asleep to a story or some gentle music. Music, in particular, can be very soothing and some studies indicate that it can have a profound effect on the nervous system. Obviously active music or frightening stories will have a negative impact on sleep, but lullabies or child-friendly books on tape can lull many highly strung children off to sleep.

Babies and very young children seem to respond to "white noise," perhaps a hangover from the soothing sounds of the womb. As ridiculous as it sounds, you might want to invest in a white noise tape, or turn a radio to a static-only setting, to help your child drift off.

Some children find it difficult to fall asleep in the dark, whether they are frightened, feel lonely or just like the comfort of seeing their environment. In these situations, a nightlight can be useful. However, a study led by Professor Richard Stone of the Scheie Eye Institute at Pennsylvania University in Philadelphia, Pennsylvania, found that children under two who sleep with a light on are five times more likely than children who sleep in the dark to grow up short-sighted and needing glasses. Short-sightedness, or myopia, is the inability to focus on distant objects, and it may be a risk factor for blindness in later life. It is caused by excessive growth of the eyeball, which grows particularly quickly before the age of two. Scientists believe light at night may stimulate the eyeball to grow.

Music and sleep

- A variety of studies have shown that soothing music has the ability to reduce stress hormones, while lively music can encourage them.

- A study on the effect of music on preschool children concluded that soft music (in this case lullabies) relaxed restless children, and it took significantly longer for children to fall asleep in silence than it did while listening to music.

- Studies into the effects of music therapy indicate the following conditions can be improved: allergies, asthma, dyslexia, migraine headaches, back pain, anxiety, insomnia and diabetes. If your child suffers from illness that is affecting sleep patterns, it may be worth investing in some classical music tapes to ease symptoms and improve sleep. For more on music therapy, see chapter 10.

- In the U.S., a study reported the effect of the sound of heartbeats on young children. Slower beats produced a relaxation response, while quicker beats induced anxiety or agitation. Since that time, "heartbeat recordings" have been used successfully in the treatment of a wide range of health conditions, including impaired sleep in children. See Resources, page 438, for details of how to order tapes with or without musical accompaniment.

Nightlights can, of course, be turned off after your child has fallen asleep, but when he does waken in the night (as part of the normal sleep cycle), he will be more likely to stay awake and find it difficult to drift off again in the dark. Some parents find it useful to provide a child-safe lamp that can be switched on and off as required, making it clear to children that it should be used only when absolutely necessary. Many children sleep better knowing that they have some control should they waken. The best advice, however, is to get your child used to sleeping in the dark, which will establish good patterns in later life.

Keep the room on the cool side, and layer covers as required. If your child habitually kicks off his covers and wakes up cold, you might want to invest in a pair of fleece pajamas with feet, or a sleeping bag. Children are more likely to wake up if they are too hot than they will be likely to waken from cold. Young babies can be swaddled for warmth and comfort (see below) and older children will soon learn to pull up a duvet cover or blanket if they are chilly.

Never banish your child to his bedroom or bed as a form of punishment. Some children do need to have a "time-out" as a form of discipline, but if they begin to associate their bedroom with being naughty, they'll be much less likely to sleep well or, indeed, want to go to bed. Save bedrooms for sleep and quiet time.

Establishing good habits

In the early days, your baby's sleeping habits will be dictated by her need for food or comfort, and it is best to fall in with her needs for the first few weeks. No baby will benefit from being left to cry, or from having a strict regime imposed on his natural schedule. While it may seem horrendous to be woken repeatedly throughout the night, these weeks do pass quickly and it won't be long before you can start to set up a routine that works for you and your family.

The only form of communication that a young baby has is crying. There may not be anything obviously wrong, if she's warm enough, has a dry diaper and has been fed. She may just want some company, or the comfort of being held. Try to go with these demands for the first month or so. She'll learn that she can rely on you and will feel more secure and confident when she is alone, in the knowledge that you will come when she needs you. Babies who are left to cry will never understand that you are too tired to soothe them; they'll simply feel miserable. They may learn to stop crying at night, but it's a fairly sorry lesson for a baby to learn, and you'll have peaceful nights at the expense of your child's security.

Most babies fall asleep during feeds, and in the early days this is acceptable, as long as she is getting enough nourishment to allow her to sleep for longer than an hour or so. If you've got a sleepy baby who drifts off the moment a breast or teat is placed in her mouth, try to keep her awake, and wake her up to burp her before placing her in her crib to sleep. Falling asleep while feeding is not a good idea for older babies. When they waken naturally in the night, they'll automatically look for the same source of comfort and will cry until they get it.

Sleep associations

All children need to learn to fall asleep by themselves and to get back to sleep if they waken in the night. If they are fed and rocked to sleep every night, these are the very things that they will need to fall asleep. Sleep associations need to be introduced early on and maintained throughout childhood as part of a routine. Rocking and a warm drink are lovely parts of a sleep routine, but they should be undertaken before your child goes to sleep. Offer a drink, rock them while you sing a song or read a story, but put your child to bed awake. You can stand over the crib and talk to them for a little while. You can also return to the room every few minutes to reassure your baby that you are there. Some parents find it useful to stay in the room—putting away clothes, tidying toys or simply reading—for a few minutes so that your baby can hear the comforting sounds of activity.

Contrary to some theories, your child will want to hear the sounds of the household as he falls asleep. If he's left alone in a dark room he can feel very lonely and isolated. He may learn to fall asleep in these circumstances but, again, he'll be more likely to waken with any sudden noise. What you want to do is encourage your child to sleep through the sounds of normal family activities.

Sucking to sleep

Some "sucky" babies seem to need the comfort of suckling in order to get to sleep. It's not unusual, nor is it problematic. Many people have "oral" fixations, chewing pencils, biting fingernails or even smoking, and babies can have this inborn need for oral satisfaction. If your baby has fed well and still seems to need the comfort of suckling, she may be happy to suck fingers or even a pacifier. Pacifiers have had bad press over the last few years, and many parents feel that they have many negative attributes, including being associated with dental problems in later life. However, it is fairly clear that the ultimate role of a parent is to satisfy a baby's needs. If your baby needs the comfort of suckling, by all means introduce a pacifier. Most of them are now designed to reduce orthodontic problems, and as long as they are kept scrupulously clean, they will not harm a baby. In fact, they can be a godsend for parents whose

The family bed

Some children and parents find that the answer to problem sleep is sharing a bed. It's a controversial subject, and many people think it is inappropriate or even distasteful to sleep with children. First and foremost, it is irrelevant what anyone else thinks. If it works for you, go with it. All children grow up and become independent, and you will not be harming that development by sleeping with your child. In fact, many children feel more confident and secure, particularly if they are light sleepers who need the comfort of regular contact. They will eventually want their own space, and you can let them make that decision on their own. Our society places too much emphasis on independence. Pushing a child to do something that neither you nor he feels comfortable with will never inspire security or self-esteem. Children become confident and independent when they feel good about themselves, when they feel loved, secure and accepted. Many experts believe that sharing a bed encourages those feelings. It's normal and natural for a young child to want to be with a parent all the time, and she may even find it easier to fall asleep and stay asleep in your bed, even when you are not there. Your smell and the knowledge that you will be there when they waken can make sleep much more restful for many young children. Children are young for such a short time, and nothing will be gained by pushing them toward independence too quickly. Let their needs dictate the way you choose to do things.

The answer is to set up routines and arrangements that benefit your child and your own lifestyle. If you don't feel comfortable, ask yourself why. Ultimately, we all want what is best for our children and if this makes a difference to emotional health, go for it.

babies simply cannot settle without something in their mouths. Research from the Netherlands also shows that they can prevent SIDS (cot/crib death) in susceptible children, probably because they stimulate the child to suck throughout the night.

In the early months, your baby may lose her pacifier in the bed and call you to replace it. This will obviously disrupt parental sleep, but the process of finding the pacifier can be much shorter than breastfeeding or preparing a bottle in the middle of the night, particularly if your child simply wants something to suck. By six months, most babies can find their pacifier themselves, and it's a good idea to leave a few in the bed. Other babies will use their fingers or thumbs for comfort. Try not to discourage these activities in young children—they are an instinctive form of self-comfort and show that they are learning to look after themselves.

Naps

Paradoxically, regular naps will help to encourage good nighttime sleep habits by ensuring that your child doesn't become overtired and unable to settle, and by making falling asleep a routine part of life. Your baby or child will be much more likely to accept bedtime, and missing household activity, if she is used to it. Furthermore, babies and young children do need a great deal of sleep and it is unlikely that they will get enough in the nighttime hours alone. Regular sleep establishes a good sleep/wake cycle that will ensure their needs are met. To help your baby fall asleep at a reasonable hour, don't let him nap past 3 or 4 P.M. Ideally (although not always possible), try to ensure that at least four hours elapse between the end of an afternoon nap and bedtime. Make nap times a part of a daily routine, and your child will soon learn to know what to expect and will feel comforted by the regular routine.

Bedtimes

Most babies should be asleep between 7 and 8:30 P.M. Any later, and they'll become overtired and find it difficult to fall asleep. Many babies and toddlers do not seem tired late at night and, like some adults, get a second wind, appearing hyperactive and full of energy. This is, however, a clear indication that your child is overtired and needs to be settled. Most parents find that settling babies before 8:30 P.M. can make a big difference. In fact, if you have a baby or toddler who finds it difficult to get to sleep, try bringing the bedtime forward by a half-hour. It sounds ludicrously simple, but it works in the large majority of cases.

Signs of sleepiness

It can be difficult to assess when a child is ready for bed, and it's important to learn to recognize signs of sleepiness. In young babies, pulling ears, crying, rubbing eyes or even developing dark circles around the eyes are an indication that they need some sleep. Try to act quickly when you see these signs. If you wait it out, they'll be much less likely to settle. Older children may become tearful, overenergetic and demanding when they need some rest. They may not seem remotely tired, but a burst of energy signals that sleep is required, and you should head into the bedtime routine as quickly as possible.

Waking your child

Some children do need to be wakened in the morning. Although it might be tempting to let them sleep, and to assume they need more, most children will benefit from being on a regular schedule of nighttime and naptime sleep. Interestingly, the human body actually runs on a 25- not a 24-hour-clock, and without the regularity of meals and other activities during the day, we would naturally fall into the habit of going to bed and sleeping an hour later the following morning. It's not surprising that babies and young children follow their body clocks more than adults, whose days are more regimented, and you may need to wake your child to keep him on the right schedule. A child who is ill or recovering from illness may need longer sleeps, but try to punctuate them throughout the day rather than letting one sleep run on for too long.

Learning the difference between night and day

This isn't a problem that affects only babies. After periods of illness or bad nights, many older children and even adolescents can find themselves sleeping for long periods in the day and feeling alert and unable to sleep at night.

▶ For babies:

Babies can be born off kilter, and you may notice that your unborn baby has periods of activity at night, which is a sure sign that you have a night owl on your hands. When your baby is first born, go with his routine for the first little while until he has established good feeding habits. Then:

- Keep the blinds open while he sleeps in the day. Settle him down for naps at regular intervals and even if he doesn't sleep, make it clear that it's time for a rest. Wake him up after a maximum of two hours.

- If he falls asleep feeding, gently wake him and spend some time talking to and playing with him.

- Keep household activities as noisy as possible during the day, so he becomes used to the idea that it's normal to be awake during these hours.

- Invite friends and other children around to play, and ask them to hold and play with your baby as often as possible.

- Keep his chair or crib in a busy area, where he can see and hear everything going on.

- Set up a good pre-bed routine and stick to it, whether he seems ready to sleep or not.

- Put him to bed at a reasonable time, even if he's not obviously tired. Close the blinds and shut his door. Come back if he calls, but don't be tempted to play or get him back up again. Rock him if necessary and speak in a quiet voice.

- When he wakens in the night, feed, change and comfort him, but keep the lights low and talk to him quietly. Once again, return if he needs you, but don't offer any fun!

- Wake him in the morning at a reasonable hour and keep things as routine as possible throughout the day. He'll soon learn that daytime is for fun and nighttime is just plain boring!

▶ *For an older child:*

- Put a fairly rigid routine in place, and stick with it. As boring as it may seem, try to keep things even and organized, with the same activities and meals taking place at the same time every day, at least until things settle down.

- Don't let her fall asleep in the car! Hum, sing, nudge, chat—anything you have to do to keep her awake.

- If she is very tired and still has naps, settle her down at the normal time, but wake her after an hour or so. Be prepared for some irritability!

- Settle her down early to bed: 7:30 is an appropriate bedtime for most children. In fact, one study showed that 8 P.M. is the latest that any child under the age of 14 should be heading off to sleep. Weekends may be the exception, but there is mounting evidence that children are getting less sleep than they need, and an early bedtime is one of the only ways to ensure that they get it.

- If she doesn't fall asleep naturally, read a story or give her a book to look at. Put on a story tape or some gentle music. Make sure that she knows you mean business! If you allow her to climb out of bed, you'll never instill good sleeping habits. Some children are natural owls (see page 130), but they will eventually settle down at a reasonable time if you are persistent.

- If necessary, you might need to sit in her bedroom to ensure that she stays put. Bring a book and don't be tempted to engage in conversation. Many children become more relaxed in the evenings and ready to talk about any problems or concerns—or even simply about their school day. You do want to encourage this type of communication, which is why it's important to introduce a period of quiet chatting into a good bedtime routine. However, some children learn that they can get and keep your attention by bringing up concerns and will do everything they can to engage you in conversation simply to stay up later. Beware of this ploy! Spend lots of time chatting and make sure your child knows that you are available to hear anything she has to say—but not at lights-out time! Obviously, if your child suddenly wants to talk about something serious that has not been previously divulged, you'll have to bend your rules. But stay calm, open and positive, and let her know you will discuss it more fully in the morning.

- Introduce a star chart for children who stay in their beds. Offer plenty of praise when they go to sleep at a reasonable time.

- Wake her up in the morning at the normal time. She may be tired, groggy or irritable, but it will help to establish the right kinds of patterns.

- See below for other ideas about how to deal with children who can't or won't get to sleep.

When sleep becomes a problem

There's no doubt that many children have sleep problems, whether they are caused by a poor bedtime routine, late bedtimes, nightmares, inactivity during the day or even a food allergy. These are not considered clinical sleep disorders, which we'll look at in chapter 11. Most problems can be addressed by putting a good routine in place, and by setting up a series of activities that encourage good, restful sleep. Here are some of the most common problems.

Refusing to go to bed

Most children clue in to the fact that the fun doesn't stop when they go to bed, and they may be reluctant to miss out on anything, particularly if they have older siblings who are permitted to stay up later. As tempting as it is to cave in and allow them some extra time, you won't, in the long run, be doing them any favors. Consider these ideas:

- If you don't already have one, put a bedtime routine into action and stick with it. Bedtime routines should always be pleasurable and as unrushed as possible, and if your child enjoys the winding-down period, he is less likely to feel that he is missing out on the action.

- Offer choices so that your child feels in control: let him choose his pajamas, a cup for his water, a story and even time of bedtime (within an agreed period of time).

Offer incentives, such as two stories or a quiet game of cards or a puzzle with a parent, if he comes when you want him to.

- Show him the clock and put him in charge of remembering when it's time to go up. Given a little responsibility, children normally rise to the occasion and are scrupulously honest.

- Set up a star chart. If he goes to bed without a fuss, he gets a star. If he stays in bed, he gets two. You can agree on an appropriate reward for a full chart.

- Use the choices and consequences technique (see page 183) to encourage your child to get to bed on time. For example, "If you come now we'll have time for a long chat and a story, but if you make a fuss there'll be no time for fun and I'll be cross." Children will respond when they are empowered and you can guess which option they'll choose.

- Make sure there isn't any real reason why he doesn't want to go to bed. Is he having nightmares? Is he genuinely afraid of something? Try to spend some time talking to your child each night to allay any fears. Promise to come back into the room in five minutes to check on him, and make sure that you do. Ensure that he feels confident that you will come if he needs you.

- Practice some advance planning to counter any delaying tactics. The usual ones are another story, another glass of water, a trip to the bathroom, another kiss goodnight, a hug . . . you name it. If your child knows the routine, he's gone to the bathroom, chosen his own story or stories and has a drink by his bedside, he'll be less likely to find a reason to get you back. If he's toilet training, you'll have to agree to bathroom trips, but make it clear that you are not falling for a planned escape. If he claims to be hungry, make a small snack a part of the bedtime routine.

- Make his bedroom a sanctuary, with cozy blankets and a familiar cuddly toy. Tuck him in and make sure that he is comfortable and content. Stay with him for a few minutes so that he doesn't feel that he is being "sent away."

- Wind down well before you want him to go to bed. If he is in the middle of watching a television program, or playing a game with a family member, he's not going to leap at the idea of leaving it all. Make sure that the television is off, and that all fun has ceased at least 20 minutes before you want to have him in bed.

- Make it clear that the rest of the family is not up to wildly fun activities while he goes to bed. Explain that you'll be eating dinner, ironing, helping another child with homework, or just reading. If he knows that there isn't anything exciting at hand, he'll feel happier about being on his own, perhaps with a good story tape or a book to read.

- Above all, be firm and consistent. If you give in once, you'll be setting the stage for recurrent battles. While it's never a good idea to show anger at bedtime, which may cause your child to have a troubled sleep, you can make it clear that you don't find his actions remotely amusing—without losing your temper.

- Praise, praise, praise. When he goes to bed when you ask, make a big fuss and show him how happy and proud you are. When he argues or refuses to go to bed, ignore the behavior that you don't want to encourage. Go through the normal bedtime routine, but don't be tempted to battle or argue, which only provides the attention that he might be seeking.

Daisy

From the very earliest days of her life, Daisy liked comfort. She was unhappy if she was left on her own, and night wakings became increasingly commonplace. She needed to suckle or to be rocked in order to settle, and, most importantly, she wanted to be held. Daisy's mother had had a long labor, and although Daisy had not been in distress, she had clearly been through a fairly traumatic experience. After several months of disrupted nights, Daisy visited a cranial osteopath, who gently manipulated the bones of her skull. He believed that the long labor had caused pressure to build up, which could be partly responsible for her poor sleeping habits.

The difference was dramatic. The first day, she slept on her own without being held, and at night she wakened less frequently for feeds. She still wanted the comfort of her parents when she wakened, so they decided to take her into their bed at night. From that point on, they had no problems. She woke for feeds, but otherwise slept through the nights. Her parents were slightly concerned about how it would affect their sexual relationship, but they've learned to be more imaginative when it comes to location and they reserve the bed for sleeping instead.

Can't fall asleep?

If your child will go to bed, but can't seem to get to sleep, you'll have to adopt a different approach:

- Is your child genuinely tired? All children need sleep, but they may not be physically tired enough to get to sleep. Make sure that he is waking early enough, getting enough exercise in the day and that nap times are not pushing bedtime further on.

- Consider the fact that he may be overtired. Extreme activity in the evenings is a good sign that he's past it, and he will, under those circumstances, find it more difficult to get to sleep. Move his bedtime forward by a half-hour, and make sure the bedtime routine is soothing.

- Add a few drops of lavender oil to his nighttime bath. This will help him to relax naturally, and will be calming, particularly if he is overtired. A drop on a hanky, tied to the bed or crib post will have the same effect.

- Offer a warm drink—milk or chamomile tea—as part of the bedtime routine to soothe and relax.

- Don't be tempted to allow him to leave his bedroom. If he is a child who genuinely needs less sleep, he still needs to learn how to fall asleep himself and to keep himself occupied quietly in his bed. Offer a selection of books to look at, or put on a story tape. Make it clear, however, that bedtime is time for sleep and not play. He should learn to stay in his bed, without playthings, and he will soon learn to fall asleep on his own.

- If he's a big television watcher, make sure the television is off at least an hour before bedtime. Research indicates that increased TV viewing at bedtime is associated with sleep disturbance, especially where children have TVs in their bedrooms.

- Again, make sure that nothing is worrying him. If he's under stress for any reason, he may not be relaxed enough to get to sleep. Children are not different from adults in this respect, and their minds may be swimming with unwanted thoughts when it's time to switch off. Try to take time to talk things through as part of a routine, and keep it calm and positive. Work out strategies to make things easier and let your child know that you are on his side. If you can ease his mind in any respect, he'll feel that his burden is shared and he'll be more likely to relax into sleep. See page 386 for ideas on coping with childhood stress.

- Babies and very young children may just want the comfort of you and your voice. While it's not a good idea to remain with a child every night until he falls asleep, as this can set up habits that are difficult to break, it is useful to reassure your child or baby that you are close by. Let her hear you moving around in the hall outside the room, and come in every five minutes or so to smile and give a reassuring pat. Don't be tempted to get her out of bed, no matter how heartbreaking it might be, and try not to lose your temper. Remain calm and consistent and your child will soon get the message that you are there when she needs you.

Night waking

All humans wake in the night as part of a natural sleep cycle. Most of us go back to sleep without even being conscious of waking. But some children and even adults find it difficult to go back to sleep and will need encouragement to do so. Babies who had colic, or who breathe through their mouths and snore, are more likely to waken at night. Similarly, at around eight months, separation anxiety sets in, and you may

Crying to sleep?

Many childcare experts recommend leaving your baby or child to cry it out. There are many variations on this theme, and some advice is better than others. Several studies show that leaving a child to cry (systematic ignoring) reduces night waking by up to 30 percent in two to three weeks. For parents of poor sleepers, this may appear to be the ideal answer to the problem.

The main message, however, is faulty. No child will benefit from being left to cry. She may eventually fall asleep, out of misery and exhaustion, and will believe that she is unworthy of your attention. No matter how disrupted her sleeping patterns, a child will not feel secure or sleep well if she is left on her own. This is particularly relevant for babies, whose only form of communication is crying. If you fail to respond, she will learn not to cry for attention, but you will have broken a key channel of communication. Not surprisingly, many children who have been left to their own resources at night in this manner are enormously attention-seeking during the day. They need constant reassurance that they are important. There is little point in working to raise your child's self-esteem all day, only to undo it by leaving her bereft in the evenings.

Every parent needs to focus on the child, not the parent's own lack of sleep. Rather than "teaching" behavior without considering the emotional ramifications, it is a much better option to nurture a child's happiness and self-esteem, which will make her confident enough to be independent—to go to sleep on her own, and to fall asleep again when she wakens. You certainly can teach a child to go to sleep by ignoring her, but she learns through negative behavior and by feeling that she is somehow inadequate. This is not a message that any caring parent wants to give.

The answer is to find a middle ground. Many children cry because they know that it upsets you and gets instant attention. What you need to do is to acknowledge their upset, but be firm and consistent in dealing with nighttime crying. Come when they call you, stand over the crib or bed, and offer plenty of reassurance and comfort. Don't pick them up or try to ease the situation by playing or reading another story. Make it clear that you are concerned about their unhappiness, and let them know that you will come when they call. They will eventually learn that you mean business at bedtime, and that tears will not persuade you otherwise. If they start to cry when you leave, go back in and say "good night" again. Stay for a few minutes, and then leave as before. Call out to them from elsewhere in the house and return as required, but don't be tempted to pick them up. Sing a song, fold laundry in the bedroom. Be positive and friendly, but keep it low-key. Don't make your child feel guilty for not wanting to sleep on her own. It is natural for children to want to sleep with someone else there, and they need consistent love and attention to ensure that they don't begin to associate sleep with abandonment.

find that your good sleeper suddenly demands your constant presence. Childhood is a period of enormous development, so don't be surprised if your child suddenly starts waking at night during periods when big milestones have been met. For example, if your child has recently learned to walk, roll, crawl or even talk, he might waken in the night, remember his newest achievement and want to try it out again. He may be overstimulated by the excitement of the day, and find it difficult to settle and to stay asleep. Try to be patient during these periods, which will happen frequently throughout childhood. At these times, it's all the more important to implement good winding-down routine. Remember to praise your child for sleeping, as well as for achievements throughout the day. If he feels good about himself at bedtime, he'll be more likely to sleep.

Don't be tempted to let your child cry it out when he wakens (see page 134), which will lead to feelings of abandonment and even panic. What you want to do is to ensure that your child feels confident and happy enough to settle himself back into sleep. In the early days babies cry because they are hungry, uncomfortable, cold or even just lonely. It's easy to see that a baby who has spent most of the day with an adult, being carried, fed, changed and played with, will find it difficult to be on his own. In some cases a "family bed" may be the answer (see page 126). If that isn't an option for you, you'll need to find other ways to provide the necessary reassurance:

- Providing a comfort object, such as a favorite blanket or cuddly toy, can help. Many children just want the reassurance of the familiar when they waken in the dark.

- Babies often jerk themselves awake (a natural reflex), and you can avoid this by swaddling them tightly in a receiving blanket at bedtime. It can be very frightening for a young baby to find himself in an open space, when he is used to the tight confines of the womb, and certainly many children benefit from swaddling in the early days, to make them feel more secure.

- Try placing one of your T-shirts or your pajamas near your child's face. If he wakes and can smell you, he may not feel so frightened or concerned by your absence.

- Older babies who can sleep through the night without a feed shouldn't suddenly need one, and it can set up unhealthy sleep habits if you suddenly introduce a nighttime bottle to comfort a crying baby. Your child will learn to associate drinking or suckling with going to sleep and will not be able to do it by himself without the aid of his bottle. If your child needs a drink in the night now, change to water and keep a beaker or bottle where he can reach it, beside his crib or bed. He may be irate that his warm comforting drink has been changed, but he'll soon realize that it's not worth waking for cold water unless he is very thirsty.

- Don't take your child out of his bed or crib unless he is very distressed. He'll need the comfort of knowing that you are there, but he will not benefit from learning that crying fits will get him attention. Praise your child when he lies down on his own, and encourage all of his good sleep habits. Make a point of mentioning how well he did to family members the next day. Children who live with encouragement learn confidence and when they waken at night, they will think proudly that they can get to sleep again, particularly if there's the bonus of all that familial praise the following day.

- Some children seem determined to cry unless they have a particular parent there to comfort them. This can be a difficult situation, and you can end up feeling

Tips for tired parents

It's difficult to be patient and comforting when you are at the end of your tether, no matter how much you love your child. Sleep deprivation can lead to irritability, mood swings, tearfulness and a feeling of being unable to cope. To get through difficult periods, it is essential that you take time to focus on yourself and your own needs. Some of the following tips may help:

- Try having your baby in your bed with you. If you are breastfeeding, you will soon be able to feed him without really waking. Babies who sleep in their parents' bed often wake much less than other babies as they get older, and it may help him to feel secure.

- Go to sleep early yourself, after your baby's early-evening feed—if you wait for the last feed and he doesn't waken until later, you have wasted valuable time. You might even want to wake your baby before you plan to go to sleep, and feed him then, in the hopes that you might get at least a few hours of unbroken sleep at the beginning of the night.

- Feed your baby as soon as he wakens, so that he doesn't fret and wake up completely. He certainly may cry himself back to sleep, but if he was hungry, he will only waken again, and disrupt you once more.

- Find ways for both partners to help. Express some milk, if you are breastfeeding, so a middle-of-the-night feed can be undertaken by your partner. Have a bottle ready in the refrigerator for just that purpose. Try to take turns with the waking, so that at least one of you has a good night's sleep.

- Don't be tempted to get up and have a drink or eat after you have settled your baby. Get in the habit of going right back to bed, and perhaps read a little or have a warm (not hot) bath if you are finding it difficult to get back to sleep.

- It may help to move your baby's bed out of your bedroom, if he is sleeping with you—particularly if you are a light sleeper and are disturbed by snuffling and his movements in the crib.

- During difficult periods, ask a friend or relative to watch your baby for an hour or so in the afternoons and take a nap. A 20-minute nap is the ideal length of time and can leave you feeling refreshed and calm. Better still, sleep when your baby sleeps. Don't worry about the housework—it will still be there when you waken.

- Make sure you have some "me" time. Having a cup of tea and reading a book or the newspaper while your baby is napping can help you to relax.

- Working parents find broken nights increasingly untenable, without the option of a mid-afternoon nap. If you fall into this category, you might want to investigate the possibility of taking a catnap (or power nap) at lunchtime. Or try going for a walk in your break. This can go a long way toward reducing tension and boosting energy levels.

- Get some support. If you can't work through the problems within two weeks, you might need some specialist help from your doctor or a local sleep clinic. Just talking things through with friends or other parents can also make you feel better.

- Remember that almost all sleep problems are short-lived, and if you can stay calm and in control during bad times, you will be much more likely to get your child through things easily. If you are kind to yourself, it'll be much easier to cope.

exhausted and tied to your child, and guilty when you have to be unavailable. From the earliest days, ensure that both parents or even other family members play a role in settling a child back to sleep. Get a babysitter in early on, and make sure she is aware of your tactics. Every child needs to learn to settle by himself in different situations, and keeping some variety teaches them to do so. If this problem already exists, try coming in with your partner several times, or with an older child.

Adolescents and sleep

Adolescent sleep has become a topic of great concern, spawning a number of conferences worldwide to address the problem. As a group, adolescents appear to be among the most sleep-deprived in our society. Why does it matter? Sleep deprivation can impair memory and inhibit creativity, making it difficult for sleep-deprived students to learn. Teens struggle to learn to deal with stress and control emotion, and sleep deprivation makes it even more difficult. Irritability, lack of self-confidence and mood swings are often common in a teen, but sleep deprivation makes them worse. Depression can result from chronic sleep deprivation. Not enough sleep can endanger adolescents' immune systems and make them more susceptible to serious illnesses. Judgment can also be impaired, and given that many teens are for the first time being given freedom to make their own decisions, and to drive cars and bikes on the roads, this can pose a serious safety risk. Adolescents are involved in some 55 percent of traffic accidents, and most appear to happen when they are on their own, at night. Experts believe that drowsiness and inadequate sleep is at the root of the problem.

New research indicates that teenagers appear to run on a different circadian clock than children and adults. In a nutshell, puberty appears to cause a change in the mechanisms that trigger when the adolescent needs to go to sleep and to arise. Forcing the adolescent to get up early does not seem to alter the cycle. The result is that the adolescent who is "out of sync" becomes sleepy and moody.

▶ *Top tips for sleep-deprived adolescents*

- Keep an eye on your child's activity levels. If she's playing sports every day after school, practicing an instrument, has a part-time job and takes part in too many activities or clubs, you may need to encourage her to drop something. Many adolescents enjoy being busy, but if it's disrupting sleep, you'll need to make changes. Stick to a reasonable schedule that allows time for homework, fun and adequate rest.

- Make sure your adolescent is part of the family routine—eating regularly, enjoying some free time and going to bed at an appropriate time. If his bedtime is running later and later, strike up a deal and let him choose a more appropriate bedtime.

Explain the importance of sleep for good academic and sports performance, and if he's struggling with moodiness you can mention the idea that sleep has now been linked with mood swings. Reward his efforts.

- How early does your child start school? Some schools have begun opening earlier for adolescent classes, and this has been identified as one of the main problems with the sleeping habits of today's youth. If an adolescent gets less than about 6.5 hours of sleep, she will be 50 percent more likely to doze off or suffer lapses of concentration during morning classes. In other words, she won't be learning anything. Talk to your child's principal about reasonable start times.

- Keep an eye on his diet. If he's drinking coffee or a lot of cola in the evenings, his sleep will be disrupted and he'll find it difficult to get to sleep. These should be avoided from noon, if possible. Point out to your child that alcohol can also disrupt sleep.

- Intense studying or computer games before bed can be stimulating.

- Avoid arguing with your adolescent just before bedtime, which can make her feel stressed, under pressure and less able to sleep.

- Keep the television and the lights off when sleeping, and open the blinds as soon as the morning alarm goes off. This can help to create a more acceptable sleep/wake cycle.

- Limit weekend sleep-ins to no more than two or three hours later than the usual waking time, or the body clock will be disrupted.

Adolescent sleep facts

- In a survey of over 3,000 U.S. high school students, 85 percent got inadequate sleep, with 26 percent sleeping less than 6.6 hours. As a result, some students were found to nod off in ten-second microsleeps, missing important facts during lectures.[1]

- In a U.S. study, students achieving A's and B's went to bed earlier on both weeknights and weekends than those with D's and F's. High achievers averaged about 35 minutes more sleep per day than low achievers.[2]

- Ninety-nine University of Arizona students who reported high daytime sleepiness and irregular sleeping schedules were asked to limit their sleep to 7.5 hours per night for a four-week period, and were randomly assigned either to continue to sleep as they had been or to observe a regular sleep schedule. Students who regularized their sleep reported that they became more alert in the daytime, fell asleep faster and slept more soundly.

- Research by the University of Pennsylvania's Division of Sleep and Chronobiology suggests that teens who stay up very late on Friday and Saturday nights are noticeably more sleepy during the week even if they go to bed at a more reasonable hour during the week.

- A broadscale study in the U.S. showed that irregular sleep scheduling can be as damaging as sleep deprivation. In girls it related to more days off sick from school; in boys, more serious injuries were reported. Those who slept longer on weekends and less during the week reported more weekday sleepiness.

Be positive!

As dreadful as it seems at the time, few sleep problems last more than a couple of months, and being patient and understanding will help you to provide the emotional support your child needs to become secure enough to develop good, healthy sleep habits and to sleep well throughout the night. Short-term dramatic measures rarely work. You may upset your child and damage his confidence, making sleep an "issue" that goes on to haunt him—and you—in years to come. Working through difficult periods calmly will set up good sleep hygiene habits that will be with him for life. Sleep is a natural part of living, and all happy, healthy children will benefit from restful sleep that leaves them balanced and full of energy.

chapter seven

A Natural Environment

Everything your child eats, drinks and breathes contributes to her overall health. As important, however, is your child's home environment—the atmosphere in which she grows and is nurtured into adulthood. Your child's environment can affect her physical and emotional health. It can also affect something much deeper than that—her spirit. In chapter 8 we'll go into detail about the concept of spirit, but for the purposes of this chapter it is important to understand the idea that we are all made of and surrounded by energy. The energy in your home can affect your child's own energy patterns, which can make a big difference to her overall health.

There are many things you can do to make your child's environment positive and healthy, from choosing household chemicals that have the least impact on your child's body to ensuring that the atmosphere is conducive to happiness and well-being. Let's start at the beginning.

A toxic world

Our natural environment is a place corrupted by pollution, chemicals, drugs, processed foods and a buzzing, demanding energy that keeps us on the run from morning to night. The human body has an amazing capacity to adjust and evolve according to the pressures placed upon it, but the world has undoubtedly changed faster than our ability to adapt, and even the strongest among us succumb to the pressures of our environment.

Apart from joining the green movement, which works toward making the world a safer, healthier place to live, there is little we can do to change what lies beyond our doors. We can recycle, choose products that do not harm the environment, walk instead of drive, and invest in companies that have ethical policies, but until this movement becomes a way of life, we can have little control over our world. Take part in the movement for change—we all have a stake in making the world a better place for our children both now and in the future. We can't undo the advances of technology, but we can ensure that they do as little damage as possible to the world around us.

Even more importantly, however, we can make our homes places in which the effects of the outside world can be balanced. We can create a healthy nurturing environment where our children can recover and become strong.

One of the most important elements to consider is the idea of toxic overload. The body is designed to cope with a certain number of toxins—those naturally occurring in foods, for example. Toxins are either neutralized, transformed or eliminated by our bodies. The liver helps to transform toxic substances into harmless ones; the intestines break down protein, carbohydrates and fats, while the kidneys filter waste from the bloodstream. We also eliminate toxins through our skin, when we sweat, and our lymphatic system clears debris from our blood. The immune system is also involved—fighting off bacteria and other invaders.

If our children have a healthy diet, rich in fresh fruits, vegetables and whole foods, the detoxification process will be working at a good level. However, too much junk food, pollution and everyday stress can mean that the process is impaired. What happens is a condition called "toxic overload," where we have taken in more toxins than we can get rid of. Uneliminated toxins are stored in the tissues, and they can harm overall health on a daily basis, and sow the seeds of future illness.

And it isn't just diet involved here. Every chemical to which your child comes in contact has to be dealt with—or "detoxified"—by the body. If your child uses medication to control eczema, or asthma, for example, those medications place a strain on the body. When your child walks to school, or sits in a stroller on the way to the store, he breathes in carbon monoxide that poisons his body. Scented shampoos and soaps, cleaning products, perfumes, radiation from televisions, computers, cell phones, electricity masts, pollution, smoke and even ordinary household dirt and dust are dealt with by your child's body on a daily basis.

Don't get me wrong. The body is set up to do just that—to protect itself from toxins that can harm it. What happens, however, is that as more and more demands are placed on your child's body, an increasing amount of energy is required to deal with them. This is the same energy required for other body functions, such as breathing, digestion, fighting off infection, thinking, moving, developing and growing. These processes are necessary for life, and our children's bodies are simply not designed to cope with the stresses placed upon them. Toxins build up, and body systems work ineffectively. This is one of the most common causes of low-grade niggling disease on a daily basis (insomnia, fatigue, irritability, headaches, digestive disorders, skin problems, poor concentration and susceptibility to common ailments, for example), and in the long term it can be responsible for broadscale immune system failure and a host of debilitating diseases.

What's the answer? There are two steps to take. First and foremost, you want to make your children's home environment as toxin-free as possible, to ease the stress on their bodies. Secondly, you can work to detox your children on a regular basis, to ensure that toxins causing illness do not build up, ensuring that they can deal more effectively with the pressures of the world around them.

Zap your house

Many parents who have children with allergies will understand the concept of an allergen-free home—which involves taking steps to remove substances that can trigger allergies in susceptible children. What you may not know is that all children will benefit from this approach, whether they suffer from obvious allergies or not. Anything that triggers allergies in susceptible children also puts strain on the bodies of healthy children. They may not suffer from allergies, but these substances still need to be dealt with by their bodies, requiring energy that could be better used in the context of overall health.

Cut the chemicals

Consider the products you are using in your home. A new report entitled "Multiple Chemical Sensitivity Recognition" was recently published by the British Society for Allergy, Environmental and Nutritional Medicine. The report urges the government to tighten the regulation of chemical use, including stricter controls on the authorization of new chemicals, and the removal of persistent chemicals from food. The authors found that exposure to chemicals can not only cause allergies and fatigue in susceptible people but also lead to a condition called "multiple chemical sensitivity," which means developing a severe allergy to chemicals in everyday products. Allergies are still not fully understood, but we do know that they represent a profound breakdown in the immune response, which recognizes ordinary foods and other substances as invaders. Given that so many of our children are now immunized (see page 213), which can dramatically affect the immune response, and taking into consideration the number of chemicals used in everyday life, these allergies—some of which can be completely debilitating—are likely to become more common, and more dangerous.

What can you do?

- Solvent-based paints, varnishes, cleaning fluids and sprays, glues and chemical treatments all have the potential to cause a reaction in children's sensitive skin or airways, and they need to be dealt with by the body whenever there is contact. Avoid solvents wherever possible.

- Buy emulsion-free paints and other home-improvement products from specialist suppliers (see page 440).

- Throw out most of your cleaning products. Use only environmentally friendly products, which use the least noxious chemicals and pose the least threat to your child's health. What can you use instead? Good old-fashioned soap and water, or washing soda and water, are your best bet. We have been misled into believing that we need special antibacterial products in order to make our houses clean enough, but this is a fallacy (see page 149) and can actually do more harm than good. If you have young children and are concerned about contact with too many bugs, use plain bleach instead. Clean windows with vinegar and water; wash your kitchen floor with lemon essential oil, fresh lemon juice, soap and water; use an environmentally friendly, nonbiological soap powder for your clothes; and clean the bath with tea tree oil mixed with soap to naturally fight fungi, viruses and bacteria.

- The healthiest carpets are hessian-backed and not treated with pesticides (such as permethrin or mitin FF), which can give off a vapor and soak through to the surface, affecting your children's skin (and health!).

- Many dish detergents are biodegradable. Choose a brand that is naturally scented (or unscented) and use it in place of most household detergents. If you are concerned about bacteria, use a drop or two of essential oils, such as lemon, tea tree and lavender, in the bowl.

- Polish furniture with beeswax and a little lemon essential oil.

- Freshen your air with a drop of peppermint, lavender, lemon—or indeed any other—essential oil in a sprayer full of water.

- Clean your oven with stainless steel wool and bicarbonate of soda (and hot water!). It is effective and will not cause irritation.

- Naturally bleach white clothes in the sunlight, or add washing soda to your wash. Bicarbonate of soda (baking soda) can remove many stains, as can soap and water and a little elbow grease. A mild bleach solution is not dangerous occasionally, but put your clothes through another wash cycle before your child wears them.

- What about personal hygiene? Soap and water are the best options, although young children do not need anything more than water, with a drop of a gentle essential oil, such as lavender. Use a little olive oil if you want to soften your child's skin. Choose a mild, unscented shampoo and conditioner (again, environmentally friendly, or one of the new organic products is best) or make your own.

- Choose moisturizers that are natural and have not been tested on animals. Don't buy brightly colored, heavily scented products. You can buy a number of gentle products for babies or, again, make your own. For example, you can add two or three drops of essential oils or flower essences to about six tablespoons of cream or lotion. Smoothed into the skin, these creams will moisturize and heal, according to the herbs, essences or oils you have chosen. If an ointment is required, boil 2 cups (450 ml) of pure olive oil and 2 oz (50 g) of beeswax for a few minutes over low heat. If you are using dried herbs (chamomile or hypericum, for example), add a handful of finely chopped and pounded herbs to the solution before boiling. Press through a muslin bag to remove any traces of herbs, and pour into heat-sterilized jars, where the ointment will solidify. If you want to use an essential oil or a flower essence, add it just after taking the oil off the heat.

- Choose a natural toothpaste flavored with lemon, mint or fennel. These are widely available, and will keep your children's teeth and gums clean and healthy without the risk of fluoride (see page 148), artificial sweeteners (in toothpaste, yes!), flavorings and other chemicals designed to make them more tempting.

- Pests in the house? Don't be tempted to use highly toxic bug sprays. Many essential oils, including tea tree oil, lavender oil, lemongrass and rosemary act as natural insecticides. Add three drops of each to about 18 fl oz (500 ml) of water and use as required. Use tansy to repel ants, or use dried mint, chili powder or borax to kill them. Products containing chlordane are dangerous, as this chemical is a suspected carcinogen. Many insects (including cockroaches, moths and rodents) dislike sage. Tie garden or wild sage in bunches and hang around the house, or on the porch. To prevent moths, grind together: 2 tbsp (15 ml) each cloves, caraway seeds, nutmeg, mace and cinnamon. Add and mix in 12 tbsp (180 ml) orris root powder. Place in cotton or muslin bags in cupboards, drawers and trunks. For mice or rats, place several drops of peppermint oil on a cloth and wash around doors and windows, and cracks in the foundation of your home. If you know you have mice, soak a cloth in peppermint oil and leave it near their nest. They'll soon vacate the premises!

- If your cat or dog has fleas, don't be tempted to use pesticide sprays, which are toxic and contain lindane, dichlorvos and carbaryl. If you have no choice, treat your pet outside. Vacuum all carpets and soft furnishings carefully and wash what you can in boiling water. Spray tea tree and eucalyptus oils diluted in water (six drops of each in 14 fl oz (400 ml of water) onto furniture and carpets (test an area first, to ensure it doesn't mark). Use an herbal flea collar on your pet, and shampoo with a mild baby shampoo to which you have added one drop each of mint, eucalyptus and tea tree oil. This will help to repel fleas. If your pet does have fleas, add a drop of each of these oils to some olive oil and comb through your pet's fur with a fine-toothed comb. Crush the fleas or drown them. Wash the oil away with a mild shampoo.

Detox your child

Luckily, children have had much less time than adults to build up a seriously dangerous store of toxins, and a "spring clean" before beginning a healthy eating plan, and once or twice a year thereafter, can make a big difference. Detoxing releases stored poisons and helps to encourage the functioning of a healthy elimination system.

Most people will be surprised to hear that children need to detox. Most children look the picture of health, despite an often unhealthy diet, and it is hard to imagine that there could be anything sinister afoot. In fact, most children do not need the type of full-scale detox that adults do—and it would be dangerous to even attempt to limit their diet to such an extent. Detoxing kids involves a gentle cleansing of the body, to boost energy, aid concentration, improve digestion function and absorption of nutrients, boost a sluggish elimination system and restore life to their cells.

Do my children need to detox?

The answer is almost certainly yes. If you can honestly answer yes to any of the questions below, a detox will benefit your child—even if he is only mildly toxic:

Yes

- Does your child eat junk food of any sort? ☐

- Does your child eat processed foods or refined products, such as white bread and pasta? ☐

- Is your child under any stress (such as exams, parental divorce, changing schools, playing competitive sports)? ☐

- Is your child in contact with cigarette smoke, either at home, at friends' homes or at a carers'? ☐

- Does your child smoke or drink any alcohol? ☐

- Does your child drink carbonated drinks, or any sweetened drinks, apart from pure juice, milk and water? ☐

- Are any of the fruits, vegetables, meat, milk or grains you serve not organic? ☐

- Does your child have asthma or eczema, or suffer from frequent skin rashes or hives? ☐

- Does your child take medication regularly? ☐
- Has your child had antibiotics in the last six months? ☐
- Do you live in an area with high levels of air pollution? ☐
- Is your child overweight? ☐
- Does your child seem tired, but have difficulty sleeping? ☐
- Does your child suffer from frequent constipation? ☐
- Do you live in a city? ☐
- Do you live in the country, near farms that use chemicals of any sort? ☐
- Do you use household cleaning products? ☐
- Does your child use a cell phone, or watch a lot of television? ☐
- Does your child crave sweet foods? ☐
- Does your child suffer from frequent headaches or abdominal upsets? ☐
- Does your child have mood swings linked to blood sugar (after school, before breakfast or after sports, for example)? ☐

The number of "yes" answers indicates how toxic your child will be. More toxic children will experience more symptoms during the detoxification process. These can include mild diarrhea (anything more should be reported to your doctor), headaches, irritability, pimples, smelly breath and fatigue. Don't be alarmed. Symptoms are a healthy sign, indicating that their bodies are eliminating stored toxins.

Caution: This program is safe for all children over the age of four. If your child has a health condition, show the program to your doctor before undertaking any of the recommendations. Children under the age of four will not be harmed by any part of the program, but it is unnecessary to detox before this age.

The plan

- For three days ensure that everything that your child eats is unrefined. That means whole foods that have not been processed in any way. All foods should be fresh and natural. Include whole grains, fruits, vegetables, brown rice, lean meats, dairy products with no added sugars or flavors, legumes, nuts, seeds and plenty of water.

- Children should be given *only* water, organic milk and fresh, diluted juice (preferably freshly squeezed) to drink.

- Candy, chocolate and all processed or refined foods are out.

- Avoid fats apart from a little organic butter and olive oil.

- Follow the food pyramid on page 23 for the appropriate number of servings of each of the main food groups. Make sure your child gets enough of each.

And:

- Before breakfast every day, serve fresh grape juice (white or red) with a squeeze of fresh lemon. If your child doesn't like the juice, she should have a handful of fresh grapes. Grapes help to speed up the metabolism, and cleanse the liver, kidneys and other eliminative organs.

- Make sure your child has at least five of the following fruits or vegetables each day—raw, if possible: pears, grapefruit, apricots, apples, pineapples, melons, papayas, bananas, beets, cabbage, carrots, celery, cucumber, lettuce and fennel. These all help the detoxification process. Avoid tomatoes and spinach while detoxing; they can irritate the digestive tract.

- Every day offer at least one serving of steamed brown rice, served without salt or fat.

- Avoid condiments as much as possible (although a little ketchup, for example, won't harm the detoxification process unduly).

- Make sure your child drinks at least one glass of fresh water before every meal. You should aim for between five and eight glasses each day.

- Add fresh garlic to at least one meal a day. Garlic is an excellent blood cleanser, and it stimulates the digestive organs.

- Give one acidophilus pill between meals. They are now available in vanilla flavor, which is more appealing to children. Acidophilus balances the intestinal flora (natural bacteria) in the gut, which helps to encourage healthy digestion and elimination, and to insure against future toxicity. If you can't find the pills, offer a little fresh, live, plain yogurt. Don't be tempted to sweeten it. If your child finds it unpalatable, mash in a little overripe (black) banana, which will not alter the healthy bacteria levels.

- If your child is hungry throughout the day, offer fruit, unsalted nuts (for children over the age of five), brown rice crackers (with sesame seeds, if possible), raw vegetables, seeds or dried fruits.

Three days is enough for most children; indeed, one is enough for some. If your child is highly toxic, you might want to repeat it once a month for, say, three months. Don't be tempted to do it any more often. All children will benefit from a yearly spring clean—after the holiday season, for example, when they've had too many candies or fatty foods. Some experts recommend undertaking a cleansing program once a month, for one day.

The fluoride debate

If you've been brought up to believe that fluoride in toothpaste and fluoridation of water is the answer to preventing dental caries in children's teeth, you might be surprised to hear that this practice is the subject of much controversy. First and foremost, many parents believe that fluoride should not be forced upon a community. Secondly, there are literally thousands of studies linking fluoride with serious health risks. For example, large amounts of sodium fluoride can result in dental enamel of the teeth mottling (dental fluorosis), as well as causing weakness in tooth structure. This is especially the case in those who are undernourished, which scuppers the argument that poorer families especially need fluoride in water. The most alarming side effect of excess fluoride is a condition called skeletal fluorosis. It is believed that the longer fluoride is taken (particularly if it as at unacceptable levels), the more risk there is of developing this condition. In terms of preventive medicine, it is something all parents should take note of. It's also worth mentioning that symptoms have appeared in the pediatric population, which means that many, many children are getting too much. The symptoms of phase one skeletal fluorosis include sporadic pain and stiffness of joints, with minor osteosclerosis of the pelvis and vertebral column (also symptoms of arthritis, which is increasing in the population as a whole). Phase two is described as chronic joint pain, arthritic symptoms, slight calcification of ligaments, increased osteosclerosis of bones, with or without osteoporosis of the long bones; and phase three, limitation of joint movement, calcification of ligaments in the neck and vertebral column, crippling deformities of the spine and major joints, muscle wasting, and neurological defects with compression of the spinal cord.

What should you do?

- If your drinking water is fluoridated (with an industrial by-product of aluminum and phosphate production), find out to what extent and consider drinking bottled water instead. Fluoride may naturally occur in mineral water, but you can look for brands with lower levels. You can also be comforted that this is naturaliy occurring fluoride from the earth, and not the equivalent of effluence.

- Ditch the fluoride toothpaste. Your child should be getting more than he needs in his diet, and in beverages. If you do go for a fluoride toothpaste, use only a tiny dab, and make sure your child spits and doesn't swallow the foam.

- Don't choose brands that are too appealing to children. Chances are they'll eat the toothpaste, or be tempted to swallow when brushing.

- Never, ever use a fluoride supplement unless advised by a dentist, doctor or natural health practitioner, and even then, ask why.

Supercleaners cause superbugs

You aren't doing your child or the environment any favors if you go on an antibacterial kick. Many households use antibacterial products for everything from washing clothes, dishes, carpets and hands, to putting antibacterial products in the bath and spraying it in the air. There is a certain comfort to be gained from keeping everything germ-free, particularly if you have little ones about.

Don't be fooled. One of the reasons food poisoning has increased so dramatically in recent years is because antibacterial products and antibiotics have been overused in the food chain, and in the processing and packaging industries. The products designed for home use are powerful antibacterial agents, and they wipe out "good" bacteria as well as dangerous bacteria. Good bacteria helps to balance the population of more dangerous bacteria, but it is not as resistant and can be more easily destroyed. On the other hand, the bacteria responsible for illnesses is stronger and constantly mutating. With no healthy bacteria to balance their growth, these bacteria are able to develop a resistance to many of the products we are using in our homes, which makes them stronger and much more dangerous in the long term.

Secondly, some scientists believe that exposure to some infectious agents (bacteria and viruses included) in early childhood may help to prevent the development of allergic reactions, such as asthma and rhinitis, an inflammation of the lining of the nose. This is because the immune system becomes accustomed to dealing with foreign invaders. Without that exposure, the immune system remains weak and vulnerable.

There are many experts who support this view, pointing to the fact that children are cleaned so clinically that their immune systems are never given a chance to develop and mature.

The answer is to ban antibacterial products from your home, except under the following circumstances:

- If one of your children (or you) suffers from a contagious disease such as hepatitis, impetigo or even salmonella, use an antibacterial handwash.

- Take a bottle when you travel abroad to a foreign country. Your children will not have built up immunity to foreign bugs, and this can help to prevent infection.

- Use an antibacterial handwash after visiting a farm where children have petted the animals.

- An antibacterial handwash in the bathroom can help to halt the spread of infection, particularly if your child is new to toilet habits, or if there is a cold or other infection in the house. All children should get into the habit of washing their hands regularly—after a trip to the bathroom and before meals. Good hygiene doesn't mean overzealous scrubbing.

- If you do want some antibacterial action in your home, use natural bactericides, such as essential oils, which do not damage healthy bacteria, and have immune-boosting properties. Tea tree or lavender are good choices. Add four to five drops of each to a full natural liquid soap pump 11 fl oz (about 300 ml).

- The best choice for reducing harmful bacteria in the house is ordinary bleach. It will wipe out populations of bad bacteria, while leaving the good bacteria intact.

- Sterilize a very young baby's bottles and pacifiers, but use soap and water for toys and anything else with which they are in contact. Don't continue sterilizing past the age of about five or six months. Children do need to be in contact with bacteria, viruses and even fungi if they are to develop strong immunity.

Dust and mites

One of the most common allergens in young children is the dust mite. Dust mites are microscopic and they live by eating particles of dead skin that we all shed on a daily basis. The mites are not, however, the big problem—it is their excrement that causes an allergic reaction in some children.

No matter how clean, freshly painted or new your house is, dust mites will be found in carpets, curtains, sofas, beds, cushions, pillows and all soft furnishings. They like warm conditions, so they have become much more common since the advent of central heating and double glazed windows. Your child's bed is a breeding ground—one study showed that the average mattress (a lovely warm and moist place for dust mites to gather) contains in the region of two million mites.

What can you do?

- Throw out as many soft furnishings and carpets as you can (maintaining a certain level of comfort, of course!). Strip wooden floorboards, use blinds instead of curtains, and use wooden furniture for your children.

- Keep soft toys out of your children's bedrooms (apart from one favorite toy), and wash them regularly in very hot water (see below). If they are not washable, put them in the freezer for a few hours to kill any mites.

- Dust your home on a daily basis, using a damp cloth rather than a variety of fancy sprays. You can polish less frequently.

- Keep your home cool and dry by opening windows as often as possible, and keeping the heat down, particularly at night.

- Dry your clothes outside whenever possible, as humidity from the dryer or from clothes drying on radiators can produce the ideal breeding ground for mites.

- Vacuum your floors and soft furnishings as often as possible, but make sure that your vacuum is effective. You'll need a good air filter system, or the dust sucked in will be coughed right back out again. Some of the newer vacuum cleaners with a plastic reusable section replacing a bag claim to be much more effective than the traditional vacuum cleaners, and much more hygienic. Check out their claims before you purchase one.

- Wash all bedding on a weekly basis to kill mites, and wash duvets and pillows once a month. Add a drop of tea tree oil to the rinse water to act as an insecticide. Bedding will need to be washed at temperatures above 131° (55°C) to be effective. If you want to dry clean them, find a "green" dry cleaner who uses fewer toxic chemicals, or simply take the duvets and pillows to a laundrette and tumble dry on the highest setting, with a rag soaked in lavender and tea tree oil to freshen and kill any parasites.

- Cover pillows, mattresses and duvets with allergen-free barrier covers that are now widely available and less expensive than they used to be. If you really can't afford it, double up sheets, pillowcases and duvet covers.

- It was once believed that synthetic duvets and pillows were better than feather, but this has now been refuted. A study showed that levels of cat and dog allergen, both major asthma triggers, were found to be seven and eight times higher respectively in synthetic rather than feather pillows. Earlier research by the same team found that synthetic pillows also contained higher levels of dust mite allergens. Feather pillows were encased in a closely woven fabric, to prevent feathers protruding. This was thought to help keep dust mites and allergens out. The researchers believe a pillow's casing may also be a key factor in reducing allergies and asthma symptoms.

Keep out the damp

Moisture can increase the population of viruses, bacteria and fungi in your home beyond acceptable levels, particularly if your home is centrally heated with little ventilation. All of these critters thrive in a warm, damp environment, so it is important to keep damp at bay. Moisture also breeds mold, and mold spores are allergens.

- Fix leaky roofs, rising damp (which seeps up through the foundations of a house) and leaky pipes.

- Ventilate kitchens and bathrooms, and ensure that your clothes dryer is ventilated outside the house.

- Dry clothes outside if possible, and not on radiators (see above).

- Keep the windows open on dry, sunny days and give the house a good airing.

- Consider investing in a dehumidifier if your house is damp.

Additives in food

Below, we look at some of the various additives in detail (and for more on chemicals in food, see chapter 3).

Labels

Obviously, reading every label of every food we buy would mean spending a day a week in the supermarket, but it's a good idea to read the odd label. You might be surprised by what you find. Many of the foods that we consider healthy simply aren't. They've got so many things added to them that they've become chemical cocktails.

All additives are rigorously tested to ensure that they fall within safety limits. The problem is that children, like all of us, tend to eat a lot of the things they like. A high intake of any particular additive could take children's intake above the acceptable levels. Nor has there been any research into the combinations of chemicals, and while they may be "safe" in small dosages or singly, we don't know what they might do when they are taken together. Finally, we need to ask ourselves what "safe" means. If something can cause illness or death in large doses, is it really all right for our children to have it in moderation? I think the answer is no.

What we need to aim for is a diet that is as free from chemicals as possible. If there are eight ingredients in a batch of homemade chocolate chip cookies and the store-bought brand contains 32, you'll know which one is better for you. Choose foods with the fewest number of ingredients and additives, and you'll be ahead. Choose natural, unrefined foods, and you'll be doing the best you can.

Flavors

Unless the flavor is preceded by the word "natural," it's a chemical, and it's worth avoiding. Natural-identical flavors are not natural. Don't be fooled. Flavors are not normally listed on food products because they would reveal the "secret recipe" of the product.

Emulsifiers

These are used to prevent ingredients from separating (for example, oil and vinegar and even milk). Emulsifiers are, at the moment, considered largely benign, but it's worth watching out for research showing anything to the contrary. Many emulsifiers are synthetic, and may contribute to toxic overload (see page 141).

Stimulants

Many drinks and now some foods contain stimulants, the most common being caffeine. Apart from tea and coffee, caffeine is found in cola drinks, chocolate and even headache pills. Caffeine excites the brain by stimulating the heart and circulation, and by increasing adrenaline levels. It would be difficult to get enough in food or drink to cause death, but stimulants like caffeine are not recommended for children in any quantity. They can cause digestive problems, headaches, anxiety and depression, and they may interfere with crucial stages of development.

Colors

Food manufacturers have backtracked on this one. At one time, all sorts of foods were filled with extra, artificial colors, but these were the first to be implicated in food additives scares, and manufacturers have taken note. You can now find many products without "artificial colors," and you should seek them out.

Some of the colorings that should definitely be avoided for adults and children alike are: Curcumin, Tartrazine, Quinoline Yellow, Yellow 2G, Sunset Yellow, Cochineal, Carmoisine/Azorubine, Amaranth, Ponceau, Erythrosine BS, Red 2G, Patent Blue V, Indigo Carmine, Brilliant Blue FCF, Green S/Lissamine Green/Acid Brilliant Green, Caramel, Black PN, Brilliant Black BN, Carbon Black, Vegetable Carbon, Brown FK, Brown HT/Chocolate Brown HT, Lithol Rubine BK/Pigment Rubine. They cover most colors in the rainbow, and are the most likely to appeal to children.

Stabilizers

These improve the texture of foods. Many are natural, such as lecithin. Again, there is no direct link between stabilizers and ill health, although carageen has been put on the additive hit list by various authorities.

Fillers

These are substances added to products to thicken, absorb water and bulk out the food. These are empty calories with few, if any, nutrients. Avoid them if you can. Fillers include corn starch, rice flour, soy flour, gelatin, pectin, vegetable gums and various types of starch. Are they dangerous? Perhaps. A 1998 study showed that modified starch (which is corn starch that has been chemically treated) caused loose stools in infants. That may not seem significant, but any diarrhea in infants can lead to dehydration fairly quickly, and to loss of nutrients essential for growth.

Preservatives

There's no question that preservatives have a role. Most foods would go off rapidly without them, and potentially deadly diseases such as botulism can be prevented by their (prudent) use. There are, however, some that have been associated with health problems, and worsen symptoms of complaints such as asthma. The preservatives in question include Benzoic acid, Sodium benzoate, Potassium benzoate, Sodium sulfite, Sodium hydrogen sulfite/Sodium bisulfite, Acid sodium sulfite, Sodium metabisulfite/Disodium prosulfite, Calcium hydrogen sulfite/Calcium bisulfite, Biphenyl/Diphenyl, 2-Hdroxy-biphenyl-2-yl-oxide/Sodium orthophenylphenate, Hexamine, Hexamthylenetetramine, Potassium nitrate, Sodium nitrate.

Sweeteners

We discuss sugar as a separate issue (see page 38), but there are other sweeteners apart from sugar. Artificial sweeteners are the number one thing to avoid. You may cut down on calories, and possibly tooth decay, but they are potentially dangerous. Saccharin is linked to cancer in rats, while aspartame (Nutrasweet) has been linked with the growth of malignant brain tumors. Aspartame is 200 times sweeter than sugar, and it is used in many low-calorie and no-calorie drinks, as an additive in foods and as a sweetener for hot drinks such as tea and coffee. Apart from obvious cancer fears, adults have reported dizziness, headaches, epileptic-like seizures and menstrual problems after consuming aspartame. Is aspatame something that you would feel comfortable allowing your child to consume? Researchers from King's College in London are currently investigating the links in a three-year study. That should be enough to put off most parents.

Flavor enhancers

The big one is MSG or E621. Used in a variety of products, including Chinese food, sauces, and a wide range of ready-prepared meals, MSG has been shown to over-excite—even kill—brain cells. Given the potential risks to children, baby manufacturers in the United States, European Union, United Kingdom, Canada, Australia and New Zealand have been forced by law to stop adding it to their products.

Antioxidants

These are not the same thing as the antioxidants we take for health (see page 284). These chemicals prevent damage to the product caused by air. Watch out for Propyl gallate/Propyl 3, 4, 5 trihydroxybenzene, Octyl gallate, Dodecyl gallate, Dodecyl 3, 4, 5, trihydroxybenzene, Butylated hydroxyanisole BHA, Butylated hydroxytoluene BHT. These should not be consumed by children or adults, as there are health risks associated with them.

Vitamins and minerals

Don't be fooled by unhealthy products with added nutrients. Adding vitamins to a carbonated drink does not make it healthy. In fact, the chemicals contained in it far outweigh any benefits that the nutrients might offer.

The verdict

Avoid additives as much as possible. Some are necessary to keep food fresher, but you'll be much better off serving your children fresh, natural foods, both to keep the toxin levels down (see page 40) and to prevent reactions that can cause ill health.

Techno trauma

It's not just chemicals that can have an impact on your child's health. All parents need to be aware of the dangers of too much technology. We'll go into the emotional effects of technological advance in chapter 8. Here, however, we'll examine the physical effects.

Electromagnetic (EM) fields exist in most households, and they are derived from extra-low-frequency AC electrical wiring and appliances. There is increasing controversy about the possible health risks from the radiation in these EM fields. Like everything else, some children and adults are sensitive to their effects, while some are not, but everyone seems to be affected to some degree.

Electrical appliances at the center of the storm include microwave ovens, electric blankets, televisions, computers and cellular phones. New research appears on an almost daily basis refuting or disputing claims that EM radiation causes health problems, so it's an impossible situation to assess with any validity. My feeling is that if there is considered to be any risk, then parents need to be made aware of the situation in order to make choices:

- A number of studies have reported higher childhood leukemia in homes where EM fields were higher than average. Another showed that high appliance use leads to strong EM fields that are associated with an increased risk of cancers in all children.[1]

- Using a VDT screen has been linked to miscarriage and birth defects, and televisions are much the same as VDTs.[2]

- Another study suggests that EM fields may reduce the production of melatonin, a hormone that maintains the normal daily rhythms of the body, including the sleep and wake cycle. Reduced levels of melatonin are associated with depression.[3]

- Cell phones are also the subject of intense controversy, with conflicting studies appearing regularly. A recent study suggests the microwaves generated by cell phones may damage the ability of white blood cells to act as the "police" of the body, fighting off infection and disease. A new study published in May 2000 indicates that cell phone use by children should be discouraged. Sir William Stewart, the scientist behind a recent study into cell phone safety, confirmed that he would stop his own grandchildren using them. Although Sir William's report says there is no current evidence of a health risk to either adults or children, it says children should be discouraged from making "nonessential" calls on cell phones until further research is completed.[4]

- The ten-month Stewart inquiry report recommends a precautionary approach, and claims that the use of cell phones is not totally "without potential adverse health effects." Stewart said, "There's some preliminary evidence, and I emphasize very much preliminary evidence, that emissions from mobile phones may cause in some cases subtle biological changes."[5]

- It is thought children could face more potential health risks from cell phone emissions because their skulls are thinner and their brains are still developing. The reports suggest that children should use cell phones only for essential calls. I suggest that they should not, on the basis of this new research, use them at all.

- A study showed that the rate of death from brain cancer among people who held cell phones to their head was higher than those who used phones away from their head, although an even newer study shows that headsets increased the damage caused by radiation even further. In their relatively short history, cell phones have been blamed for causing all manner of ills, including cancer, headaches, memory loss, high blood pressure and strokes.

Moving away from EM radiation, the overuse of computers can have other health effects. Many studies show that they can disrupt sleep, but on top of that, new evidence is emerging that schoolchildren could fall prey to repetitive strain injury (RSI) caused by the misuse and overuse of computers. The RSI Association, based in London, England, is concerned that many pupils do not have the correct workstations and equipment to help prevent the condition. Indeed, campaigners are concerned that children risk serious damage by using computers while sitting at traditional desks at school. They add that even greater numbers of children may be putting themselves at risk by the way they use computers at home.

What's the answer?

It's easy to be overcautious and to suggest that children be banned from anything emitting EM radiation, but that would not be practical in our modern world. What you can do as parents is to keep an eye on the research, and take in any new safety guidelines. There will always be research proving and disproving different theories—that's the nature of the beast—so you need to make decisions based on the best information you can find. Again, if there is any indication that an appliance can cause ill health, it pays to take note. We do know that the strength of an EM field is decreased (rapidly) when you put distance between the source and your child, so rather than ban everything electrical, consider the following.

▶ Top tips for reducing EM radiation

- Most televisions emit very low levels of ionizing radiation, but if you have an old set, you might want to consider replacing it with a low-radiation version.

- Ensure that your children sit at least 6 feet (2 m) away from a television set, and if they are playing on a computer game, use a remote control that can be set well back.

- Limit the number of hours that your child spends in front of the television (see page 101). Obviously increased exposure means increased EM radiation.

- Don't use electric blankets on the bed while your child is sleeping. Warm the bed by all means, but turn it off and remove it before your child goes to bed.

- Turn off electrical appliances when not in use.

- Discourage your child from standing in front of a microwave oven when it is in use.

- If your child spends a lot of time at a computer (for school work or while playing games) make sure he takes frequent breaks. You might consider a screen that can help to reduce radiation.

- To prevent RSI, ensure that your child's workstation is appropriate. He should be sitting above the keyboard, and the VDT screen should be set at eye level or above. It's worth investing in an ergonomic station, particularly if your child spends a lot of time at the computer. Encourage your child to take regular breaks from activity, changing to an activity that is more physical (running up and down the stairs for a few minutes should do it!)

Living under a high-voltage power cable?

- Researchers in the U.K. say they have found significant evidence that could explain the long-suspected links between high-voltage power cables (pylons) and childhood cancers. A team at Bristol University found that there were "mechanisms" that increased exposure to environmental pollutants near high-power sources. The study showed an increased risk of exposure the nearer a person moved toward the cable.

- One U.K. study found that migraines were much more common in people living within 500 yards (500 m) of an overhead power line.

- Research carried out in Russia, the U.S. and the U.K. indicates that people living near such power lines are more prone to nonspecific symptoms such as fatigue, palpitations, weakness, eye pain and ear noise.

What can you do?

- You can demand that high-voltage cables are moved from the vicinity of your home. Contact your local electricity supply company to find out who is responsible for the cables. Talk to your local government and get the support of other residents in the area.

- As dramatic as it may sound, you may want to consider moving. Although research into the effects of EM fields on health is in its infancy, what we do know now is enough to concern most parents.

Let there be light!

The home environment can greatly influence our children's ability to absorb vital energy into their systems and thus directly affect their well-being and quality of life.

Natural light is necessary for health on all levels. For example, the endocrine system, which is governed by the pituitary and pineal glands, requires light in order to function properly. These glands control the release of hormones into the body, which are closely linked to moods and emotions. Many holistic practitioners also believe that natural light (living light) is necessary for the soul or "spirit." Like plants, children need natural, living light in order to thrive and to grow. Whether this works on an energy level or not is unclear, but we do know that children who live in an environment with little light fail to thrive. Many therapists believe that we absorb energy (or chi) from light and air, and that failure to get this energy results in an impaired sense of well-being, and ill health. Lack of natural light appears to be one of the causes of "sick building syndrome," and sufferers of SAD (seasonal affective disorder) experience emotional and physical symptoms during the winter months when there is lower light. Symptoms disappear in as little as two days when they are treated with full-spectrum light.

No form of artificial lighting can match the healing effect of natural sunlight, so try to ensure that you get natural light into your house from outside.

▶ Top tips for letting in light

- Keep windows clean and check that they all open.

- Design window treatments to allow the maximum amount of natural light into the room.

- Draw curtains back as far as possible and keep blinds up during the day.

- Move away any plants or objects that obstruct light coming into your home.

- Use mirrors opposite windows in rooms with low light levels.

- Use low-energy lighting or full-spectrum lights where possible, which are second best to the natural thing.

- Create skylights, atriums and sunrooms where you can, so that you can enjoy the benefits of sunlight.

- Most importantly, however, make sure your child gets plenty of sunlight every day. Slather on the sunscreens and put on sunshades if the sun is strong, but make sure that she gets a chance to absorb the energy of natural light as often as possible.

Creative color

The world is full of color, and it is impossible to imagine what life would be like without it. Throughout the ages, many great civilizations have extolled and benefited from the use of color as a powerful healing agent. The ancient Greeks, for example, had "color healing" temples, and the Chinese utilized color for diagnostic purposes. There has fairly recently been a renewed and growing interest in the effects color has on the mind and body. Each color has a specific vibration that your child's mind and body can take in on various levels. Blind people can learn to tell which color they sense under their hands.

Color for health and well-being

Research has begun to validate the importance of color in the treatment of disease. For example, contemplating blue light has been shown to lower blood pressure, by calming the autonomic nervous system, while red light causes it to rise. Color therapists claim that every subtle change in color affects us on every level of our being, and this is corroborated by research physicists who state that the cells of the body are made up of contracted light. By definition, cells made of light will respond to color.

Color your world

The colors your choose for your environment will obviously have an effect on your child's mood, health and sense of well-being. Having a knowledge of the therapeutic qualities of colors can make a child's home environment a place to nurture her learning skills and personality, while providing her with a safe haven in which to play and grow.

Colors can be used to calm or to stimulate, according to your individual child's needs. They can encourage sleep, or they can make an environment more conducive to learning. The colors your child chooses will say a great deal about his personality. There is some evidence that children are instinctively drawn to colors that will help to balance them. For example, a withdrawn child may choose red, or a hyperactive child might choose a pastel blue. Try it out at home.

Color therapy doesn't need to involve a therapist (although you can certainly take your child to see one—see chapter 10—if he suffers from a health problem). Parents can be aware of the colors they use for their children, for their clothes, their meals and for their bedrooms. Some color therapists believe that babies should not wear bright colors until they are a year old, and that the traditional white baby clothes are the best option. It is believed that the very delicate and still vulnerable aura (the energy field surrounding the body) of a child can be destroyed by colors that are too bright, and that this natural protection against outer influences will be weakened.

A guide to the therapeutic value of colors

red	physically stimulating, action-oriented, warm, cozy, vibrant, antidepressant
pink	emotionally soothing and calming, gently warming, uplifting
peach	digestive aid, warm, secure, glowing, creative, stimulating
yellow	uplifting, happy, bright, mentally stimulating
green	harmonizing, relaxing, cooling, calming, restful to the mind
blue	cool, relaxing, calming to the mind
turquoise	refreshing, cooling, calming to the mind, youthful
violet	dramatic, formal, spiritual, creative
brown	nurturing, earthy, supportive, practical

Paler tones of these colors will have a milder action, while richer, deep tones will have a more powerful effect.

What color for your child?

If your child is ill, with a high fever, or even chronically ill, choose pastel blue pajamas to cool and relax. If your child wears red pajamas, for example, you would enhance your child's dynamic state and make him more uncomfortable. On the same principle, parents could chose blue colors for a hyperactive child's environment, but red colors to stimulate the dynamic energy in children who are quiet and withdrawn.

▶ *Top tips for choosing colors in your young child's room*

- Strong, bright colors have the effect of shocking a baby's inner vibrations. This could make the infant unsettled and restless. Bright, intense colors such as primary red, yellow and orange can stop a child sleeping well, as well as cause her to cry.

- Strong, contrasting colors and bold patterns are also likely to be overstimulating, so for a small infant choose soft tones of yellow or cream, peach or pink, which are emotionally soothing and comforting.

- Green is calming but can be cold when used as a wall color, especially in a cold or dark room. If you do use green, make sure it is a soft, light tone.

- Blue on its own can also be cold and, according to color therapists, may make the child susceptible to colic and colds. Blue is a good color for an overactive child, but will not offer much emotional or physical support. Therefore, it is a good idea to use blue on the walls, making sure there is a contrasting warm color in the curtains and other furnishings. Pink, peach, apricot, pale almond, white and lavender are all nurturing colors, that can make your child feel more secure.

- To stimulate your child, hang brightly colored mobiles above his crib or play area, but remove them when it's time for sleep.

- Shells, bamboo, wood or metal wind chimes can bring gentle reassuring vibrations to the nursery.

- The colors of the child's bedclothes and bedding have a direct effect on her physical and psychological well-being, as the subtle color vibrations permeate our aura while we are asleep. Unless the child is well-balanced and outgoing, be careful not to have strong, large or geometric patterns on curtains, blinds or walls. These shapes can send off jarring vibrations. Removing these negative vibrational patterns from the room is the best thing you can do to help your child get a good night's sleep.

- If your child has trouble sleeping, consider using a soft nightlight with a pink or peach glow near the crib. These color are warm and nurturing, and according to color therapists, give out vibrations of love and security.

- A soft yellow-tinted light bulb also gives a friendly light. You can change the light bulb from time to time, especially when a child cannot sleep or is suffering from a childhood disease like chicken pox or measles. Blue works best for any hot condition where the child is running a temperature or has itchy skin.

Colors for older children

- Children grow and develop fast, and as they explore their world they become attracted to brighter colors. Don't be surprised if your child has a strong idea about what color he wants in his room. If they are all bright—reds, yellows and blues—compromise by adding accessories in these colors, which will not overwhelm a child while sleeping, or keep him from sleeping.

- Keep the walls one solid shade of a color that best suits your child's needs—or stick with a soft cream and add accents of color in the curtains, carpets or pictures.

- Color can stimulate your child's inquiring mind and encourage emotional development, so choose carefully. In a study area, choose color that stimulates without distracting, so that he won't be tempted to fall asleep, but he won't become too hyperactive either! Try to introduce wall colors that are less visually exciting, and stay away from busy patterns and wallpapers, especially strong geometric shapes, which emit disharmonious vibrations. Various shades of blue-green work well in a study/bedroom, and contrasting warming colors would be better if confined to bedcovers, curtains and blinds, cushions and rugs.

- If your child has a brightly colored room it may be possible to create a quiet corner, where the colors are more muted and quiet. Pale yellow-cream contains yellow energy to gently aid the mental processes, helping logical and clear thinking, while at the same time is not too disturbing.

Colors for adolescents

- Not surprisingly, most adolescents have a firm idea of what colors they want around them, and it is a good idea to give them fairly free rein. If the rest of your house is more restrained, they can relax or rejuvenate in other rooms, if that's required. Again, however, if a strong color is chosen, it is important to have a calming corner of the room, where your child can read or relax. In a bright red room, for example, you could set up a cream screen in the corner, with pale yellowy-cream beanbag chairs and cushions.

COLOUR THERAPISTS claim that the colors used in television sets are synthetic, not natural, and they interfere with our own vibrations, throwing our whole being out of balance. Children who watch a lot of television will be more susceptible to these bad vibrations that aggravate any health, learning or emotional disabilities. The answer? Keep television to a minimum, and turn it off if your child is not actively watching.

- A teenager may use her bedroom for entertainment and home study, as well as sleep, so would need a more warming and uplifting color scheme than a bedroom used solely for relaxation and sleep.

- Color therapists believe our auras become more brightly colored as we get older. So, as a child grows up, her pastel-colored aura becomes stronger, as pinks turn to reds, pale greens turn to bright greens, and pastel blues turn to bright blues. Orange-red predominates during puberty, which may explain why adolescents are so drawn to bright colors in the red spectrum.

- According to some color therapists, you can tell a lot about your teenager by the colors she chooses. For example, red expresses sexual development and intense energy. Pink shows a great need for love and affection. Blue suits a quieter nature and a search for a calm, soothing atmosphere, especially if there is tension in the home, or at school. Green shows a need for individual space, and time to reflect and develop ideas and ideals.

Feng shui fun

Feng shui (pronounced *fung shway*) is the art of living in harmony with your natural environment, thus allowing a natural flow of energy, or chi. Feng shui means "wind" and "water." Dating back at least 4,000 years, feng shui is widely practiced today throughout China and by successful businesses in the East, as well as in the West where its benefits are now being increasingly recognized.

It's a complicated discipline, and a small section in a book cannot do it justice. Trained feng shui experts (it takes six years to become a master) claim that do-it-yourself feng shui is impossible in a broad context. It's rather like a mechanic examining a sick child and giving a diagnosis and then treatment. Having said, that, however, there are many principles that can be absorbed into your family home, which can make a dramatic difference to the way your children feel.

Clear the clutter!

One of the main principles of feng shui involves being tidy, to avoid adding to the imbalances of your environment. Clutter traps chi, which then dies, and you live surrounded by dead energy. It is particularly dangerous at foot level, according to practitioners.

It's easy to believe that clutter can consume energy. Any parent who looks into a child's playroom after a busy day will feel a distinct sensation of energy being drained. And if you have piles of things you are meaning to deal with building up around the house, you'll understand the concept of wasted energy. The task preys on your mind, makes you feel guilty and continues to do so until the job is done. Think again about the feeling you get after successfully clearing out cupboards, rooms or drawers. There is a renewed sense of purpose and vitality, equating to energy moving once again.

▶ *Top feng shui tips for children*

- Clear away toys at the end of the day, and leave plenty of free surfaces for chi to flow across. A room should have a sensation of movement within it—of air and energy flow. If you enter a room and it appears stagnant, it's time to make changes.

- Make sure that your child's bedroom isn't littered with unfinished tasks distracting him from good restful sleep, or his homework. Encourage good organizational skills, teach your child to throw out things that are useless, unused or unnecessary, and to keep a sense of order in his environment. When he is younger, you'll need to do this for him, but he will learn from your example.

- Don't fill a room with decorations and toys. Clear spaces are important for chi to flow. Envision yourself in the most peaceful room you can imagine. Is it full of clutter? Not likely. Most of us imagine a clear, white room, probably empty except for a few simple pieces of furniture. Bear this in mind when furnishing your child's room. While all children need some stimulation, feng shui is all about the art of balance. In other words, balance hard and soft materials, dark and light colors, and areas of light and shade.

- The best position for your child's desk is in the corner opposite the door, where the two walls act as protector and make your child feel in control. Try to ensure that your child's desk faces the door, but not directly. Feng shui experts say that the incoming chi could be overpowering. Never place your child's desk with her back to the door, for concentration could "slip out the door."

- Wind chimes and bells can be useful in dark corners and long corridors, particularly if your child's room is at the end of a hall. These attract and invigorate chi.

- Ensure that your child's doorway is not blocked. Obstructions will prevent good chi from reaching your child.

- Lighting should be natural wherever possible, but both dim and strong light are considered unhealthy by feng shui practitioners. Ensure that your child's room is properly lit at dusk and in darkness, and shaded from harsh sunlight in the daytime.

- Mirrors in the bedroom are believed to have an unsettling effect because they intensify the energy reflected in them. For example, if you place a mirror opposite your child's bed, it reflects stimulating energy back while he sleeps, which can cause restlessness. If your child needs a mirror, keep it in a cupboard or cover it at night.

- The head of your child's bed should not be against or underneath a window. She needs something solid behind her to encourage a feeling of security and to enable her to relax.

▶ *Improving the flow*

You don't have to believe in the concept of energy to see it in action. Here is a simple trick to "clear" a space of past or unhealthy vibrations. If you feel that your environment is negative in some way—perhaps you've had that feeling since you moved into the house, or perhaps it is something that has occurred more recently—you can get the chi moving again, and dispel old energy.

You can practice this technique in one room of the house, but it would be better to give the whole house a once-over. The idea is to "clap" away old energy, moving in the direction that energy (chi) would normally travel, in order to encourage new, fresher, healthier energy to take its place.

If you don't believe it works, try this first: enter the first room and ring a bell. Listen to the sound of the bell and try to hold a memory of it.

- Now, starting at the entrance to your house, room or flat, hold your hands in the air and clap loudly, walking as you clap along the hall to the first doorway.

- Continue clapping and enter the room, walking to the right in a large circle around the room's circumference. Clap up and down into corners, but keep moving.

- Move out of that room and into the next, clapping all the time.

- Continue in exactly the same manner until you have reached the top/end of the house or flat and then clap your way back to the entrance and out the front door.

- Outside the door, focus on and clarify what you want from your life, and set it into a positive affirmation. For example, "I will have a peaceful house with no violence or unnecessary arguing. I will have a calm household where we will all feel happy and comfortable together." Once this is fixed in your mind, re-enter.

- Ring your bell again, in the same room in which you rang it the first time. Listen to the sound. It will sound clearer and more distinct. If it doesn't, try the exercise again.

This may sound unlikely, but I can guarantee that it works. With my five-year-old son in tow, we clapped our way around our house (my son ringing the bell occasionally for the sheer pleasure of it) and back out again. Neighbors watched in amazement as we appeared from window to window clapping happily, but we persevered. When we re-entered the house, the atmosphere was decidedly different. It felt lighter and somehow clearer. We rang the bell and it had a more definite sound.

For the next few weeks guests to our house looked around upon entering and asked if we had repainted, moved furniture or had a clear-out. Something was different, and that difference was tangible.

If you have an argument with your child, use this technique in the room in which it occurred. You'll probably both end up laughing, but it can clear the air—literally!

Do you need a feng shui consultation?

It isn't as expensive as you might think, and consultations normally include a survey of your home, a long discussion of the problems you are facing, a written report outlining suggested changes and follow-up visits.

What are some of the reasons you might need to make changes? Feng shui experts suggests that you ask yourself the following questions:

- Do you feel as if your home doesn't "feel right" and you have been unable to come up with a solution?

- Is there disharmony in the family that can't be explained?

- Are your children particularly difficult and/or not doing well at school?

- Do a lot of accidents happen at home?

- Do you or your children suffer from stress or find it difficult to shift bad health?

The answer may be an imbalance in your life, or even due to vibrations inherited from previous tenants or outside influences. A feng shui practitioner can address imbalances, clear away past vibrations, and ensure that the energy moves through your household, your family's bodies and your life in a positive way.

This chapter touches on only some of the ways that we can make a difference to our children's environments. The theory behind the disciplines may seem diverse and unrelated, but the concept remains the same. The healthiest atmosphere for your child is one in which he will thrive. It involves addressing external factors that will affect his health, such as toxins and chemicals, and taking steps to ensure that he is growing up in an environment with good, positive energy that will work on all levels to improve well-being. Use color and light to make your home a sanctuary in which every member will thrive and find peace. Clear out the rubbish, the least natural elements and the negative atmosphere, and you'll notice a big difference in the way your child feels, develops, concentrates, sleeps, works and plays.

You don't have to refurnish your home, move house or throw out everything artificial. Any change you make will be a step in the right direction. It's all about balance—balancing the natural with the unnatural, the dark with the light, the good with the bad. Create an environment that is comfortable and welcoming, a home in which you feel confident that you are doing the very best you can for your child. Using an antibacterial spray after clapping your way around the house isn't going to undo the positive effects, nor is choosing a red duvet cover for a baby going to mean a lifetime of poor sleep. Select the techniques and tips that are most relevant for your household and your family, and adapt them to suit your lifestyle. Your home is your child's castle—her own natural world, where she learns many of life's most important lessons. If the atmosphere is positive and the approach is as natural as possible, you'll do a lot to balance a toxic outside world.

chapter eight

The Key to Happiness: Emotional Health

W hat do you want for your children? It seems an easy question to answer, and the same response will trip off the tongues of most parents: I want my child to be happy, to be successful and to be healthy. Most parents, and certainly any parent reading this book, want the very best that life has to offer for their children, and many go to extreme lengths to prepare them for a magnificent future: swimming lessons, dancing, hockey coaching, French lessons, good schools, music lessons, bank accounts, extra tuition, and holidays and outings designed to stimulate young minds. This is the preparation that we give our children for life, and if we are particularly diligent, we can ensure that every minute of their waking life is spent absorbing something that will make them better—no, wait—the best. Success as a parent seems to be gauged by the extent to which we are able to prepare our children's young minds and bodies for the future, by giving them everything we did or didn't have in our own childhoods.

Looking at this scenario, it becomes clear that some very important elements of childhood are being discarded in order keep the bandwagon rolling. Where is the relaxation, the fun, the development that comes from an unsupervised exploration of time and environment? How can a child be emotionally and spiritually balanced in a world where dealing with stress is the answer to a serious and growing problem—emotional stagnation and spiritual disquiet? Our children are under enormous pressure—stress, if you like—which manifests itself in the same way as in adults: ill-health, fatigue, irritability, tearfulness, an inability to relax and a dependence upon adrenaline to get them through the day. But dealing with stress, from a holistic point of view, involves much more than a little cranial osteopathy or a drop of lavender oil in the bath. Short-term measures are effective solutions for short-term problems, but we are looking at a situation that has become a way of life for many children, and it is frightening to think what the future might hold.

Many parents will protest that emotional health is a high priority, and have proved it with their wallets—buying one or more of the hundreds of books now available on emotional intelligence and self-esteem. In fact, self-esteem has become a kind of buzzword over the last few years to the extent that many parents now fit emotional coaching, a sort of litany of emotional-intelligence training sessions, into their children's hectic schedules, to give them an emotional vocabulary and to ensure that they become well-rounded adults. Temper tantrums are treated with time-outs, stubborn children are reasoned with until both child and adult are blue in the face, and even toddlers are taught to *feel* their emotion, and to express it in graphic and subsequently applauded terms.

Don't get me wrong. If we ignored emotional health completely, our children would be incapable of getting up in the morning, given their demanding lifestyles, so it's a good sign that parents are embracing the idea that there is another aspect to raising children apart from forking out cash to keep them on the treadmill. But I question the motives. Self-esteem appears to be the miracle cure for all kinds of problems, from poor behavior and lack of concentration, to depression and low grades. In other words, it's become yet another tool for molding children to become model citizens of the future—hardworking, accomplished, successful, multiskilled, clever, educated, musical, refined. What this approach fails to take into consideration is the uniqueness of children. Every single child is different, with a multitude of features that makes each one special. But so much of the attention paid to emotional health appears to be aimed at helping our children to conform: a highly-strung child needs to be calmed; a quiet child needs to be brought out; a poor student needs to concentrate; an academic needs music lessons or extracurricular sports to round him out.

Empowerment is another tool that's become a feature of emotional training. It's a good philosophy—giving a child some control over her world—but again, it's being misused. We empower children to make them powerful. The bottom line is that when we say we want the best for our children, we mean that we want them to be the best.

This chapter looks at the importance of emotional health from another angle, and it goes further, to take into consideration the effects of emotional health and stability on our children's spirits. I'm not talking New Age philosophy here—I simply mean that every child has a right to be himself, to have confidence in who he is, to be comfortable in his body and his mind, and to use that supreme sense of contentment and self-knowledge to find a path in life that will bring him happiness and, above all, peace.

Many of the terms used here are the same as those used in other books—self-esteem, discipline, empowerment, for example—but I want to look at them in a new light, and focus on finding ways to apply them to your child with every one of her unique attributes. No one method works for every child, and all parents need to explore and experiment in order to find ways to encourage their children to find a sense of inner peace and happiness. Forget about the traditional signposts of "success," such as a top job, lots of money, a big house and lots of material trappings. You will be a successful parent if you can nurture the qualities in your child that make her unique. She will be successful if she loves life and chooses a path that brings her happiness.

Emotional health

In chapter 9 we look at the importance of emotional health on a physical level—how state of mind affects the body. Here, however, we'll look at how to ensure that our children are emotionally healthy, and what that means in terms of their lifestyles.

It's impossible to define emotional health in a way that applies to all children. Some children are naturally exuberant, and others find contentment in quieter pursuits. Some children whistle and sing in the morning; others prefer to curl up with a good book, or to daydream. No one of these scenarios is "correct," and it's important that you don't try to create a lively, bubbling child from an introspective dreamer. What you can do, however, is look for signs that all is not well.

▶ Check your child's emotional health

Answer the following questions honestly:

	Yes	No
1. Can my child tell me how he is feeling? (This means can your child express his feelings—at bedtime, in a quiet moment, or in the throes of an argument—without being prodded?)	☐	☐
2. Does my child exhibit signs of stress (see page 386)?	☐	☐
3. Does my child seem listless or withdrawn on a regular basis?	☐	☐
4. Does my child laugh less than he used to?	☐	☐
5. Does my child smile or show delight less than he used to?	☐	☐
6. Does my child become frustrated easily, and want to give up?	☐	☐
7. Does my child push himself too hard, to be the best, the top of the class, the best player on the field or the winner of the prize?	☐	☐
8. Is my child reluctant to take on new challenges or activities that he would normally enjoy?	☐	☐
9. Does my child become extremely upset if criticized or corrected?	☐	☐

	Yes	No
10. Does my child put himself down regularly?	☐	☐
11. Is my child overly critical of others?	☐	☐
12. Does my child try too hard to please people (teachers, friends, family members)?	☐	☐
13. Is my child clingy?	☐	☐
14. Does my child suffer from inexplicable fears, or is he afraid to face new situations?	☐	☐
15. Does my child need continual approval?	☐	☐
16. Does my child boast?	☐	☐
17. Is my child aggressive or attention seeking?	☐	☐
18. Is my child impatient and unappreciative?	☐	☐
19. Does my child suffer from a series of low-grade infections, abdominal pains or headaches that cannot be explained, but appear regularly?	☐	☐

If you answered *yes* to the first question, and *no* to all the others, you have a supremely balanced child and you are unlikely to need to read this chapter. Chances are, however, that you will have a blend of *yes* and *no* answers. This isn't a test, but it provides a basis for understanding the signs of emotional ill health, which can impact on your child's life in many ways.

What you want to do is aim to ensure that your child is emotionally balanced, so that she feels good about herself, feels confident in new situations, doesn't feel a need to be the best or to get the most, is patient and, above all, likes herself. No child will ever be perfect, and there will always be times when she experiences dips in confidence, has feelings of low self-worth, loses her temper and lashes out, and even becomes depressed. Like physical health, emotional health can slip and soar. In the same way that you can take steps to boost your child's immune system, in order to encourage her body to fight off hostile invaders, you can boost your child's emotional health, to help her get through the multitude of new situations that will face her throughout life.

Should we worry?

In the U.S., as many as one in 33 children and one in eight adolescents suffers from depression, according to the U.S. Center for Mental Health Services. Thirteen percent of U.S. children between the ages of 9 and 17 suffer from an anxiety disorder, while a MECA Study (Methodology for Epidemiology of Mental Disorders in Children and Adolescents) estimated that almost 21 percent of U.S. children aged 9 to 17 had a diagnosable mental or addictive disorder associated with at least minimum impairment.

As many as 10 percent of children and adolescents have some sort of mental disorder, with half of those (i.e., 1 in 20) suffering a clinically diagnosable condition, according to the first ever U.K. government survey.[1] The survey involved face-to-face interviews with 10,500 parents of children aged 5 to 15, and 4,500 children aged 11 to 15. Emotional disorders include a wide range of problems such as overanxiety, phobias, panic attacks, obsessive-compulsive behavior and depression. Behavioral disorders include awkward, troublesome, aggressive and antisocial behaviors. More boys than girls were identified as having disorders.

▶ *Helping redress the balance*

No child is perfect, and all have their own individual idiosyncrasies. In certain situations, you'll need to adapt your game plan to take into consideration their personality and character traits. Here are some ways to help a child who may be considered "more difficult."

- **Shyness:** The child who is shy or clingy should be introduced to new situations gradually. Talk about what's coming beforehand and then allow him to proceed at his own pace. Don't be tempted to force him to be, extrovert, or shove him into the limelight. Avoid, also, speaking for her. Let him take his time, and develop self-confidence in his own abilities and strengths.

- **Overenergy:** Consider how stimulating every situation may be in advance, and make sure you allow time for letting off steam and cooling down. Keep things particularly calm at home, allowing space for energy to be distilled, but moments when quiet is encouraged.

- **Strong-willed:** Try to avoid inflexible confrontations. Make your position known early on; but be open to negotiation. Usually you should state your position gently but firmly, and do not allow her stubbornness to prevail over what you know is right. Look for an occasional situation where her position can be shaped to be acceptable, and praise good efforts and persistence. Remember that later in life a strong, determined character will be applauded.

- **The rebel:** Some children find it difficult to fall in with expectations (even those that are fair and reasonable). He may have trouble going to sleep, eating his dinner or even toilet training. Don't despair. Put good routines in place for the whole family and ensure that your child takes part in all of them. Ensure that he goes to bed at a reasonable time, even if he doesn't sleep, and ensure that he sits at the table, even if he doesn't eat. Take him to the lavatory, but don't force him to go. Eventually he will become used to the pattern of daily life and settle in.

- **A moody child:** Some children do naturally have emotional highs and lows. There are many ways to balance these with natural remedies (see page 175), but on a practical level, consider the following: try to let her act out her moods for a while, and then distract her by involving her in other activities that you know she enjoys. Try not to let negative moods overshadow the rest of the family's fun. When she comes round, show extreme pleasure and she'll get the message that being happy is much more fun.

- **Highly strung:** You may have a high-energy, overexuberant child who is extreme in every way. He yells, barges into conversations, interrupts and generally ensures that you know he's there. You will, no matter what, need to adjust your tolerance level. You can't create a mouse from a lion, and when your child is older you will be able to channel this energy more effectively. Pretend if you have to! You can control volume, and overreactions, and stop activities until he settles down. You can also explain that some people find noise and energy alarming. He can learn to control himself in some situations, but leave plenty of space for letting off steam.

- **No change:** Some children find new situations and change completely disruptive, and at worst they can develop something approaching a phobia. Some children adjust slowly to new situations, and others simply cannot face them. The best thing that you can do is to provide regular routines in your home, so that they have a basic level of security. Be as consistent as you can be. When a new situation is expected, talk about it well in advance, pointing out exactly what to expect and what your child can do in different situations. Focus on the positive aspects of change whenever you can.

The importance of self-esteem

Parents can have a direct impact on their children's self-esteem, and it is worth looking at how you interact with your children on a daily basis. A child with low self-esteem is not necessarily the product of poor parenting. There are many factors in this big bad world that can affect the way your child views himself, but from the very first words you utter to your child, you can encourage or discourage a positive self-image.

When a child is born, he trusts his parents completely. He asks questions about his world, and they are answered. Parents are the all-powerful source of knowledge, and children learn by watching and listening. You tell your child that the sky is blue. You tell him that 1, 2, 3 is counting. You tell him that shoes go on feet. You tell him that nighttime is for sleeping. You tell him that cats have kittens, that books are for reading, that a cow says "moo." He believes you, and this belief is validated by the fact that the outside world seems to be in agreement. His grandmother gives the same response to his questions; his nursery school colleagues all believe the same thing; his babysitter confirms that cows do say "moo." His trust is complete. Everything you say will be taken seriously. He will believe you.

Take this one step further. In the throes of a chaotic day, your child feeds his toast into the video player. You lose your temper and shout "How could you be so stupid?" Or your child runs into the street to collect a favorite ball: "How could you be so disobedient?" you cry. Think of some of the things we say to our children: you are a very bad girl, you are a spoiled brat, you are silly, badly behaved, jealous, dumb, impossible to control, selfish . . . You get the picture. When we are angry, upset, frustrated, busy or just exhausted, things come out that we don't intend. This is obviously the source of much parental guilt, and we make it up with kisses and cuddles and even apologies later. But stop and consider this: your child believes everything you say. If you tell him he is stupid, even in a burst of anger, he will believe you. If you tell him he is selfish, he will think it's true. Every time we use negative words to define our children, they take them on board and file them away for future reference. No child will remember a particular incident, or be traumatized for life by being called stupid, but these occasions form faulty bricks in the foundation of his self-image. No matter how much you try to make up for it afterward, if you have said something, your child believes it, even if it is on an unconscious level.

No parent can ever be completely calm, or show a level of self-control approaching sainthood, particularly with small children about. What is necessary, however, is to learn to think about how to say things in order to prevent labels from becoming self-fulfilling prophecies.

▶ *Top tips to boost your child's self-esteem*

- Change personal attacks to more general messages about behavior. You love your child, she's bright and clever, but her *behavior* is unacceptable. So, instead of your child being naughty, her *behavior* is naughty. Instead of your child being selfish, she is acting in a selfish way. This has the effect of distancing the criticism and making it more constructive. Children can accept that they are behaving badly (which can be changed) more easily than they can accept a damning critique of their personality or character (which cannot).

- Consider whether the behavior or action is really that bad. For example, if your child fed his toast into the video, he or she probably had a very good reason for

Emotional ups and downs?

Your child may suffer from negative emotions from time to time, or as a feature of her personality. Apart from working on self-esteem, you may want to take steps to right minor imbalances that might be causing her emotional state. One of the best ways to do this is by using flower essences (see page 254):

- If your child is jealous, perhaps with a victim mentality and a feeling that she has been hard done by, you may consider holly flower essence, which enables her to feel happy for others, even if she is having problems herself.

- If your child is an artistic dreamer who becomes absent-minded, inattentive and easily bored, consider clematis, which can recall him from his dream world and focus his attention on everyday life.

- For a child who constantly seeks the reassurance of others because she does not trust her own judgment or intuition, try cerato, which gives her the ability to believe in herself.

- For children who are perfectionists, who find it hard to tolerate or understand the shortcomings of others, use beech.

- For children who are gloomy for no reason, in periods that seem to last for months, try mustard.

- Try gentian for the eternal pessimist, who is easily discouraged, even when he is doing well. This encourages perseverance and provides the will to succeed.

- For a child who is shy, nervous and blushes easily, try mimulus. This remedy helps to give courage.

doing so. Ask him why he did it. Children do all sorts of things as part of the developmental process, and they learn by trial and error, and by example. He's probably never seen you push your breakfast into that slot, nor has anyone ever told him that he shouldn't do it. So, why not? Let's see what happens. Try not to be too judgmental. There are very few children who are willfully naughty without good reason. If he isn't harming himself or others, try to understand rather than lash out. You'll be a lot more likely to teach your child what is acceptable if you are calm.

- Change the emphasis from attack to explanation, from *you* to *me*. For example, if your child runs into the street, say "I was very frightened. I was worried that a car could come along and run you over." Or if your child throws a tantrum in the middle of the supermarket, say "I feel very sad and upset when you do this, and I am worried that people will think you are a naughty child when I know how nice you really are." By explaining, rather than attacking, and drawing attention to your concerns rather than her shortcomings, your child will have a better understanding of what is and is not appropriate behavior.

- Find something positive about your child in every situation. For example, "You are such a caring boy. I am shocked that you would drown the hamster in the bath." Or, "You are such a smart girl, and I am surprised that you would rip up your brother's painting" or even "You are so organized, I was worried when you came home so late." By ensuring that your child knows that you think he is good, fundamentally, he won't experience a loss of face, or faith in himself.

Praise, praise, praise

In our society there is far too little praise. Everyone is too busy to stop and appreciate, to comment on the little things that make us feel good about ourselves. Think of a typical child's day: he's rushed through breakfast and into clothes, out the door and off to school. He comes home with a new painting, and you glance at it and say "Hey, that's pretty" and urge him to do his homework. He might have a music lesson to fit in before dinner, and then there is the ubiquitous battle over what he will and won't eat. Everything is running late, so bathtime is just a quick splash, and if there's time for a story before bed, things are looking up. Lights out and most parents breathe a sigh of relief.

Look back at your child's day. How often did you praise him? How did you make him feel good about himself? Probably not much, and maybe not at all. If he was overexcited, grumpy or "difficult," you probably blasted him. He may have been disciplined, but he probably hasn't been praised.

I can't overstate the importance of praise. Praise produces a warm feeling inside that makes your child think: I am all right. He learns to feel good about himself, to appreciate, and to see good in the world around him. He feels loved, and valued, and worthy of your attention. He sees that he can do good, and that you will recognize it, and him, for his efforts. He learns to like himself and he develops confidence.

Fit praise into your day as often as you can. If you praise only good marks, he may become obsessed with schoolwork as a way to please you. If you praise only his efforts on the basketball court, he may drive himself too hard to get your attention. If you never praise him, he will continue to do whatever gets your attention, which probably means "naughty" behavior. If, during a day, the only time you give your child your full attention is when he won't eat his dinner, slaps his sister, plays his music too loudly, or spends hours on the telephone, you can guarantee that these behaviors will be repeated. Negative attention is better than no attention at all, and all children thrive on attention.

Be liberal with your praise. From morning to night, notice and dwell on the good things about your child's behavior, his actions, his personality and his views.

Tape-record your family

One of the best ways to analyze the way you interact with your children is to tape-record a typical day (or a few hours). The purpose of this exercise is to examine honestly how you speak to your children, and how they respond, so don't put on your best behavior and make it sound good. No one needs to hear this but you and your partner. Choose a time when things are busy and you are under pressure—first thing in the morning, for example, or the period leading up to bedtime. If you are busy, you are less likely to be self-conscious about being taped.

Tape as much as you can and then listen carefully. How often did you praise your child? How often did you use positive language? How does your child respond when you are under pressure? Many parents find that their children are appalling just when they need them to behave well—when you have an important telephone call to make, there is someone present whom you want to impress (a grandparent, perhaps), you are under a lot of pressure at work and need time to think, or time is simply running short and you have other commitments. Why is this? Children sense anxiety and tension. It has to do with an exchange of energies. If you create a negative energy, they respond in kind.

Creating a positive emotional environment involves a lot more than praising and using encouraging language. You have to take the pressure off yourself and your family environment by relaxing and accepting that some days and times will be better than others. Allow extra time for when things fail to go exactly to plan, and keep calm. It can be enormously frustrating to work to a tight schedule when your children have their own agenda. Try to find a happy medium, where your children are not rushed and you don't feel anxious, and then try to find ways to let off steam, so that your own frustrations are not taken out on your children. A parent who nurtures himself as well as his children will be more balanced and able to cope with the demands of family life. If your tape recording shows periods when things become negative, try to make changes. Change routines, so that they are less stressful. Cut down on activities if you are always on the run. Make rules (see page 181) to define what you expect from your children, to give scope for plenty of praise. And then try to incorporate praise into every interaction you have with your child. Above all, praise yourself. Parenting is hard work, and if you can keep the status quo, you've done a good job.

Self-awareness is one of the cornerstones of positive parenting, and if you can begin to understand how you are interacting with your children, you can take steps to improve it.

Praise him for eating his cereal, even if the fruit remains untouched. Praise him for putting on his shoes without being reminded, even if they are on the wrong feet. Praise him for getting his gym bag to the front door, even if he forgets it on the way out the door.

Praise his artwork, his homework, his mediocre spelling test results, his appearance, his memory, his organizational skills, his sense of humor, his silly jokes and really mean it. Show interest in him and his world. Be thrilled for his achievements, even if they don't live up to your expectations. Use both general and specific praise, so that your child has plenty to feel good about, even when one aspect of his life slips. If your child gets a C grade, but his teacher says he's really trying, make a fuss. If your child fails everything, but he gets a glowing personal report, focus on the fact that he is a nice, popular child. Praise everything good about your child and what he does. If he feels good about himself, if he believes you like him, flaws and all, he will develop self-esteem that will spill over into every part of his life.

Most importantly, however, praise your child for just being himself. Praise his appearance constantly. Children will define their bodies by how others perceive them. If you make them feel that they are attractive, you will improve their confidence and their self-image. Fat children, skinny children, adolescents with acne, babies with chicken pox—everyone needs to feel that they are lovable and nice to look at. You won't create a big-headed child by praising appearance, you'll simply ensure that your child feels comfortable in his own skin.

If you haven't been as lavish with praise as you might have been, it's never too late. Your child may appear suspicious at the outset, but he will feel proud and flattered underneath. Soon, it will become a way of life, and your child's confidence and self-image will slowly grow, when he knows that he has your unconditional love and approval.

Physical affection

Nurturing touch plays a strong role in infant and child development, and research suggests that it continues to be important as a way of communicating love and caring between parents and their older children. Most parents continue to share some level of physical closeness with their daughters during the growing-up years, but this can change dramatically with sons. Most parents (mothers in particular) of boys find that this nurturing physical contact with a son grows more awkward and less frequent by around age eight or nine, but the shift is perhaps most dramatic when he moves into adolescence. Many children naturally withdraw, particularly in front of their friends, and this is something we have to expect and respect. However, it doesn't mean that we should give it up altogether. Like many other aspects of parenting, physical closeness remains important throughout a child's life. As she gets older, a parent is one of the few people who can give a child the emotional comfort of physical warmth in a nonsexual context, and children need to experience physical tenderness if they are to be able to be physical themselves as adults.

A child who is not touched will feel ignored, ashamed, unworthy of attention, inferior and misunderstood. That child will feel lost, alone, unsure and unhappy. Touch has a language of its own. It can offer reassurance and love that go beyond words. A pat on the shoulder, a warm embrace, a gentle massage, tousling hair or stroking a much-loved little face can communicate acceptance and affection that tell your child how you feel about him. Don't demand affection when you need it. Watch for signs that he needs a little reassurance and make it natural. An attention-seeking child may just need a little of just that—quality attention. Sit down together with a book and put your arm around your child. If he's watching television, stroke his feet. If he's struggling with homework, give him a hug. If he cries, don't expect him to be more mature. Get down there and be physical. There is safety in physical affection, and all children will benefit.

This brings us to the question of bodies. Children need to feel good about their bodies and themselves, and physical affection can provide reassurance that they are attractive and lovable. No one touches things that they find distasteful, and if you fail to touch your child, he will get the message that he is something with which you would rather not be in contact, even if this is on a subconscious level. Touch raises self-esteem and it costs nothing to give.

Disciplining with confidence

Only an idealist would think that praise will make your child a perfect person, and even children with high self-esteem and confidence need guidelines for behavior. One of the most important jobs a parent has is to teach life lessons to her child, and behavior is part of that. For people to live together in harmony, there has to be a basic level of respect for others. You need to respect your child, and she needs to learn to respect you, herself and everyone else around her. Teaching respect is the art of discipline.

First and foremost, consider your expectations. You cannot make a lively child into a quiet conformist, and you cannot turn a dreamer into an outgoing conversationalist. One of the most important things to remember is that you are working with a unique personality, and your expectations have to be geared to those characteristics. A lively child should not be "controlled," but taught appropriate behavior in various situations. A shy child should not be expected to hold a long eye-to-eye conversation with an adult, but she can be taught to be polite.

Parental expectations are crucial to discipline, and you need to assess whether they are appropriate before passing them on to your child. If you expect your child to behave beautifully in all situations, your expectations are probably too high. Children have abundant natural energy, and while it can be channeled, it should never be suppressed (see page 190). Many parents feel the need to control their children because of the way they will be perceived by others. "Bad" behavior is too often considered to be a sign of poor parenting, or lack of parental control. What nonsense!

The best parents are those who allow their children some free rein, some scope to be children, some freedom to be themselves, while still respecting the rights and needs of others. What children need is guidance, and an understanding of the world around them. You can teach children that they must keep their voices low in the library, or that they should not interrupt when adults are speaking without saying "Excuse me," or that jumping on the sofa can upset many adults who are proud of their homes. What you need to do is provide your child with an understanding of how other people feel and think, and what will be expected of them in certain situations. No child knows instinctively how to behave, and with even the best guidance, there will always be times when emotion overtakes logic, or exuberance overtakes wisdom, or temper overtakes self-control.

Be realistic in your expectations, and praise every good part of a job well done. You can't expect a three year old or even an adolescent to behave immaculately at all times, and nor should you. Make allowances for age and temperament, and make sure you have made clear your expectations before every situation. If they let you down (which they inevitably will, from time to time), then you need to consider forms of discipline that will get the message across in the most positive way possible.

▶ *Top tips for using discipline*

- A highly strung, rambunctious child will probably not respond to a quiet word in the corner. Gear your discipline to your individual child. Maybe time-out is appropriate for this type of child. He may long to be part of the action, and even the threat of a few moments alone on the stairs will be enough to calm him down.

- A less confident, quiet child might be devastated by the thought of time-out, or away from you and the rest of the family. In this situation, a quiet word in the corner, explaining why behavior is unacceptable just might work. Whatever you do, don't assume that a method is appropriate for your child without trying it out first.

- Prepare your child in advance of every situation by letting her know what you expect. If she knows the game plan, she can make choices accordingly.

- Set up some household rules. Sit down with your child at the table with the whole family and work out what is expected from every family member (see page 181).

- Give warnings! If your child is behaving badly, don't slam down a punishment. Give him a warning of what is to come. In our household we use the soccer disciplinary system of red and yellow cards. Yellow cards are a warning. A red card means big trouble, and a prearranged penalty. We have only ever got to red-card stage two or three times over the past two years, so it is a system that definitely works.

Family rules

Establishing expectations can have a dramatic effect on your children's behavior, and you will need to sit down as a family, with all members from nursery-school-age upward, to decide what is and is not appropriate. Focus on problem areas. For every rule, decide upon the behavior you would like to see. Here are some examples:

"I won't play my stereo loudly past 10 P.M. I will respect the fact that other people in the family need to relax and sleep."

"I won't make a fuss about getting dressed in the morning. I will get dressed before I watch cartoons or eat my breakfast."

"I won't fight with my brother. I will treat my brother the way I would like him to treat me."

"I won't come home after 10 P.M. [adolescents]. I will phone if I am running late, and I will always tell my parents where I am going to be."

"I won't have a tantrum if I don't get a treat at the supermarket. I will choose a treat in advance and not ask for anything else."

"I won't argue about doing my homework. I will do my homework after school."

"I won't suck my thumb throughout the day. I will suck my thumb only at bedtime."

- For every rule that is satisfactorily maintained, offer a "reward." Obviously it would be impractical to give a treat for everything done properly, but there are many ways of rewarding children. One of the best is a star chart, where a star can be given for everything done well. Ten stars can mean money (allowance) or a magazine. Twenty stars can mean a small toy. A hundred stars can mean a family day out to a theme park or the beach. Encourage your child to choose what would be the best reward for consistently sticking to the rules. While it may seem extravagant, we had almost two months of literally stellar behavior for the new Manchester United soccer shirt. It was worth it!

- Remember that these rules will soon become a way of life, and you can drop them when they do so. Family rules need to be updated constantly in order to be effective. There is no point in giving stars for getting dressed in the morning if your child has been doing it successfully, of his own volition, for a month. Change the rules, dropping and adding, as your child grows and develops.

- For rules that are broken, a penalty will need to be determined. Encourage your child to choose her own penalty. You'll find that children are much harder on themselves than you will ever be! For example, losing playtime on the computer, missing out on a trip to the library, giving up an after-dinner treat. Whatever your child

HOLISTIC HEALTH FOR BODY, MIND, AND SPIRIT

chooses (within reason), let it stand. You can consider a time-out, if that's appropriate for your child, but she will need to agree that it's a suitable punishment. Try to keep the penalty in line with the rule.

- Remember that praise will encourage respect of the rules. For every success, also offer praise and show your pleasure.

- Parents need rules, too! If the whole family is to take part, your children must be allowed to expect certain behaviors from you, too. Ask them what changes they'd like to see! If you lose your temper easily, one of your rules could be to avoid shouting. It's all about respect for one another, and you need to show equal determination to please them. Choose your own reward—a week without shouting could mean some time to yourself on a Sunday morning to read the papers in peace. And what about a penalty? This is where it can become good fun! My children suggested that I should not be allowed to have a glass of wine with my dinner if I broke our rules.

- Children have a terribly strong sense of justice, and they will take things very seriously if you encourage them to do so.

- Make it fun! Don't go wild, but choose, say, five or six rules for each member of the family, and talk about them at length. Make sure everyone is happy with the rewards and the penalties, and hold family meetings from time to time to reassess.

- Make sure you are communicating on the same level as your child (see page 185). You can shout till you are blue in the face, but if you aren't on the same wavelength, she may not be getting the message.

- Try not to shout. It can be hard to control your own emotions in the heat of a frustrating or distressing situation, but it can turn up the temperature and make things much worse. Some children are terrified when their parents shout, and others just develop a thick skin, which means the decibel levels continue to rise over time until everyone is shouting to get a point across. Shouting also creates negative energy that can compound a situation. Try to be calm and positive wherever possible, and if you have to, remove yourself from the situation completely. If you are going to lose it, count to ten, and try again.

- Don't use physical violence, whatever the problem (see page 188).

Power and discipline

Respect your child and give him choices. Allow him to have some control over his environment and his own behavior.

- Let your child choose the way he behaves. In the middle of a temper tantrum, for example, offer a choice: "You can stop shouting and screaming now, and I will be able to finish the shopping and we'll have time for a trip to the library. You can continue to shout and scream, I will be mad, and we will be too late to do anything other than go home. Which do you choose?" Give your child time to think, and then respond accordingly. Whatever you do, be consistent. If you say that you won't have time for the library, don't go. If you say that you will, you must make the trip.

- For an older child, this method works in a variety of situations: "If you do your homework now, you can watch 20 minutes of television after dinner. If you don't do it now, you will have to go to bed straight after dinner." Whatever the situation, give a choice and let your child know the consequences of either one.

- All children need to know that you or another adult (teacher, baby-sitter, police officer, whatever) are in authority. That doesn't mean you have to be authoritarian; it simply means that your child must learn to respect people in charge. You must establish early on that he has rights and choices, but within certain guidelines. No child will benefit from being allowed to run wild. Emotional health and freedom must always take place within the confines of a structured environment. Children feel much more secure when they know where they stand—at any age—and giving too much freedom (see page 196) can be alarming. Being rude or argumentative are behaviors that suggest disrespect, and every child needs to learn that they are inappropriate in every situation. Children do need to be given license to debate and to ask questions, and you must be willing to negotiate on the basis of a sound argument. However, it is important to be consistent, to stick to the family rules, and to ensure that your child respects your authority to make overall decisions.

- If you do have a problem with lack of respect for authority, empowering your child can help. If he feels that he has some control, and some scope for making choices and decisions, he will be less likely to challenge you on everything. For example, if your overall rule is that your child must dress herself in the morning, and you face a battle every single time, use choices. Do you want to get dressed before your breakfast or after? Do you want to wear socks or tights? Allowing choice makes her feel that she's in charge to some degree. You haven't changed the rule—she still has to get dressed—but you have given her some personal power.

- It works for older children, too. If your child regularly refuses to do his homework, offer choices. If we do it now, I can help you, or you can do it on your own after dinner. Do you want to do it now or in 20 minutes? Do you want to borrow my computer or do you want to write it out? Present it as an accepted fact that the homework *will* be done, but offer him some choices as to how, when and where.

- Remember that discipline is not about control. No one has the right to control anyone else. It is about guidance and respect, and teaching your child how to behave and to act, in every situation. Use praise, rules, choices, star charts, rewards, penalties and chats to indicate what is acceptable and what is not. Allow your child to make choices based on knowledge of what will happen when she behaves appropriately and what will happen when she does not. Focus on the good, and ignore the bad (see below).

- Model appropriate behavior. If you shout and lash out in anger, you can expect your child to do the same. If you constantly lose your temper, interrupt your child when he is speaking, show little respect for his view or needs, you cannot expect him to act any differently. If you adopt a calm, reasonable approach to dealing with your children, they will learn that this is the way to behave. Children who live with fairness learn that there is justice.

- Above all, give your child an outlet (see page 190), and don't expect her to be angelic all the time. Everyone needs to let off steam. Children in particular need to be allowed to be children. Don't expect adult behavior in a child. Children do not have the self-control or the same sense of propriety, or even an understanding of societal expectations. As your child grows older, she will learn, through you, and

---

Encouraging good behavior

Apart from using praise and rewards, you do have another powerful tool at your disposal: ignoring what you don't want to encourage. When a child learns that living by the household rules, and showing respect for others, wins him praise and plenty of positive attention, he'll be more likely to repeat his actions. If he learns that behaving in a naughty way gets no response, he's much less likely to bother.

- If one child is annoying a sibling while she is trying to do her homework, ignore him. Praise the sibling for managing to concentrate with all the distractions and focus all your attention on her. If he gets no response, the child doing the annoying will probably give up.

- If your child tries to shock you by swearing or using aggression, calmly point out that it is not acceptable behavior, and focus all your attention elsewhere. In other words, ignore her. If she doesn't get the expected response, she'll try something else. Used in conjunction with plenty of praise, this is a very useful technique. However, it is crucial that you offer plenty of attention for the good things—hugs, stars, rewards, praise, for example. If the only time you focus your attention on her is to address negative behavior, she'll be bound to do anything she can to hold your attention, even if it causes you both distress. Unacceptable behavior should be met with little interest or, in the extreme, prearranged penalties.

through the reactions of everyone else around her, what is appropriate. Until then, let your children be children. Delight in their boundless energy, their imagination and the way they view the world. Don't stamp out that natural enthusiasm for life. Give it room to blossom within guidelines that your child understands and accepts.

Communicating with your child

The cornerstone of any relationship is communication, and it is important that you take time to establish communication that you both understand. Look back on your day. Have you had any real interaction? Many days are spent chivvying children along, asking questions but not really listening to the answers, expressing your viewpoint without really understanding theirs. When was the last time you sat down and had a satisfying conversation? And when you did speak to your child, did you get the message across satisfactorily, and was he able to put forward his own message?

In even the most hectic lifestyles, it is important to make time for conversation and interaction. Make it part of a bedtime routine, when your child is relaxed and calm. If you get one child on his own in the car, ask questions and show genuine interest in the response. Give every child a chance to speak at the dinner table, and have a rule about hearing everyone out before interrupting. Encourage communication, whether it is positive or negative. The expression of emotion can be daunting for many children, and it is crucial that you give them space in which to do so, and that you offer a nonjudgmental, reassuring ear.

Children need to learn to communicate without being afraid of the repercussions. If your child confesses that he's broken a window, eaten his brother's chocolate, ruined your best shirt or even, in the extreme, tried a recreational drug, don't blast him. Honesty is extremely important to successful long-term communication, and if your child believes that he can tell you the truth without a lecture, argument or punishment, he will continue to do so throughout his life. If your child has done something serious, let him know how you feel, but stay calm. If he has broken a rule, ask him how he thinks you should deal with it. Most children will willingly offer a suitable punishment, given the authority to do so. They will feel less chastised if they have had a part in the proceedings, if they have been the instigator of justice.

Are you on the same level?

Communication is an art, and there are many theories about how it can be undertaken to best effect. One of the most useful tools for communication is NLP—neurolinguistic programming.

NLP looks for patterns, and one of the earliest patterns noticed in humans is a tendency for the eyes to look in a certain direction when thinking in a certain way. More

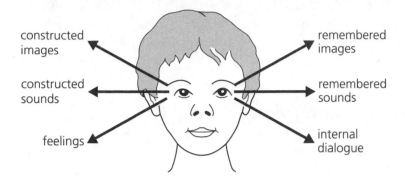

constructed images

constructed sounds

feelings

remembered images

remembered sounds

internal dialogue

specifically, people generally look up and to the right when thinking about a remembered image, up and left when constructing an image, directly right for a remembered sound, directly left for a constructed sound, down and to the right when having an internal dialogue with themselves, and down and left when experiencing feelings.

This may seem complicated, but watching your child's face can provide information about how she is thinking, which can be an important indicator of the approach you should take when communicating.

Let's put it into practice:

- If you ask your child a question and she turns her eyes to the immediate right or left, she is using auditory constructions (sounds and the sounds of words). She will therefore respond to aural cues. For example, if you have an aural child, saying "I see what you mean" will probably not have the same effect as saying "I hear what you are saying." Auditory children need auditory cues: listen, hear, register, tune in, sound out, recall, verbalize, voice and orchestrate. Match your words to the sensory system most indicated by your child's actions.

- If your child turns his eyes up to the right or the left when he is thinking or responding, he is using visual constructions (pictures and images). He will respond to visual cues. For example, saying "I see what you mean" is better than saying "I understand what you are feeling." If you ask your child to tidy his room and he looks up to the left, he is probably remembering what his bedroom looked like, or seeing himself cleaning it, and balking at the thought. If you say, "You will feel much better when your room is clean," he will probably resist. If, however, you appeal to the visual, you will be speaking the same language: "You will feel much more organized when your clothes are away, there is space on the floor and your toys are in their boxes." He will be able to *picture* this scenario, which will be much more appealing than a vague sense of feeling good.

An emotional vocabulary

Children need to be taught to express themselves, and they need to learn the vocabulary to do so. Boys in particular have been much neglected on the emotional interaction front. In fact, if you ask the majority of boys "How do you feel about that," you are likely to get nowhere. They might talk about how they approached a problem, or divulge a plan for setting something right, but most boys do not easily express emotion, largely because boys are characteristically different from girls in their emotional expression, and those differences are enhanced by a culture that supports emotional development for girls and discourages it in boys.

As they get older, most children are discouraged from outward displays of emotion, and they learn that it is better to hide feelings than to incur the teasing or wrath of a tired parent, sibling or peer. Without emotional literacy, children are left to manage conflict, adversity and change in their lives with a limited emotional repertoire. They are, effectively, faced with inexplicable, confusing and even frightening situations and change that they do not have the tools to address or express.

▶ *Top tips for teaching your children to express themselves*

- From an early age, help your child to express himself. Start by expressing your own emotions: I am feeling sad, tired, excited, happy, frightened ... and explain why. Children learn by example, and if they see that it is acceptable for parents to express themselves in emotional terms, they will much more likely to do so themselves. Emotion is a part of life, not a sign of weakness or imperfection.

- Help your child by giving her the words: you must be feeling very disappointed; that must have made you very sad; I can see that you are excited; you must feel proud of yourself; you should be thrilled; it's no wonder you are feeling angry. Teach her how they are used.

- If your child is reluctant to express himself, encourage him. For example, you must be feeling very cross about being overlooked for the football squad ... and then let him expand upon this. Use the words that he needs to learn: proud, happy, excited, angry, frustrated, confused, distressed, sad, lonely, jealous. Let him know that it's OK to feel even negative emotions, as long as they are expressed rather than used in aggression or withheld, which can be damaging.

- Share your own experiences. If your child is having a difficulty in any situation, try to find a similar situation that you experienced as a child (or even adult). Describe the way you felt, and ask how your child would feel in the same situation (even if you know full well she's feeling that way now). If a child learns that it is acceptable to feel, she won't be ashamed to admit it.

- Most importantly, however, listen! There is no point in encouraging honest emotional vocabulary in a child if you brush it off. If you teach a child to express feelings, you must acknowledge them, offer reassurance and spend time finding ways to make your child feel better about himself and a situation. For example, if your child says that he is sad because his sibling is going to a party and he is not, don't say, "That's ridiculous! You've been to three parties this month and he's been to none." Accept and validate his feelings. Show understanding: "I would be upset, too. It's hard to see other people having fun when you've got nothing planned. Why don't you and I do something nice together instead." If your child tells you when he feels jealous, don't become angry or judgmental. Accept his feelings and let him know that they are normal.

- Much aggression is caused by an inability to express feelings. When we suppress emotions, they have a tendency to boil over from time to time, and, in children in particular, they can come out as violence and physical loss of control. Most aggression can be curtailed by regular expression of feelings.

- Looking down to the right side of the body indicates kinesthetic tendencies: body sensations, emotions, smell and taste. If your child won't eat her dinner, you will probably get nowhere if you describe a dinner that will appeal to her visually, nor will you convince her to eat if you tell her that it will be healthy. Try using appropriate language: "You'll feel happier when you eat this. It tastes delicious. Do you remember the pasta we had at Grandma's? It smells the same and you remember how much you loved that."

Recognizing whether someone is seeing, hearing or feeling allows you to match the sensory system he's using and communicate with him much more easily.

Physical punishment

Physical punishment has no place in the upbringing of any healthy child. However, no parent can ever maintain full control, and there may be times when you lash out in anger. This type of physical aggression is, however, much less serious than a planned physical punishment. If you give your child a clip around the ear in a moment of complete and utter frustration, admit that you've lost control. Apologize and explain that you felt so angry you just couldn't help yourself. He'll understand that you don't consider it acceptable behavior, and he'll be less likely to use violence himself. But if you use violence in a premeditated way—spanking a child as a form of discipline, for example—you are sending conflicting and negative messages. I have seen parents bite their children "to teach them how it feels," after that child has bitten a sibling or a friend. What an extraordinary contradiction this presents. You cannot teach a child that violence is unacceptable and then use it yourself.

If you were physically punished as a child, how did you feel? Angry, embarrassed, invaded, distressed or frightened? Did you lash out or did you withdraw? Did you feel intense rage or hatred for the perpetrator, or did you feel guilty and unworthy? This is an important exercise. Most of us have been hit at some point in our lives, and the feelings we experienced are the very ones that we will create in our children if we use violence. No positive feelings ever come from physical discipline, and you can undo a great deal of good work by degrading your child in this way.

There are times when children completely lose control and become hysterical. If you are absolutely unable to get through to your child on these occasions, you may feel they need a short slap on a wrist to come round. As a one-off, last-ditch effort to restore calm, this might be effective and even necessary, but it should never be a means by which you can expect to control your child. You may stop the hysteria and the negative behavior, but you do so by shocking your child and decreasing her sense of self-worth.

If you find that you are losing your temper and resorting to spanking too often, look at your own life. It may be that you are under too much pressure. Take time for yourself. Remove yourself from the scene. Ask for help. Nurture yourself—read a book, listen to some calming music, get a massage, go to bed early, order a take-out dinner instead of cooking. Leave the laundry and forget about the ironing and watch television instead. Give yourself a break and try not to feel guilty about being less than perfect. Parenting is the most demanding, unpredictable and thankless job you may ever do, and it's important that you feel good about yourself in order to do it well.

When you feel yourself losing control, count to ten. A surge of adrenaline takes ten seconds to disperse, and if you can hang on for that long, you are much more likely to exhibit some self-control. Try as hard as you can to see the humor in a situation. If you can laugh, you will be doing a great deal to diffuse a situation. Try to see things through another's eyes—you have an angry teenager who refuses to bend. You are standing face-to-face, glaring at one another and engaged in a shouting match. Try to see the funny side. No one can win this situation, and locking horns can be exhausting for everyone involved.

Alternatively, just give up. Throw up your arms and admit defeat, and explain that you cannot cope anymore. Most children will feel rather alarmed by instant victory and will immediately begin offering concessions. Children challenge authority as part of growing up, and they rebel in order to test their power and their boundaries. They don't actually want those boundaries to shift, leaving them in an unknown situation. They simply want to see how far they can push you, and they want the attention that comes from an interaction of any sort—negative as it may be. If you suddenly change the script, they will be flummoxed and may hastily retreat. This isn't a method to use on a regular basis, for no child needs to be empowered to the extent that negative behavior offers rewards, but it can work occasionally to break a deadlock, and to prevent things from spiraling into fury and even violence.

Giving children an outlet

Today's children are expected to conform from a much earlier age. They attend school earlier, their lives are packed with activities and there is much less time for play and relaxation. Not surprisingly, this can cause an enormous amount of stress in a child, and it can be reflected in his overall health, well-being and behavior.

In Victorian times, children would be expected to sit in a room without speaking, while adults carried on with their conversations, showing little regard for their young guests. Thankfully, times have changed and most children are encouraged to take part in conversations and the family routine. But remember, Victorian children would have been shoveled off to the nanny or the nursery on a regular basis, where they could play and relax and be normal children. Today, we offer little opportunity for children to be children. They are expected to conform to an ideal—not making a fuss, not interrupting, concentrating at school, on the sports fields, on their homework, eating their dinner and getting dressed without a murmur, bathing quietly, and going to bed, where they are expected to fall asleep immediately, and sleep through the night.

Where is the outlet? At what point are children offered the opportunity to express emotion, to unload tension, to let off a little steam, to be children, with a natural buoyant energy and spirit?

I've heard countless parents complaining that their children are so good at school, but a complete nightmare in the home environment. If this picture seems familiar, take heart. Your child has learned appropriate behavior for the school environment, and she has probably worked very hard at concentrating and keeping her emotions and enthusiasm in check for an entire school day. In the comfort of her own home, she is able to let down her defenses and let out all that energy that has been bubbling inside during the day. This is the way it should be! A child's home is her castle—the place where she can be herself without expectations or judgment or punishment.

That's not to say that naughty or rebellious behavior at home is always appropriate, but you must allow some leeway. If your child comes home in a state every day, he needs an outlet and it is up to you to provide it. Organize some fun exercise. Throw him out in the backyard to run and explore. Laugh, tell jokes, wrestle, play, relax—anything that lets the energy flow. Don't expect the rigid routine of school to be followed by an equally rigid routine at home. Certainly, a routine will help your child to feel secure, but time has to be allowed and, indeed, encouraged, for fun, high spirits, laughter, shouting, cheering, crying or just lying about. If you child is exhibiting signs of stress, he does not have an appropriate outlet, and you will need to create one.

The same goes for a preschool child. If she sat through your efforts to get the house in shape, waited while you made telephone calls, has been in and out of the car and the shopping cart, and behaved angelically at lunch with friends, you cannot expect her to be relaxed, happy and calm. She will also need an outlet—time for herself, to express herself, to let her natural energy flow. Just as adults need time for themselves, children need space and freedom to be themselves. Never expect adult behavior and self-control from a child. If she can learn appropriate behavior in certain situations, you've done a good job. The rest of the time, you need to gauge your expectations accordingly.

The concept of spirit

Children need space and peace in order to blossom and grow. They need understanding, compassion, freedom, love and unconditional acceptance. They need to feel good about themselves, to feel comfortable in their skins, happy with their lives and content with their lifestyles. They need to be able to find happiness in the world, and they need to be able to find peace within themselves.

Our children's lives are enormously overscheduled, and our expectations provide an intense pressure that can stunt their emotional and spiritual growth. In chapter 9 we look at the idea of a vital force—the living energy that animates us all. This forms part of the concept of spirit, which is as important to overall health as emotions and physical well-being.

Many of us have an instinctive understanding of spirit, a sense of our own life force and being. We may be sensitive to the energy of others, and aware of the impact of our own energy. As parents, we can witness the impact of negative energy on our children: a baby becomes anxious and cries when her mother is distressed; a child throws a temper tantrum when his father is rushed and under pressure. Many mothers claim that their children are most badly behaved when the mothers themselves do not feel they have the resources to cope—at the end of an exhausting day, in the lead-up to menstruation, while trying to get dinner and the house organized for guests. Did you ever stop to think that it is not the children who are the source of the problem? Parents transmit energy, negative and positive. When you are feeling calm, your children respond by acting calmly. If you are wound up, they will be too. Think of a birthday party where lots of little children share a communal high energy. It can take a great deal of time for your child to "come down" after exposure to this type of energy. If your child witnesses something shocking or negative (a parent being hurt or involved in an accident), a negative or fearful energy will pervade and have its effect on your child.

When we give out negative energy, we get it back. When we offer our children love and positive energy, they pass it on. Watch the effect of a positive encounter—the way energy has the effect of rippling outward. Smile at your child for no reason, and he will smile back. Smile at a stranger, and the same thing happens. Radiate peace and love, and your child will absorb it and pass it on. Spirit is all about having a positive energy that can transform your child's life into something positive and fruitful.

Spirit is a kind of life energy. Some people call it a soul or "the spirit," but you don't have to be religious to understand the concept that there is a unique and conscious entity that inhabits and animates the human form. Spirit is seen in terms of love and light and peace. It involves a fundamental personal belief and power, which affects the way your child lives his life on a daily basis. Spirit is what makes your child individual, and it is something that we all share.

Spiritual awareness involves self-knowledge and a fundamental acceptance of who we are. Encouraging your child to become aware of spirit is a path to peace. It is a kind of awakening or rediscovery. It is the place where your child can find peace and be secure. Drawing upon spirit, children can gain the ability to overcome obstacles, tolerate situations, discriminate between right and wrong, cooperate with others, and rediscover peace.

Your family and spirit

The family is the school of the spirit, a dynamic, changing, unfrozen set of relationships that provides the bedrock for growth, for self-understanding, for maturity and for life. The lessons learned within the family environment feed and nurture the spirit, allowing peace and love to blossom. On this basis, children go out into the world, and are able to share this peace and love. They'll be the kind of people that others find comfortable and energizing. They'll see good in the world, and they will want to be a part of it. They'll *create* good and happiness because they are good and happy themselves.

The family is the cornerstone of single culture in the world, and it is the basis upon which future generations are created. The happiness and unity of your family will have long-term ramifications on your child's future.

Think about your child's life. How much time is there for positive interactions, for personal growth? Most of us have allowed the stresses and technological advances of our modern lives to overwhelm the significance of our families. We build our households not around interactions, but around distractions: the television, the video, the stereo, the computer. These are the technologies that absorb our energies, and suck the life from our families. We no longer have the time to be a parent, a lover, a sibling or a child; we replace crucial relationships with toys, with material goods, with an overemphasis on "success," and with a noisy environment. Spirits need peace to grow and the warmth of a loving environment to develop.

Technology is a part of our lives. Few of us would want to live without it, but it is important that we create a balance in our children's lives. Television is an important way of keeping in touch with the world, and it is a part of popular culture. If your child is banned from watching television, she will be at a social disadvantage and she may become obsessed by not having or doing what everyone else is doing.

The key is balance. Time for technology and time for peace. Time for doing nothing and time for the PlayStation, the Game Boy or the computer. Keep your television off when your child is not watching it. Turn off the radio occasionally, and encourage a healthy silence. Watch television together as a family, using it as a source of discussion and interaction. Set guidelines in advance, as part of family rules, so everyone knows where they stand. Bend the rules for a special hockey game or program, but make it clear that it is an exceptional case. Never use your television as a baby-sitter. No child will benefit from being in contact with the television all day long, and they may pick up on things that are inappropriate for their level of development and maturity. Children grow by interaction, by watching, by learning through experience. This is seriously curtailed by focusing on only one activity, such as watching television, playing on a game console or sitting at a computer. Balance means using technology to help your child grow and develop where appropriate, but using other tools to teach and involve your child as well.

From dependence to independence, children need guidance and understanding to reach maturity. They need the interdependence of the family to achieve peace and self-knowledge. When stages of development are overlooked or underattended, you compromise your child's spiritual health, and unnecessary and negative elements enter the picture: fear, guilt, anger, loss of confidence and insecurity. If your whole household is too busy to register change and growth, to recognize changing needs, everyone will suffer. As parents, we need to pay close attention to our children's development, and to provide the appropriate stimulus, comfort and interaction that they need at every stage. Babying a child who is long past that stage will cramp his spirit; giving a young child too much freedom and responsibility will do the same. It's important to match your expectations and your lifestyle to the needs of your child, in order to ensure spiritual health.

▶ *Top tips for creating a spiritually healthy family life*

- Spend time together. If you can't manage it every day, block off time to be together as a unit. As children get older, they will want to have a say in activities and you should encourage this as part of their individuality.

- Try to eat at least one meal together every day. An alarming survey recently revealed that a large proportion of children *never* sit down with their families to eat.[2] Not only does this have enormous repercussions on nutrition (see page 93), but many children do not, as a result, have any time to interact with families— a crucial part of family life.

- Keep the atmosphere calm and loving. Every family member needs to ensure that he is dealing with negative elements in his life (dealing with stress, upset, trauma, emotional problems) to ensure that it does not impact on the family environment. As a unit, you can work together to ensure that every family member is happy and supported in times of trouble. The positive effect of that communal energy will have an overwhelming effect on a child or other family member with problems.

- Encourage time alone! Don't insist that your child be by your side for every moment of the day. Encourage responsibility and freedom (see page 196), and give time for growth and learning by experience and experimentation. Let her dig in the backyard, water the lawn, splash in the kitchen sink, read on her bed, make a magnificent snack, mess up the family room—have fun!

- Balancing work demands, time for taking care of ourselves, and time for relationships and family can be a juggling act of immense proportion. In a spiritually happy family, every member needs a voice. As a unit, you need regularly to determine your priorities and values. Regularly asking yourselves what is important in your life and why this is a good exercise in personal development. Then, compare these priorities and values to how you are living your lives. Set realistic goals and know your limits. No one has more than 24 hours each day in which to live, work, love, learn and rest. Trying to squeeze in too many activities and responsibilities usually means cheating someone or something else. Make time for the important things in life.

- Watch your child carefully for signs of emotional ill health, which will impact on his spiritual well-being (see page 170). If your lives are overscheduled, cut them back. If he isn't getting pleasure from his activities, change them or leave them altogether. If he's under pressure at school, talk to his teacher and make sure that your expectations are not compounding the problem. If he's generally unhappy or seems out of balance both physically and emotionally, consider using a suitable flower essence (see page 254) or homeopathic remedy (see page 268) to help.

- Take the emphasis off the material, and balance a technologically busy life with an appreciation of the natural world. Take walks together, watch a sunset, get a bird-feeder. There is an amazing world out there that your child can appreciate and grow through. The natural world is full of a vibrant energy that can help to restore spiritual weakness.

- Don't instill a desire for material possessions. Many people with nothing material are perfectly happy. Many parents struggle to give their children everything—the newest technology, trading cards, bikes, toys and games—at the expense of family life. As the old saying goes, the best things in life are free. Your child will benefit far more from your presence, affection and interaction than from a lot of material goods that keep you working all hours of the day and night. Professor Jonathan Bradshaw of York University has been studying the relationship between family wealth and a sense of mental well-being in children aged 11 to 15. The study measured poverty in a number of ways including income, lack of possessions and whether a family was on income support, and found that children's levels of sadness, worrying or happiness weren't affected by these variables. Professor Bradshaw said there was no doubt that poverty had a terrible effect on children, but he said it was not necessarily the most important factor when talking about children's mental health. "The key determinates of children's mental well-being are relationships with parents and peers, rather than the level of income they are living on," he said. This type of research confirms the fact that wealth does not equate with well-being. The well-being of three of the richest countries—Germany, Japan and the U.S.— is less than that of many less wealthy developed nations, such as Ireland, Finland and Australia. Furthermore, surveys have consistently found little change over time, despite increases in wealth. The U.S., for example, is much richer than it was in the mid-1900s, yet about the same numbers say they are happy today as then. What we are seeing is the fact that material possessions do not equate to happiness, and there's no reason to believe that children are any different.

- Encourage friendships in your children, and welcome their friends to your home. Children need experience in dealing with their peers, and they learn how to be themselves in the company of others. Children should be encouraged to be self-aware in order to have confidence in themselves. Peers and friends are an important part of this process, as children will be faced with new and different situations in which they must use their own resources. Remember that human beings cannot truly live happily in isolation. Your child may eventually choose a relatively solitary path, but it is still his relationships with others that will largely define the quality of his life. Ultimately the health of all of your child's relationships depends upon his relationship with himself—his spiritual awareness.

Parental time

Leisure time and levels of stress are inversely proportional—the less leisure, the more stress. Stress-reduction experts ask patients to fill in a chart to see what their work/leisure ratio looks like. They are asked to think of their lives (excluding sleep time) in four compartments (work, family, community and self) and then to assess what percentage of their time and energy in an average week goes into each part. There is cause for concern when work is over 60 percent and/or when self is less than 10 percent. It's hard to be a giving parent if you never get anything for your self. Self-directed activities can include exercise or recreation, relaxation, socializing, entertainment and hobbies.

Having time to yourself decreases stress levels, making you a more confident and relaxed parent, so the whole family will benefit.

Creativity and spirit

Your child's mind is a wonderful workshop of imagination and creativity. If she is given freedom to explore her creativity, she will gain confidence and develop the art of being original. By being creative, children are able to express the most fundamental aspects of their being.

Does your child have any scope for creativity in her life? Is there time to muse, to think, to explore and to experiment? Are her questions, suggestions and views given your full attention and validated? Does she have time to draw and paint, or to listen to music, or tinker on the piano?

Creativity is essential to spirit. It is an outpouring of conscious and unconscious thought that represents our children's most basic instincts, beliefs, emotions and concerns. If we stifle creativity in our children, we stifle their most important outlet. Creativity is a kind of rapport with the outside world that doesn't necessarily require words.

Don't be tempted to force the creative process. Children are most creative when they are given time and space and freedom. Offer the tools—music, books, paper, pens, paint, clay—and allow the time. Leave the rest to your child. Praise his efforts, ask questions about what he is saying, showing or doing. Encourage an outpouring of effort. There is no question that creativity (music and art, for example) can have a dramatic effect on overall health (see page 247), and part of that effect is due to its spiritual implications. When a child has a vehicle for self-expression, and the confidence and encouragement to use it, his creativity will grow with the light of his spirit.

Personal freedom

The message of this last part of the chapter is about space and time to grow. Another aspect of this idea involves personal freedom—giving your child some responsibility for his own life on a day-to-day basis. Everyone needs some control over her environment. Think of how you, as an adult, feel when you experience powerlessness. For example, you may be in financial difficulties. Your bank refuses to help and you have creditors pounding on your door. You feel powerless and frightened. You may feel angry and rebellious. You may even feel trapped and depressed. Whatever you feel, you can bet that your child feels much the same when she is given no freedom or when she has no power over her life.

Giving personal freedom involves allowing your child to do things that are appropriate for his age and his level of maturity. At some stage we all have to let go of our children—let them take that first walk to the shops on their own, take a bus ride or a bicycle ride by themselves, drive a car, light the fire, cook a meal, use a sharp knife. As parents we need to assess when the time is right, and to offer our children some freedom. With freedom comes a sense of responsibility.

We've already discussed empowering children in their daily lives by giving them choices. Taking this one step further, we need to give them freedom.

▶ *Top tips for giving your children freedom*

- In every part of their day, offer some time that is their own. Allow them to choose what they want to do and let them do it. Give them choices (within the confines of a safe family environment, with household rules) and give them the freedom to enact them.

Are you living through your child?

As parents, we may become dependent upon our children for our own self-worth. We may not encourage their spirits to flourish or their individuality to develop. They bear the weight of our expectations, our need for success, our misspent dreams, our concerns about reputations and appearances. We suffocate their spirits by trapping them within the confines of our own insecurities. In extreme cases, we love our children not for who they are, but for what they achieve, and what we want them to be.

If parents radiate competition and expectation, children believe this is the right way to live. Children compete for parental attention, reflecting the values of their parents and the lessons they have demonstrated to those children at a very early age. This is a breeding ground for conflict, separation, argument and the breakdown of the ability to connect, to cooperate, to be united and to love.

Let your child be himself. Accept his strengths and his shortcomings and celebrate his uniqueness. Filling his life with piano lessons and sports if he hates them will not encourage healthy growth or happiness. Pressuring your child to do well at school when he clearly isn't a shining star will do nothing but pass on dissatisfaction, which will compound the situation. Our society places too much emphasis on the trappings of success, and children have become a sort of accessory. We tend to believe that if we have a clever, bright, athletic, musical child, we are OK parents. You may have a child who is a little star, but the credit for those achievements belongs to him. Let him bask in his own light. On the other hand, your child may not be academically brilliant or good at anything in particular. Don't try to re-create him. He may never go to university, but he may be a great people person. Reanalyze your interpretation of success. Health and happiness are the best things we can want for our children, and they do not have to be the best in order to achieve those things.

Think carefully about what you didn't do as a child, at places where you feel that you were not encouraged to be a success. Are you using your child to fulfill those dreams? If you never made the hockey team and always wanted to be the school's athletic hero, are you hoping that your child will take your place and do it for you? If you never went to university, and failed to find a job that you enjoyed, are you assuming that education is the key to your child's long-term happiness? Pushing a child into a mold that does not fit can damage his self-image, his self-esteem and his future. Let him be himself, and take pleasure in his individuality.

- Assess your child's readiness for responsibility by giving small bits of freedom and see how he manages. Don't present it as a "test" though. Big years for change developmentally are 3, 6, 9 and 12, so try looking at his life at these points especially and perhaps once a year in between to decide what new freedoms to offer. Allow him to walk alone to a friend's house when you feel he is ready. Allow him to choose what he wants to eat occasionally. Teach him how to cross the road and let him do it on his own. Teach him to use a knife, and give him space (and a recipe book) to make a family dinner. Give him a watch and send him off to the park with friends, telling him what is expected and when you need him to be home.

- Parenting involves teaching children to behave maturely in every situation. Giving an immature child freedom for which she is not ready will not encourage growth. She'll probably feel frightened, out of control or confused. The point is to assess your child's individual capabilities, and to offer freedoms appropriate for that. It doesn't mean sending a child out unarmed into the wide world. It means providing, as your child grows, the tools for coping, and then giving her some space to experiment.

- Give your child a little of his own money and encourage him to choose what he does with it. Money teaches responsibility (see below) and offers a little freedom in which to make decisions. Too much money can encourage materialism, but as money is a part of our world, like it or not, he will need to get used to dealing with it and it can offer him a little personal power.

- Give responsibility. Get a pet and make it your child's own responsibility. Buy a plant, or give your child a section of the garden to call her own. Leave her in charge of a younger sibling for ten minutes while you make a telephone call. Responsibility encourages emotional and spiritual growth. It encourages children to use their own resources in order to cope. If you smother your child and withdraw her responsibility, reducing her time for freedom to suit your own schedule, she will never learn to rely upon herself, to take pleasure in her own achievements, to feel the glow of completing or looking after something successfully. She will never learn to make her own decisions, and when she does leave home, she will not have the confidence she needs to find a path that will lead to happiness and well-being.

Whatever your job, wherever you live and no matter how many children you have, your children's needs must be considered and addressed. No one has ever claimed that being a parent is an easy job, and in many ways, looking after children's emotional and spiritual health is much more difficult than anything involved on a physical level. But these are the elements that are most crucial to your child's future—his happiness, his success, his ability to relax, to integrate with others and to achieve a sense of well-being and satisfaction with himself and his life. If nothing else, remember the following: children learn what they live.

Part Two
Illness and Natural Health

chapter nine

Understanding Illness

Over the past decades we have become universally fearful and intolerant of pain, symptoms of illness and ill health. There are hundreds of thousands of products now available to suppress virtually every symptom we may experience, and even the most health-conscious of us expect to see instant results from complementary therapies or remedies. This is the age of the quick-fix solution, and if it isn't quick and efficient, we complain. No one has time for anything less than perfection these days. And, most worryingly, this ideology has been extended to health and health care.

When we have a headache, we pop a pill. When our children have a fever, we dole out a syrup or fruit-flavored pill that brings it down immediately. Runny noses, diarrhea, coughs, colds, flu—there's a symptom-snuffer for everything. The end result? Good health is equated with feeling good—or, rather, not feeling bad—with little regard for what may be going on underneath the surface.

The importance of illness

There are many misconceptions about illness, and few of us really understand why it is important. Here are the main issues:

- Illness is good for us. Taking it one step further, good health is not a complete absence of illness. Obviously no one wants to suffer from debilitating symptoms, but illness works to build up the body's immunity, making us stronger and better able to deal with infections. This is particularly important for children, who are born with immature immune systems that need to develop through illness. Many illnesses are also cleansing; they provide the body with an opportunity to offload built-up toxins. Measles is a good example of this type of detoxifying illness, but a simple cold will do much the same thing.

- What we consider to be "illnesses" are, in fact, symptoms. Headaches, skin rashes, fever, runny nose, coughs are all symptoms that indicate our body is working to fight off disease. The rise in body temperature that we call fever helps to create an inhospitable environment for viral or bacterial invaders; it also stimulates the production of disease-fighting white blood cells. Diarrhea indicates that the body is flushing unwanted substances from the body. The sneezing and runny nose that accompany a cold show that the inflammatory response is in action: mucus is produced in order to discharge a virus from the respiratory tract.

- Symptoms also point to underlying imbalances. Chronic catarrh, for example, might reflect a food allergy; recurrent headaches may point to a toxic overload or high stress levels that need to be addressed. We need to welcome these messages from the body, for they are the only means by which we will know when things are going wrong.

- Taking medicines and remedies that suppress symptoms (in other words, make us feel better without addressing the cause of the symptoms) is the equivalent of turning off a smoke detector in a burning house. The noise has abated, but the fire is still burning. You can relieve the pain of a headache, but whatever is causing the pain still exists. You can suppress your child's cough, but you will be preventing the body from naturally expelling bacterial or viral invaders. Hydrocortisone cream will ease the inflammation and itching of eczema, but it has done nothing to treat the cause of the condition. Many natural health practitioners believe that suppressing symptoms drives them deeper, making conditions chronic and less treatable—by any means.

Emotional factors

Illness is more than just a series of physical symptoms. There is a great deal more involved in ill health than what is going on in the body. It's important to understand that emotional, spiritual and physical health go hand in hand—that's the underlying premise of the holistic revolution. We are more than the sum of our physical parts, and optimum well-being is based on three distinct elements: mind, body and spirit. We looked at emotional and spiritual health in chapter 8, and will focus here on how to keep our children healthy on a physical level. But the importance of these two other areas cannot be underplayed.

As adults, we can often sense when we are becoming ill—we may become irritable, emotional or tearful. We will also succumb to illness more readily during periods of stress, or following a trauma, such as a bereavement or a divorce.

The vital force

One of the main differences between conventional and natural medicine is the approach to health. Conventional practitioners treat illness as a biological or chemical malfunction of the body. The main premise of conventional medicine is that curing disease will lead to good health, ignoring the fact that pathology is individual to the sufferer, and that each of us is unique. For example, tonsillitis would be treated with antibiotics in most cases; asthma with Ventolin, steroids or the equivalent; eczema with hydrocortisone cream or another suppressive remedy. A few lifestyle changes might be suggested, but by and large the treatment offered is aimed at the average child (or adult), not the individual.

Natural practitioners believe that there is something more afoot than simply a physical diagnosis of disease. Indeed, the many elements of health—the mind, body and spirit—are taken into consideration when treating children suffering from virtually any health condition, at any level. But more than that, there is a belief in a vital or "life" force.

Different therapies and disciplines have a variety of names for this force: spirit or energy, for example. But the concept remains the same. It is the body's controlling energy. It vitalizes the physical body, and it is the link between the body, soul and mind. It directs all aspects of life: it animates our emotional life, provides thoughts and creativity and conducts spiritual inspiration. It makes us different beyond physiology.

There are well-known physical processes that keep our bodies alive, including the immune system, the brain and nervous system and the endocrine system. These are important on a physical level, and are crucial to maintaining the body's equilibrium. However, they are not the only level of functioning. Equally important is the guiding mechanism. Some complementary medical disciplines believe that energy flows through our bodies, and that illness or "dis-ease" is caused by blockages and imbalance. Others believe that it is simply a governing force that can be weakened by environmental factors (diet, trauma, stress, pollution, sleep, for example), so that it can no longer keep the whole body (that is, mind, body and spirit) balanced.

The vital force is not a material substance, such as water or air, but it is equally indispensable for life. Its presence distinguishes living things from inanimate matter. When illness occurs, it appears first as a disturbance in this natural energy long before it manifests itself as physical symptoms. This is why children appear grumpy, tired or out of sorts for some time before symptoms actually appear.

The fact that conventional medicine has not conquered illness, or indeed prevented it to any great degree, is ample proof that biology and chemistry are not enough. Most doctors will admit that the majority of medicines on the market are palliative—in other words, they make us feel better. Prozac, doesn't, for example, prevent depression. It merely makes the sufferer feel better. Ventolin doesn't make asthma go away; it allows the sufferer to breathe. Anti-Inflammatories will reduce inflammation, but when medication ceases, the condition will return.

The concept of a vital force is not New Age dogma. Many of the most ancient therapies are based on the existence of a vital energy flow. Western medicine was until fairly recently in agreement that there is an animating force, but as the focus became more scientific, the idea of a vital energy was largely dispensed with. However, the huge wealth of material amassed by scientists into the functioning of the human body is all true and correct, and they do not by any means contradict the idea of the vital force. Physical and chemical mechanisms are merely tools of the vital force, which act upon the physical plane of the body.

The concept of the vital force also helps to explain the differences between us—why some children are more susceptible to environmental factors than others. For example, some children may sail through school and exams, do well at sports and appear to suffer fewer health problems than their peers, despite inadequate sleep, a poor diet and the pressures of a competitive school or home environment. Others are knocked sideways by a spat in the playground, need hours of sleep, eat well, yet become ill more frequently and are more easily upset by something that another child would take in his stride.

Obviously, it's more complicated than this. There are inherited predispositions to illness and other elements afoot. However, the vital force is one of the most important—and oft-overlooked—elements of health and well-being. Some of the most successful treatments for conditions that cannot be cured by conventional medicine are those that address health on a holistic level, taking into consideration the mind, body and spirit, and working with the body's own energy to encourage healing.

Energy medicine

Natural remedies work on an energy level. They direct a child's energy and vitality toward healing so that she overcomes the problem naturally. They don't heal, in the same way that we might expect if we took a conventional drug, and they don't pretend to do so. Instead, natural remedies encourage the body to heal itself, by operating on a level that is above the physical. For this reason they may take longer to work, and your child won't experience an immediate relief of symptoms. She will, however, be healed on a much deeper level and experience much better overall health as a result. Many herbs and vitamins work on a physical level as well—supporting vital organs, acting as natural antibiotics or antiviral agents, for example, or even encouraging the body's natural response to illness. But the similarities between conventional medicine and natural medicine end here. Fundamental to almost every single therapy and remedy is the concept of a vital force. It's the ultimate defense mechanism, and it makes it possible for all of our other physical and emotional defenses to work. You can make a big difference to your child's overall health by ensuring that her energy level, and her vital force, is strong.

The mind-body relationship isn't the paragon of alternative medicine alone—there are literally hundreds of scientific studies that show how closely the two are linked.

Why is this important for children? We often overlook the importance of emotional health in our children. We accept that temper tantrums or crying spells or periods of sleepiness or hyperactivity are normal. We say, "He's just being difficult" or "She's hard work at the moment," rarely considering this a health issue. Instead, we should learn to read these as an indication that there is an imbalance on some level. Most parents know that a child who suddenly becomes tearful, angry or even depressed for no obvious reason is heading for illness. In fact, this negative emotional state is very much a part of the impending illness, and presents part of the picture of your child's overall health.

When there is an emotional imbalance, physical health can be affected. Similarly, physical health can impact emotional health. These factors are inextricably intertwined and as parents we need to learn to recognize changes in our children's emotional health in order to see the "whole picture."

The healing power of illness

Even healthy children need to become ill. Illness builds up the immune system, making our children stronger and more able to fight off infections of all sorts in the future. Adults are more prone to colds and other illnesses when they are stressed, anxious or depressed. Children, on the other hand, usually succumb because their immune systems are immature. Having said, that, however, every child is individual, and his ability to fight off illness will reflect his overall health—that is, his health on every level.

Bodies are designed to heal themselves, and given the opportunity they will do so. When a healthy child comes into contact with bacteria, viruses or other disease-causing agents, her immune system will respond by attacking the invader. A healthy child will present the symptoms of an acute illness—that means a high fever and probably rather dramatic symptoms, such as pain, a rash, diarrhea, a cough or a streaming nose. The difference between a healthy and a less healthy child, however, is that these symptoms will be short and sharp; they will be intense, but they will be short-lived. When the vital force is strong (see page 203), a child may be aggressive, extremely irritable, inconsolable, red cheeked or frightened when ill. Whatever the symptoms, they will be extreme and they will pass as quickly as they came. While these dramatic symptoms can be alarming for parents, and all parents should be on the alert for serious health conditions that require immediate attention, such as meningitis (see page 368), this type of reaction is, in fact, healthy.

Less healthy children—again, on an emotional or physical level—will show less dramatic symptoms. For example, colds come on slowly and seem to take weeks to pass. Fever is lower or nonexistent, there may be dull pains or aches with no distinct cause, and your child may prefer to curl up alone, seeming vacant and dreamy. The illness in this case is no more serious, but it indicates that your child's health could be improved by addressing both physical and emotional causes—and by boosting the vital force, your child's fundamental energy.

Our bodies are constantly under attack, from chemicals in food, air and water, and from stress, free radicals, parasites, hostile bacteria and even the UV rays of the sun. If they weren't programmed to fight invaders, we would all be constantly ill. In fact, our bodies do not succumb until there is a weakness present. That weakness can be caused by emotional factors (stress, aggression, jealousy, fear or any other negative emotion) that needs to be addressed, or it can be caused by physical factors, such as inadequate sleep, overwork (using resources that should be employed by the immune and other systems of the body), being run-down after a series of illnesses, a poor diet, overexertion or a combination of these things. There doesn't need to be any dramatic cause for a weakened state—in fact, many parents will notice that their children are more susceptible to illness at the end of the school year, or during an exciting holiday period, or after exams.

What we need to do is to recognize the causes of weakness, and ensure that our children are as strong and healthy as they can be by taking steps to boost their immune systems naturally, by ensuring that they are emotionally well, and addressing aberrations when they appear, also, of course, by making sure that they eat well, get lots of sleep, rest appropriately and get enough exercise.

When illness strikes, we need to take steps to work with the vital force, or our child's natural energy levels, to ensure that he fights it off quickly and efficiently. Don't be tempted to bang symptoms on the head with over-the-counter drugs. You'll mask the symptoms and it will be much more difficult to get to the root of whatever is causing the problems. Furthermore, constantly suppressing symptoms will drive illness deeper into the body, and many practitioners believe that this causes much more serious problems, where vital organs are affected. Interestingly, people who are seriously unwell—those suffering from cancer, for example, often don't present symptoms of colds or other common illnesses. The vital force has been weakened at a fundamental level, and is working much deeper in the body—at organ level, perhaps. Symptoms are a good sign, meaning that a healthy vital force is working hard to maintain health.

Let their bodies do the work

Bodies are miraculous things. They spontaneously heal cuts, bruises, burns and fractures. They sense an invader (bacteria, for example), and a rigorous defense mechanism is deployed to fight it off. More importantly, perhaps, our bodies have the capacity to remember illnesses, which makes us immune in future. All the while our bodies carry out their normal functions: developing, thinking, growing, renewing, excreting, pumping blood and digesting, while we work, exercise, play, rest or sleep.

What we do when we bombard our children's bodies with medicines of any nature is to damp down their natural healing mechanism. Instead of using the body's natural energy—its vital force—to heal, we remove symptoms, thereby "shooting the messenger"; we stop the processes that are part of the immune defense system (a cough or diarrhea, for example); and we introduce chemicals into the body that add to its toxic overload, disrupt the natural balance and, indeed, cause other illnesses.

Everyone is unique. We are all predisposed to various types of illnesses, we all have weaknesses and we all react differently to external stimuli. It's extraordinarily arrogant to believe that one medicine or treatment will cure everyone, and yet the majority of our conventional medical system is aimed at doing just that.

Boost your child's immune system

The immune system is the physical defense mechanism of the body, and it's important that it is working at optimum level to protect your child from infections and infestations, and to ensure that he heals quickly and efficiently when he does succumb to illness.

Immunity is affected by a variety of different factors, including:

- poor or inadequate sleep

- a poor diet (see page 3)

- stress (emotional, physical or environmental)

- overuse of antibiotics (see page 211)

- some drugs (including, according to a new study,[1] overuse of acetaminophen)

- exposure to toxins, including cigarette smoke, car exhaust fumes, household chemicals and anything else that requires the body to work harder

- emotional factors (including depression, unhappiness, fear, jealousy and any other negative emotional states)

- injuries

- chronic illness

- digestive disorders, such as candida, enzyme deficiencies and chronic constipation

- surgery

- overexertion

The immune system and, indeed, every other system in your child's body works more effectively when external factors are under control. In other words, ensuring that drugs and antibiotics are kept to a minimum, she eats good, fresh food and sleeps well, she takes some exercise and she is happy will do a great deal to boost immunity.

There are also a number of natural remedies and therapies designed to boost immunity, and even the healthiest children will benefit from their prudent use. The idea is not to work on immunity when your child becomes ill, but to ensure that her immune system is strong and healthy enough to resist illness, and to fight it off quickly when she does become ill. This is one of the most important aspects of preventive medicine, which is the cornerstone of the natural health revolution.

Signs of a weakened immune system

- Fatigue

- Listlessness

- Repeated infections (if your child has more than about four a year, his immune system could use a boost)

- Inflammation

- Allergic reactions

- Slow wound healing

- Chronic diarrhea

- Infections that represent an overgrowth of some normally present organisms, such as oral thrush, candida or, in girls, vaginal yeast infections

▶ Top immune-boosters

- Help your child to learn to relax and to talk about problems instead of bottling them up. Emotional health is inextricably linked to the immune response. If you see a change in your child's emotional health, try to get to the root of it. Bach flower remedies and some of the other flower essences are designed to balance negative emotions and they are a gentle, effective boost for children (see page 254). If your child is under a great deal of stress, make sure he gets enough exercise and has enough time and space to be himself. Be on the lookout for stress, and take steps to deal with it (see page 386).

- Create an environment that supports rather than puts pressure on the body. That means getting rid of some of the more toxic elements of your environment, including household chemicals and smoke (see page 142).

- If your child is chronically ill, consider seeing a homeopath in the first instance. This type of gentle medicine is ideal for children and even babies, and will work to address imbalances on all levels (see page 267).

- Breastfeed your baby. Breastmilk contains lymphocytes and macrophages that produce antibodies and other immune factors. It provides lactobacillus bifidus, the "friendly" bacteria that helps prevent the growth of dangerous bacteria. Another molecule in breastmilk actually kills harmful bacteria. In addition to providing protection against pathogenic bacteria, breastmilk contains elements that guard against viruses, fungi and parasites.

- Make sure your child washes his hands before meals, and after contact with other children who are ill. Although there is some evidence that we need "dirt" in order to build up immunity to germs (one study indicates that asthma may be on the increase because of our overzealous attempts to keep our children clean with anti-bacterial and other products), when your child is run-down, or when there is a great deal of illness about, you can prevent the spread by keeping hands clean.

- Watch your child's diet. We've already established the link between immune problems and diet, but many parents are unaware that a diet high in sugar and fat is one of the most powerful immune suppressers. Sugar consumption, especially of refined white sugar, dramatically inhibits immune function by reducing the ability of neutrophils to engulf and destroy bacteria. Neutrophils are white blood cells primarily responsible for defense against bacteria. The high sugar content in their diets means that most children have chronically depressed immune systems.

- Vitamin C is essential for the formation of the adrenal hormones and the production of white blood cells, which fight off disease. It also has a direct effect on bacteria and viruses. Indeed, a number of studies show that viruses in particular cannot survive in an environment that is high in vitamin C. Vitamin C has recently received bad press, being linked with a thickening of the arteries that may lead to heart disease, but this research is being hotly disputed and there are literally hundreds of studies that show a dramatic improvement in the immune response. The best way to get vitamin C is through a healthy diet, but supplementation is almost always necessary in our modern world. Don't overdose, but offer a good vitamin C supplement daily.

- If anyone in the house is a smoker, extra vitamin C is necessary. The same goes for children living in areas of high pollution.

- Echinacea boosts the immune system and enhances lymphatic function. It also has some antiviral properties, which can help the body to keep infection at bay. It's safe for kids, but read the label carefully. There are products specially designed for children, in fruit-flavored drops or pills. Studies show that it works best when taken on a slightly irregular basis (three or four times a week) in the lead-up to illness (when your child seems unsettled, unusually sleepy, off his food, tearful or irritable), through the duration of the illness and for a couple of weeks afterward. During the cold season, use once or twice a week.[2]

- Consider an acidophilus supplement. By increasing the "friendly" bacteria in the gut, your child is better able to absorb nutrients from food. Acidophilus also produces vitamins, some essential fatty acids (EFAs) and other helpful substances, which form part of the immune defense. Finally, healthy bacteria is one of the body's natural defense mechanisms, keeping fungi, unhealthy bacteria and other "invaders" in check. There are acidophilus pills designed for children, but if your child hates pills, go for one of the powders, which can be mixed with food or drinks.

- Every child will benefit from EFAs, now dangerously deficient in our diets. Try flaxseed oil (dribbled on foods or whizzed in the blender with orange juice), which is high in crucial omega-3 oils. EFAs are converted into substances that decrease inflammation and improve the function of the nervous and immune systems. They also work to affect mood, which is crucial to healthy immunity. Evening primrose oil, pumpkin seed oil and borage oil are also good sources of EFAs.

- Stress reduces many nutrients in our bodies—in particular, the B vitamins. It may seem ludicrous to suggest that children suffer debilitating stress, but there are many cases where this is so. If your child finds exams, a house move, school, homework, friendships, relationships or almost anything else difficult to cope with, or if he is undergoing a particularly traumatic time, such as a parental divorce or bereavement, he may well need some extra vitamins. B vitamins work together, so don't try supplementing any one at a time, unless recommended by a nutritionist. A good multivitamin or mineral pill should adequately cover the B vitamins, but for children over the age of six, a B-complex vitamin of 10 to 25 mg a day is an acceptable level at which to supplement.

- Vitamin A is one of the most important immune-boosting nutrients, working to strengthen many of the "first line defenses," such as skin, lungs and the digestive tract. A good multivitamin and mineral pill for children will contain adequate vitamin A, but vitamin A (in the form of beta-carotene) occurs naturally in brightly colored fruits and vegetables.

- Aloe vera has many immune-boosting properties, and is a good tonic, particularly in children who seem to be constantly under the weather. It is, however, very powerful, and should not be used in children under the age of about six. Read the label carefully to ensure that the product you choose is appropriate for children and follow the instructions. There are now products specifically designed for children.

- Garlic contains allicin, a chemical that is antiviral, antibacterial and antifungal. It is one of the best herbs available for fighting infection, and studies show that a garlic-rich diet helps to prevent cancer.[3] Try to add some garlic to your child's diet every day. Fresh is best, but if your child objects, choose one of the odorless capsules and drizzle over pastas or other savory dishes.

- Zinc is one of the most important minerals for immune health, and many children are deficient, particularly those who are picky eaters. Lozenges and chewable pills are available for children, or buy it in drop form and add to drinks at mealtimes.

- Don't forget the spices! Many of the more pungent herbs have antiseptic, antiparasitic, antifungal and other properties. Consider adding some of the following to your child's diet regularly: cloves, aniseed, cayenne, cinnamon and ginger, all of which have a beneficial effect on the immune system.

- Picrorrhiza, an Indian herb used in Ayurvedic medicine, is a powerful immuno-stimulant that boosts all aspects of immune function. It's safe for children, and can be added to food or drink to make it more palatable.

- Astragalus acts as a tonic to protect the immune system. Studies show that it increases metabolism, produces spontaneous sweating, promotes healing and provides energy to combat fatigue. It's particularly good for colds, flu and immune-deficiency-related problems, including cancer, AIDS and even tumors. There is also some evidence that it's effective in the case of chronic lung weakness. Never offer astragalus in the presence of fever, and always read the label.

- All children will benefit from a good antioxidant, which protects the body from free radical damage, environmental stresses and pollutants. The main antioxidants are vitamins A, C and E, and the minerals zinc and selenium. Make sure these appear in your child's multivitamin, or look for antioxidant pills prepared specially for kids.

Antibiotics

Natural medicine can have a dramatic effect on health at every level, but there are times when a struggling system needs extra help. Modern medicine offers many miracles, and one of the most effective of those is antibiotics. There is no doubt that in the case of serious illness, antibiotics can help your child to fight off an infection that she might not be able to resist naturally. The problem is that antibiotics have been and continue to be overused.

One of the key messages of this book is that a great deal of healing can take place at home. Doctors and the entire medical system are there for emergencies and cases of genuine, serious ill health. The best way to avoid ill health is prevention—boosting the immune system, ensuring that your child eats properly and has a healthy lifestyle. A child in optimum health will resist the majority of infections, but when she cannot, there are a variety of conventional treatments to fall back upon. Don't assume that antibiotics are a cure-all. They work for bacterial infections alone. They'll do nothing for a cold, for instance, or flu, or the majority of viruses that strike without warning. Several studies show that doctors often give in and prescribe antibiotics because parents demand them.

Don't fall into that trap. Many conditions can be safely treated with natural remedies, including ear infections, sore throats, tonsillitis, many types of gastroenteritis, colds, flu and much, much more. If your child is in severe pain, or seems very unwell, and antibiotics are indicated, by all means accept them, but always use them as a last resort. Here's why:

- Inappropriate antibiotic use is a major factor in the growing problem of bacterial resistance, where bacteria no longer respond to treatment with a particular antibiotic. This is a trend that may be more serious than we think. Because bacteria evolve quickly (every 20 minutes), they quickly become resistant to overuse of antibacterial agents—in particular antibiotics. This has led to strains of "superbugs," resistant to virtually every known antibiotic. Strains of resistant bacteria are almost always found in hospitals, where the heavy use of antibiotics makes them far more likely to evolve.

- Drug resistance is also allowing the return of a disease doctors believed had almost been consigned to the history books. Multi-drug-resistant tuberculosis is now a serious public health problem in countries such as Russia and in deprived inner-city areas in the U.S. and U.K. In Russia, doctors, finding all antibiotics useless against the illness, have resorted to surgery—cutting out the infected lung tissue—to halt the spread of the disease.

- Prescription broad spectrum antibiotics, especially when taken for extended periods of time, wipe out all the gut-friendly bacteria that provide protection against fungi and amoebic (parasitic) infections, help the body break down complex foods and synthesize vitamins like B12 and biotin. When the friendly bowel flora is killed off, the body has no local defense against parasites or fungi that are normally held in check. These then quickly develop and may trigger the signs and symptoms of arthritis, eczema, migraines, asthma or other forms of immune dysfunction. Other common symptoms of this bowel flora imbalance are bloating and gas after meals, and alternating constipation and diarrhea.

- Side effects of antibiotics are common, and they include diarrhea, skin rashes (some children come out in a severe rash a few days after starting a course of antibiotics), phlegm (when an infection is treated with antibiotics, excess mucus is produced and left behind. In some children this is dispersed naturally, but in others, it provides a breeding ground for bacteria, which causes a secondary infection), thrush and digestive disorders.

- Finally, antibiotics work by doing the body's job for it, which means that the immune system is not strengthened by repeated contact with infection. Suppressing childhood illness can lead to a weak immune system in adulthood. The trick is to help an ill child recover quickly and with the least amount of discomfort without suppressing the immune system.

Remember that antibiotics may kill infecting organisms, but the imbalance in the body that allowed infection to set in will still be present. In other words, your child's condition will be the same after the course of antibiotics as it was before the illness. If antibiotics are necessary, use nutritional, herbal or homeopathic remedies alongside, and continue to use them after your child seems to have recovered. This will ensure that the underlying imbalance is rectified, and will help to restore and rejuvenate, to prevent illness from recurring in the future.

Vaccination[4]

Every parent must be aware of the facts before making the decision to vaccinate her child. Although that might seem like a theoretical right, it's worth understanding the issues involved.

There is an intensifying debate into the safety of broadscale vaccination. In the U.K., many parents have made the choice not to vaccinate, or to only partly vaccinate their children. This "revolt" is, on a smaller scale, also taking place in the U.S. and Canada. Those in favor of immunization are aghast at this growing trend. Should you vaccinate your child? Here are the main features of the argument.

The importance of immunization

According to the Centers for Disease Control (CDC), vaccination is responsible for the broadscale eradication of childhood illnesses that would, and can, cause enormous suffering and even death.

Many experts believe that vaccination is one of the greatest success stories of modern medicine. As recently as the late 1980s, measles killed 17 British children in what was described as a relatively minor outbreak, which only hints at the destructive power of the virus that has been largely forgotten by the U.K. public. Indeed, the World Health Organization (WHO) claims that without MMR (mumps, measles and rubella) immunization world-wide, around three million children would die each year. According to the CDC, immunization against infectious disease has been highly successful and, in areas where there has been a good acceptance rate, has led to a large reduction in the incidence of diseases such as diphtheria, measles, German measles (rubella), poliomyelitis and whooping cough (pertussis).

So what is vaccination?

Vaccination prepares our bodies to fight against diseases to which we may come into contact in the future. Vaccination against polio, for example, stimulates the immune system to produce antibodies against the polio virus. These antibodies recognize the disease if and when it enters the body at a later date and are ready to fight it. Some types of immunization, such as those that work against polio, measles, mumps and rubella and against diphtheria, pertussis and tetanus (DTaP), are aimed at the general population, primarily at young children. Others are intended for specific people, such as those exposed to dangerous infections during local outbreaks. In many countries, including the U.S. (but not the U.K.), immunization against certain infections is a requirement for entry to school.

To keep the incidence of these diseases low, routine immunization must continue. If a large proportion of the population is not vaccinated, there is always risk of a new epidemic.

Disease decline

According to the pro-immunization front, the incidence of the diseases vaccinated against have decreased dramatically since the introduction of vaccines. Government bodies claim that these diseases became rare only after the vaccines were introduced, and they claim that this can occur only when a country has high vaccine coverage, such as in the U.S. and Canada. In the absence of immunization, these diseases would become common again, and would cause significant amounts of serious illness and potentially some deaths. For example, in the 1970s, when there was a loss of confidence in the whooping cough vaccine, and coverage fell, there were three major epidemics of whooping cough, with thousands of children being admitted to the hospital. When the vaccine coverage rose again, whooping cough declined. This situation occurred in Sweden, Japan and the U.K.

In response to the question of continuing to immunize against diseases that are on the decrease, the CDC says that these diseases remain common in many parts of the world and, if the uptake of vaccine falls, the diseases would return in the future.

The effect of decreased vaccine coverage was witnessed in Russia, which once had a well-established vaccine program where a high proportion of children were immunized. Following the dissolution of the U.S.S.R., shortages of vaccine and indifference to the need for immunization led to a dramatic fall in coverage. Since then there has been a huge epidemic of diphtheria, causing more than 125,000 cases and 4,000 deaths. The CDC claims that the only time to stop immunizing children is when a disease has been eradicated worldwide. When every country had eliminated smallpox, all countries stopped immunization.

Natural disease or vaccine?

The U.S. Department of Health and Human Services says that in most cases the immunity given by vaccinations appears to be long-lasting and effective. Government experts concede, however, that vaccines are not 100 percent effective—for example, in the case of the MMR (measles, mumps and rubella) vaccine, 5 to 10 percent of vaccines do not work, which is why a booster shot is recommended.

The problem with immunity that follows a natural illness is that the child has to have had the disease. Their message is clear: childhood illnesses can and do kill, despite the benefits of modern medicine. If a child doesn't suffer any complications, his immunity will be strong. If he does suffer complications, there is a risk of death and disablement. One study also suggests that natural measles actually damages the immune system, an effect not seen in children who have had the measles vaccine. Furthermore, there is now evidence that unimmunized children of immunized parents have much lower immunity to childhood diseases. In other words, the immunity of the population at large is lower, and the effects of a new epidemic could potentially cause mass fatalities.

Killer diseases

Apart from the usual symptoms, there are a variety of serious complications that can accompany most of the diseases currently vaccinated against. For example:

- Measles can kill, but is more likely to lead to serious complications, particularly in the very young. These can include pneumonia or bronchitis, convulsions and even meningitis.

- Mumps, characterized by painful and swollen glands in the head and neck, can cause permanent damage to the testicles, nervous system and hearing. Mumps contracted during pregnancy can lead to miscarriage.

- Rubella seems to be one of the most worrying illnesses. If a pregnant woman comes in contact with this disease during pregnancy, her baby can be born deaf and/or blind, and suffer from heart problems, brain damage and a host of other serious problems. Encephalitis is also a complication, affecting 1 in 6,000 rubella sufferers.

- Chicken pox is a relatively minor illness, but the NNII (National Network for Immunization Information) claims that it can also cause pneumonia (23 out of every 10,000 cases), inflammation of the brain (more than 1 out of every 10,000 cases), and death (less than 1 out of every 10,000 cases).

The most worrying factor for health authorities, perhaps, is that many parents have rejected the idea of immunization altogether, including the earlier DTP and polio vaccines, which have been so successful in the U.S. and across the world.

Polio destroys nerve cells and causes the muscles to shrivel and die, leading to severe disability. Since the 1988 World Health Assembly established the goal to eradicate the disease, the number of cases has fallen by more than 90 percent worldwide, from an estimated 350,000 in 1988 to a maximum of 25,000 in 1998. Good news, it appears, but doctors are concerned that money needs to be spent a little closer to home to reinforce the value of vaccinations. More and more parents are choosing to forgo vaccination (often through roundabout means, such as registering personal, medical or religious objections) until the risks are made crystal clear, and it appears that governments in the West have not done enough to reassure the population at large.

But the message from government authorities is clear: because we have lived without the daily reality of these diseases, many of us have never experienced the trauma of losing a child, or seeing him crippled by disease. We do not have the necessary motivation to see that our children are immunized, and do not understand the dangers. They believe that the dangers are even greater than they once were, because after a generation of freedom from such diseases as diphtheria, there is little or no natural immunity in the population and the reintroduction of the disease might lead to major epidemics.

The MMR Scare

The MMR has caused the most controversy, and governments in many Western countries have struggled to ease the minds of parents considering rejecting the jab. The MMR was introduced in the U.S. in 1971, almost a decade after the single vaccines were made available, and it immediately found favor with parents and doctors alike. However, at various intervals during the following years since, parents have become increasingly worried in the wake of publications suggesting links between a number of health problems that developed as side effects of the vaccine. The issue came to a head in 1998, with a study that suggested a link between MMR and autism or bowel disease. This research was subsequently denounced by government health departments, and the researchers themselves said that conclusions were drawn beyond the results of their findings, but parents have been slow to show faith in the vaccine since that time.

In the U.K., the effects have been catastrophic from a government point of view: in the second quarter of 1999, only 88 percent of two-year-olds had the vaccine, which is well short of the 95 percent coverage necessary to prevent the condition from thriving among the population at large. In the U.S., vaccination rates did not plummet to the same extent (although they were down several percentage points, to below 95 percent for most vaccines between 1999 and 2000), as regulations regarding school and day care entry ensured that parents did follow advice. However, a recent study shows that 24 percent of Americans believe that there are side effects associated with the jab, and many are unhappy with pressure to have their children inoculated.

Government authorities stress that parents reject the MMR at their peril. They point to the fact that fresh evidence published during the summer of 1999 found no evidence of a link between autism and the MMR needle, and a 2001 study confirmed much the same findings. Experts urge parents to get their children inoculated. They warn that the consequences of catching any one of the three infections could be devastating, and certainly outweigh any unproved risks associated with the vaccine. Autism is on the increase, concede the authorities, but there is simply insufficient evidence to link it to immunization. They say that the MMR vaccine is routinely given at a time when early signs of autism become evident, which may have created a coincidental link.

Should we say no?

Dr. Richard Moskowitz, antivaccination researcher and doctor in the U.S., and author of several studies and reports on the dangers of immunization, claims that we've been hoodwinked by governments, whose arguments for immunization are seriously flawed. He says that the decline of the incidence and severity of natural infections now vaccinated against remains unproved, and that it is seriously questioned by eminent authorities in the field. For example, the incidence and severity of whooping cough had begun to decline long before the pertussis vaccine was introduced. Much the same is true not only of diphtheria and tetanus, but also of TB, cholera, typhoid and other scourges of a bygone area, which began to disappear toward the end of the 19th century, perhaps partly in response to improvements in public health and sanitation, but in any case long before antibiotics, vaccines or any specific medical measure designed to eradicate them. The case of TB is of particular interest—despite mass vaccination, it appears to be on the increase.

Dr. Lendon H. Smith, author, pediatrician and spokesperson against vaccination in the U.S., confirms this viewpoint: "Many childhood diseases had tapered off before the vaccines for them had been incorporated into pediatric care. The polio epidemic of the late 1940s, for example, was waning when the drive for universal vaccination began in the 1950s."

He also claims that vaccination doesn't work to the extent that the authorities claim it does. The recent outbreak of whooping cough in the U.K., for example, affected fully immunized children in large numbers (36 percent had been fully immunized and another 34 percent had received at least one shot), and the rates of serious complications and death were reduced only slightly. Dr. Moskowitz points to the fact that in another recent outbreak of whooping cough, 46 of the 85 fully immunized children studied eventually contracted the disease, with no difference in symptoms between those who had been immunized and those who had not.

Pushing disease deeper

There are a number of studies that show how vaccination disrupts normal immune function. When we contract an illness naturally, our bodies begin to build up defenses long before symptoms become evident. An illness has to get past the skin, sneezing reflexes, respiratory secretions (mucus), tears, fever, intestinal flora and other elements of immunity before it can gain access to major organs and tissues of the body. As it passes these sites, immunity is built up against the invader. The disease itself is the peak of the "antibody response." In other words, symptoms are an indication that our bodies are fighting off the disease.

A child who gets measles, for example, will have 100 percent immunity to the disease, and the infection will have prepared her to respond even more promptly and effectively to other infections acquired in the future.

When the vaccine viruses are injected directly into the child's body, they bypass the normal immune system response. In other words, it is a fairly serious shock to the body to find itself with a virus at hand, and none of its immune responses prepared. What does this mean in practice? According to Dr. Moskowitz, vaccination, by introducing viruses directly into the bloodstream, far from preventing diseases, actually pushes the disease into a chronic form and deeper into the body, where it then attacks vital organs. He believes that the results of suppressing measles and other infectious diseases in this manner may be cancer and other chronic and autoimmune diseases.

By tricking the body with vaccination, says Dr. Moskowitz, we have accomplished what the entire immune system seems to have evolved in order to prevent—we have

Gulf War Syndrome

Why is immunization so dangerous? In 1997, Paul Shattock and Dawn Savery of the Autism Research Unit at the University of Sunderland, U.K., wrote a paper questioning the wisdom of carrying on with an immunization program that has sparked so many doubts. They take the case of veterans of the Gulf War, many of whom suffer from an extensive range of symptoms, now known as "Gulf War Syndrome." They claim that although many theories have been put forward to explain these symptoms, there can be no doubt that they were the result of the immunization programs to which the troops were treated.

The precise nature of the vaccines used to protect the troops is classified information, but the majority were immunized against at least 16 serious diseases. The effects of such an intense battery of vaccinations in such a short period of time could be serious indeed, claim Shattock and Savery, "particularly where the immune system is already compromised for any reason." The French troops, who served alongside the American and British troops (who received the same vaccinations) have not experienced the same problems—the main reason being, say the authors of the study, that they did not undergo these same vaccination programs.

In the U.S., between the ages of 3 months and around 5 years of age, children are normally exposed to 12 serious diseases in the form of up to 33 immunizations. Many experts are now beginning to question the necessity of these needles, particularly in children who are so young, and at a time when most of these diseases are no longer as life-threatening or common. Furthermore, given the experience of the Gulf veterans, there may be real danger in giving a cocktail of viruses to children whose immune systems have not ever had time to develop.

placed the virus directly into the blood and given it free and immediate access to the major organs and tissues. He claims that the persistence of the viruses in the blood for prolonged periods weakens our ability to mount an effective response not only to that disease but to other acute infections as well.

Complicated as it may sound, Dr. Moskowitz has received resounding support from many experts worldwide. He feels strongly that "what we have done by artificial immunization is essentially to trade off our acute, epidemic diseases of the past century, for the weaker, and far less curable chronic diseases of the present."

Long-term damage

Despite government assurances to the contrary, protesters are concerned by the link between bowel disorders, encephalitis, epilepsy, multiple sclerosis, diabetes and autism, among other things, and immunization. In their report, Paul Shattock and

Dawn Savery state: "There is no doubt that many parents are totally convinced that their children changed dramatically and quickly after the implementation of an immunization program."

Paul Shattock draws a link between the thalidomide tragedy of the 1960s and the current position: "When the thalidomide disaster turned up, scientists didn't run around quoting statistics about the numbers of limbless people before the drug was taken. They looked at the individual sufferers to see what they had in common and why. That's what we need to do here. The fact is that we feel there is a risk to some children, and nothing is being done to investigate that thoroughly. Instead, arguments against the research have been presented, with no new research."

NOT ONLY ARE MOST infectious diseases rarely dangerous, but they can actually play a vital role in the development of a strong, healthy immune system. Persons who have not had measles have a higher incidence of certain skin diseases, degenerative diseases of bone and cartilage, and certain tumors, while absence of mumps has been linked to higher risks of ovarian cancer.

A London homeopath who has treated many children with autism and ADD (attention deficit disorder) described one specific case where symptoms of autism arose within a few weeks of the MMR immunization. The child in question, now four, changed dramatically after the jab and his parents are convinced that the illness was the result. Despite a great deal of conventional attention, the only treatment that has shown any success was an MMR "nosode"—basically the same infectious agents contained in the immunization, but given to the child "in potency," which means in a very, very dilute form.

The homeopath has also seen many cases of asthma and eczema (the same type of incurable chronic diseases to which Dr. Moskowitz referred) arise immediately after immunization in a large number of children. By treating them with homeopathic nosodes of the illnesses against which they were immunized, she has been able to treat them effectively and in most cases cure the presenting condition.

Many critics claim that we are being seriously misled by government figures. Jackie Fletcher of JABS (Justice Awareness Basic Support)—which campaigns on behalf of parents whose children may have been affected by the MMR vaccine—gives an example: "In November 1994, 7 million children aged 5 to 16 years were vaccinated in the national measles/rubella (MR) campaign in the U.K. The U.K. Committee on Safety of Medicines states that serious reactions to the MR vaccine were very rare, but then admitted that there had been 530 serious reactions. Given that the chief medical officer's figure of 'one in a million' is usually quoted for adverse reactions and only 7 million—not 530 million—pupils were vaccinated, there appears to be something wrong with their definition of 'rare.'" That may not seem like a huge percentage, but it is higher than the risks associated with the disease itself. Furthermore, the Medicines Control Agency admitted that as few as 5 percent of adverse effects are reported, which means the numbers might be even higher.

The same problem exists in the U.S., where the FDA estimates that only ten percent of reactions to any vaccine are ever reported to VAERS (Vaccine Adverse Events Reporting System). Dr. Robert T. Chen, chief of the vaccine safety branch at the CDC, noted that in 1998 there were 7,411 reported cases of vaccine-preventable diseases in the United States and 10,236 cases of vaccine adverse events, causal or coincidental. If only 10 percent of cases are being reported, it is, therefore, very likely that there are hundreds of thousands of adverse reactions to vaccines, if not more. That percentage is far higher than government authorities are admitting, no matter how you look at it.

Anecdotal evidence?

All homeopaths and many other complementary practitioners deal with vaccine-related illness (much of it chronic, including coughs, excess mucus, asthma, eczema, allergies and other inexplicable conditions) on a weekly basis. One homeopath, Christina Head, was concerned enough to write a book about it (*An Educated Decision*), and she claims that before treatment of any kind will work effectively, it's necessary for children to undergo postvaccination cleansing, which basically means undoing the damage caused by the vaccines.

While the experiences of complementary practitioners may be anecdotal, the statistics are not:

- In the U.S., measles and rubella are resurfacing despite the shots. For example, a recent epidemic of whooping cough in Cincinnati afflicted hundreds of children, 75 percent of whom had had the DTP shots.

- In an outbreak of measles in Texas in 1987, 96 percent of the cases were considered nonpreventable, according to the Texas Department of Health. In other words, all the measles cases were either fully vaccinated, had a religious or medical exemption or were born before 1957.

- The Japanese government, in 1979, noted a cause and effect relationship between DTP shots and sudden infant death syndrome (SIDS). In response, the health department ordered the postponement of routine DTP shots until children were at least two years old. The result: SIDS has virtually disappeared from Japan. In the U.K., it claims thousands of lives every year. One study found the peak incidence of SIDS occurred at the ages of two and four months in the U.S., precisely when the first two routine immunizations are given, while another found a clear pattern of correlation extending three weeks after immunization. Another study found that 3,000 children die within four days of vaccination each year in the

U.S., and another researcher's studies led to the conclusion that half of SIDS cases are caused by vaccines.

- In 1950, before mass immunization began, the U.S. had the third lowest infant mortality rate in the world. By 1986, the U.S. dropped to 17th place. Today, they stand at 24th: many of the infant deaths attributed to SIDS.

- Many countries abandoned at least some of the mandatory vaccinations. Sweden stopped whooping cough vaccination in 1979 because of epidemics of the disease in fully vaccinated children, and due to the unacceptable side effects, including brain damage.

- In 1994 the U.S. Vaccine Safety Datalink Project monitored the progress of a half million children. Their key finding was that the incidence of seizure increased dramatically, by three times the norm, after MMR vaccinations. This was confirmed by a similar study carried out in the U.K. by the Public Health Laboratory Service, but it was withheld until the 1994 vaccination campaign, Operation Safeguard, was over.

- In the U.S., over $1 billion has been paid out in compensation for vaccine-related injury over the past ten years under their no-fault scheme.

Reporting side effects

- In 1986, the U.S. Congress officially acknowledged the reality of vaccine-caused injuries and death by creating and passing the National Childhood Vaccine Injury Act. The law requires doctors to provide parents with information about the benefits and risks of childhood vaccines prior to vaccination, and to report vaccine reactions to federal health officials. A report, four years later, showed that only 10 percent of doctors reported adverse reactions to the FDA, but in just three-and-a-half years (from July 1900 to March 1994) more than 34,000 adverse events were reported. These figures include hundreds of cases of irreversible brain damage and over 700 deaths.

- The British government has a "yellow card" system, which encourages physicians (and others involved with the administration of medicines, such as pharmacists and coroners) to report any adverse reactions to medications, including vaccines. The Medicines Control Agency has admitted that only a small percentage (around 5 percent) of even serious reactions are reported. Some doctors appear to be unaware of the system.

- Doctors in the U.K. are given incentives to vaccinate their patients. To receive an annual bonus, they need to exceed a minimum 70 percent immunization rate in their practice. And according to former Governor George Ryan of Illinois, many physicians with expertise in the field of immunizations and infectious disease have contractual relationships with pharmaceutical companies with regards to speaking engagements. Also, many medical schools and academic centers employ infectious disease specialists that perform research funded by the pharmaceutical industry.

One answer seems to be to spread out the vaccines over several years, rather than give them all together. The single measles vaccine, for example, is not available in the U.K. (the only EU country where single vaccines are not), but there is an incredibly low incidence of any problems or side effects, while the number of conditions associated with the MMR in particular seems to be escalating. In the U.S., parents can choose single dose vaccines for measles, mumps and rubella, but not, it appears, for diphtheria and pertussis.

What's the answer?

Until side effects are reported more accurately, and more studies are undertaken into the long- and short-term effects of vaccinations, we will never know the real dangers of mass immunization. However, there can be no doubt that childhood illnesses can be dangerous, debilitating and, in some cases, life-threatening. Parents whose children have died or been disabled as a result of complications from childhood diseases will argue that mass immunization could have prevented a tragedy. They may be in smaller numbers, but parents of children affected by vaccines feel equally strongly that immunization is not the answer. Parents face today an unacceptable decision—one that may affect not only their children's future health but also their lives. Parents should consider the following before they immunize their children:

1. Does my child really need this vaccination? In the U.S., the answer may be yes, if children are to enter mainstream educational systems, but there are loopholes. It's possible to present a letter of personal, religious or medical exemption, many cases of which are considered and accepted by state authorities.

2. Is my child well enough to have a vaccine?

3. Has my child had a bad reaction to a vaccination before?

4. Does my child or family have a history of:
   - vaccine reactions?
   - convulsions or neurological disorders?
   - allergies (such as asthma, antibiotics, etc.)?
   - immune system problems?

5. Do I have full information on the vaccine's side effects? Parents in the U.S. should request vaccine information statements for every single vaccine that their child is offered. Read them carefully and ask questions.

Which vaccine?

Many of the vaccines currently available have side effects that can be dangerous. Some parents are choosing to immunize only against those conditions that present the most danger, using vaccines that are least associated with side effects.

- **DTaP** (diphtheria, tetanus and acellular whooping cough [pertussis]): Side effects for diphtheria and tetanus are relatively small, and experts believe the immunization can be safely given to healthy children. Although these two illnesses are relatively rare, they still occur and there is pressure to immunize against them. Whooping cough is a different story. Although it is a serious illness and can have a dramatic effect on health, it develops slowly and responds well to a variety of conventional and complementary remedies. The efficiency of the vaccine has been questioned, as the condition has arisen in fully immunized children, and there is a higher incidence of side effects (including brain damage) than with some of the other immunizations.

- **Polio** is a serious disease, with a rapid onset. A healthy child may successfully fight off the condition, but this may not be a risk you want to take. There are few side effects to the vaccine partly, it is believed, because it is taken orally, which enables your child's body to build up a defense before it enters the bloodstream.

- **Measles** are still common, but it is no longer as severe a condition as it once was. It can be safely and successfully treated with natural remedies, and the best advice is to consider avoiding the vaccine, if you can.

- **Rubella** (German measles) is routinely offered to older girls because of the risks during pregnancy. It's not essential to offer this vaccine earlier than preteens. If your child contracts the disease before that time, remember that rubella is not normally a serious illness, and can be treated safely with natural and conventional medicine. The argument is that pregnant women could come into contact with children carrying the disease, but most women are now screened and advised to get the vaccine before conception.

- **Mumps** vaccines have a checkered history and most experts believe that the condition is not serious, provided it is acquired before teenage years (see page 372).

- **Meningitis** (Hib; also known as Zithromax) vaccines are relative newcomers and there is very little material available on the long-term side effects or damage. Worryingly, there have been numerous side effects reported by doctors in the U.K. (11,000 in the first year) and at least 11 deaths. In the U.S., Hepatitis B immunizations have been associated with 53 deaths and 828 serious injuries, but the yearly incidence of the hepatitis B disease itself is only 191 among the 38 million children younger than 10, according to a letter recently published in the *Journal of the*

American Medical Association. Meningitis is a serious illness, but it is still relatively rare. I would advise seeing a homeopath for a nosode (page 219) to boost natural immunity, or to treat any problems following vaccination.

- **Tuberculosis** (TB) vaccines (BCG) may offer little protection against tuberculosis, and there are many recorded cases of lingering illness following vaccine. Most natural health practitioners advise against giving it.

- **Chicken pox** (varicella) vaccination is, for many health practitioners, one step too far. Chicken pox is a cleansing illness and rarely serious, despite government claims to the contrary. If you have a healthy child, he is unlikely to suffer unduly from the health condition, but see your doctor if you are concerned.

6. Do I know how to identify a vaccine reaction?

7. Do I know how and why my doctor should report a vaccine reaction?

8. Do I know the vaccine's name and batch number?

Paul Shattock also suggests that parents ask for their children's antibody levels to be checked before they have the second preschool MMR shot. If there are antibodies there, there's no need to have the vaccine again. He also recommends talking to your doctor about any worries: "I think doctors are loosening up a bit, giving shots a little later, when the child's immune system is more mature. I think they are listening more to patients and taking the risks more seriously."

According to the National Vaccine Information Center (NVIC), parents should monitor their child closely after vaccination. The center suggests that you call your doctor if you suspect a reaction. If your doctor is not concerned, and you are, take your child to an emergency room. Obtain a copy of your region's mandatory vaccination laws. Become educated about vaccine requirements, your rights and legal exemptions to vaccination.

If you do decide to immunize your child, it's a good idea to get some homeopathic treatment following the jabs. All of the major illnesses currently immunized against are available in potency, and most homeopaths offer these as a precursor to constitutional treatment (see page 267). Following immunization, some children suffer an "echo" effect, which means that they never fully return to original good health. Symptoms of an echo effect include:

- swollen glands
- frequent infections

- low energy

- chronic mucus

- low-grade symptoms of the original infection (in this case, the vaccine), which can include a chronic hard cough in the case of pertussis (whooping cough), earaches and recurrent fever, thick gray mucus (in the case of polio), and a feverish cough with yellow mucus after the measles vaccine

Homeopathic nosodes will counter this echo pattern, and restore your child's physical and emotional health, and energy levels. Recent epidemiological studies show homeopathic remedies as equaling or surpassing standard vaccinations in preventing disease. There are reports in which populations that were treated homeopathically after exposure had a 100 percent success rate—none of those treated caught the disease.

Caring for a sick child

Every child reacts differently to illness, and you'll need to gauge your own child's individual needs when she is ill. Children can become dramatically ill and then recover equally quickly, which can be alarming for parents—particularly the first time around. When your child becomes ill, you may find that your household grinds to a halt. Remember, however, that most illnesses are short-lived and there is a great deal that you can do to keep your child comfortable and content. In chapter 11, we discuss the treatment for specific illnesses, including the best ways to get your child on her feet again. If your child is ill, the following tips will help her to recover quickly and with the least amount of fuss:

▶ Top tips to aid recovery

- All children need love and attention while they are ill. The mind-body relationship is a strong one, and if they feel comfortable, calm and cared for, they will recover more quickly. Forget about the housework or that urgent meeting, if you can. Curl up with your child and indulge him. Many children are frightened when they are ill, and will want constant reassurance. This is particularly common with babies, who may not want to be put down. Try to give in to your child's needs as much as possible.

- Offer plenty of fluids. Children dehydrate quickly in cases of diarrhea and vomiting, and even intense fever. If your child won't drink, offer juice popsicles or even frozen juice cubes to tempt her. Give her a grown-up cup, if that will encourage her to drink, or offer to make her a special drink in the blender, with her favorite fruits. Play Peter Rabbit and give teaspoons of cooled chamomile tea (while reading the book, of course!).

- Rest is the operative word. Although most children will want to be up and about, they will recover more quickly if they get plenty of restorative rest. Read stories, play story tapes, set up coloring books, pencils and paper, watch videos together, play a quiet game of cards, cut out paper dolls, set up puzzles, play hangman— anything to keep him calm and still.

- Keep food simple. If your child is not hungry, don't push it. Stick to easy-to-digest foods, such as soups, plain toast, boiled eggs and diluted fruit juices. Your child's energy needs to be spent getting well, not on digesting a big meal. Many children lose weight when they are ill, but most will put it straight back on again. Unless your

When to get help for your sick child

Don't hesitate to call your doctor if you are concerned about your child for any reason. Parental instinct counts for a great deal and no doctor will ever dismiss your concerns without checking your child carefully. It is always essential to ask for professional help early on, before problems become more serious. When in doubt, ask a professional, whether you choose a conventional or natural practitioner.

Get help if your child:

- becomes extremely feverish, with a body temperature above 104°F (40°C)

- becomes extremely cold, with a body temperature below 95°F (35°C)

- seems dehydrated, with sunken or glazed eyes

- has trouble breathing

- has a sharp pain in the right abdomen with nausea

- has any fever that lasts longer than six hours

- seems confused or delirious

- becomes blue around the mouth

- starts to twitch or suffers a fit

- vomits or has diarrhea for more than 24 hours (six hours in babies)

- has an unusual rash

- has a serious illness that becomes worse for any reason

- becomes unconscious

- has a headache, nausea, unusual sleepiness or dizziness, after a recent fall or blow to the head

In babies, watch for the following:

- unusually drowsy, listless, quiet or restless behavior

- when your baby consistently refuses feeds, or does not demand one, for any length of time

- the soft spot (fontanelle) on the top of the head is sunken or bulging

- when your baby cries much more than usual, sounding different from his usual requests for attention or feeding

- diarrhea or vomiting

- convulsions of any description

- trouble breathing or blueness around the mouth

- an unusual rash

child is seriously underweight, you don't need to worry about a temporary lack of appetite. Reintroduce foods slowly if she has been off her food for some time.

■ Keep his sickroom clean and fresh. Spritz lavender water in the air to disinfect, and change the sheets regularly. Air the room when he is not in it, but keep the windows closed when he is. The immune system seems to work more effectively in a slightly warmer temperature, so keep him cozy, but not hot.

■ Make sure she is comfortable, with loose-fitting clothes or pajamas. It's better to layer clothes than to put her in something too hot, particularly if she has a fever. The same goes for blankets—layers of thin blankets or sheets can be peeled off as necessary.

■ Take his temperature regularly if you are concerned. Many parents become experienced in dealing with childhood fevers and know instantly when their child is "too" hot. Until you achieve this level of confidence, take his temperature as often as you need to, using noninvasive methods if possible!

■ Stay calm, sympathetic and cheerful. Your child will pick up on anxieties and feel more frightened if you show concern. Even if you are worried, reassure her that she's on the road to recovery.

■ If your child does not have a fever, a little fresh air will do him some good. Dress him warmly and walk around the block, or just sit together in the backyard or the local park. Don't encourage playtime.

■ Some children adore the attention they get when they are ill, and while it is important to indulge her when she is genuinely sick, watch out for suspicious symptoms that miraculously appear when your child needs a little extra time or love.

■ Remember recovery time! Children will naturally want to be up and about the minute they feel better, but it is important that their bodies are given a chance to fully recover. As a rule of thumb, try to keep him quiet and calm (and away from school, if necessary) for as many days as the illness itself lasted. For most children, this will mean a day or two of extra TLC.

Remember that all children suffer from earaches, colds, coughs, fever, tummy bugs and other common ailments, and many children will experience alarming symptoms. As you become more experienced, you'll get more in tune with your child's reaction to illness, and the lead-up to it. Some children scream with pain and want to be comforted constantly; others like to heal in peace. It may take a few trips to the doctor before you feel confident enough to treat your child at home. That is perfectly acceptable, and no parent should attempt treatment until he feels comfortable doing so. As you learn to read your child's moods and changing physical symptoms, you'll soon develop an instinct for what he requires. You'll also become used to his reaction to illness, and will know what to expect. If you have a regularly inconsolable patient on your hands, you will probably be right to show concern if he suddenly becomes quiet and listless. Similarly, if your child is quiet and withdrawn during periods of ill health and suddenly becomes red-cheeked and hysterical, you might want to have him checked by a doctor.

The trick is to prevent illness by ensuring your child has a good strong immune system. When illness does strike, you want to get in early, before things become more serious.

Natural home medicine kit

As you become more confident about treating your children naturally, your medicine kit will grow accordingly. Some children respond better to remedies than others, and you may find that your natural medicine kit looks nothing like this! The following list represents the most commonly used remedies for babies and children. I've noted some of the most common conditions that each remedy can be used for, but the list is by no means exhaustive.

Keep your medicine chest in an easy-to-reach location, preferably somewhere dark. Many of the remedies need to be kept in a cool, dark place. Always keep them out of reach of children.

Flower essences

Flower essences can be dropped on a child's tongue, or rubbed into pulse points (see page 254 for more details).

Bach Rescue Remedy—for shock, trauma, injury, distress or acute illness of any sort. It will help to calm and restore.

Bach Rescue Cream—for rashes, itching, mild burns, sunburn or any skin condition, including allergic reactions.

Star of Bethlehem—for shocks of all kind, accidents, bad news, sudden startling noise and trauma.

Walnut—for change of any sort, including parental divorce or separation, a new school, adolescence, new home, new sibling.

Olive—for exhaustion and fatigue; it's good during illness and in the convalescence period.

Aromatherapy

Always dilute aromatherapy oils before use, unless specified. For a baby, one or two drops of essential oil in five tablespoons (100 ml) of a carrier oil is appropriate; for an older child, you can use up to four drops of essential oil. Keep them in a dark, cool place, away from homeopathic remedies (a different shelf will do).

Lavender oil is relaxing, antiseptic, generally therapeutic; use it for dry skin, cuts, wounds, burns, bruises, insomnia, stress, indigestion, headaches, hyperactivity, anxiety, earaches, colic.

Chamomile oil is calming, antiseptic and analgesic; use it for pain, indigestion, acne, eczema, sensitive skin, diaper rash, hay fever, toothache, sleep problems, headaches, anxiety, stress, earaches.

Tea tree oil is antifungal and antiseptic; use it for cuts, insect bites, thrush, colds, catarrh, infections, warts, head lice.

Eucalyptus oil is antiseptic, decongestant, and antiviral; use it for coughs, colds, chest infections, croup, aches and pains, flu, cuts, congestion, earaches.

Peppermint oil is digestive and refreshing; use it for muscle fatigue, toothache, bronchitis, indigestion, travel sickness, sinus congestion, exhaustion.

Lemon oil is refreshing, antiseptic and stimulating; use it for cold sores, cuts, depression, acne, indigestion, cuts.

Homeopathy

Homeopathic remedies are best prescribed on the basis of your child's unique constitution and symptom picture. However, they can be safely (and effectively!) used for a variety of acute conditions, in babies and children of all ages. For acute first aid problems in children and babies, the usual dose is 30C (see page 268). For less acute conditions, the usual dose is 6C. Take every two hours up to six doses, then three times a day.

Aconite—for fear, anxiety, restlessness, sudden illness (including a cold, raging fever, violent diarrhea or vomiting, that comes on suddenly), intense pain

Arnica—for cuts, grazes, broken skin, bruising, burns, scalds, nosebleeds, stings, sprains, dislocated joints, fractures, muscular aches and pains, eye injuries and shock

Apis—for stings, hives, water retention, cystitis, allergies affecting the throat, mouth and eyes, bites and puncture wounds

Arsenicum—for tummy bugs, diarrhea, burning discharge (from nose, etc.)

Belladonna—for fever, earache, hallucinations, sensitivity to light, noise, touch, motion or pressure during illness, complaints that come on suddenly and with great violence, intense burning, swelling, congestion with throbbing, hot head and cold extremities

Bryonia—for fractures, sprains, strains, swollen joints, heat exhaustion, colds, flu, bursting headache with nausea, illnesses accompanied by a "bear with a sore head" feeling, painful chest, dry mucous membranes, great thirst

Calendula (cream or tincture)—for burns, cuts and grazes

Cantharis—for blisters, burns, scalds, burning diarrhea, any stinging or burning sensation

Chamomilla—for teething, insomnia, severe earache, illness with bad temper, babies who are distressed when put down (during illness), anxiety dreams, severe pain, great irritability and sensitivity to pain

Euphrasia—for conjunctivitis, bruising of the eye, sore eyes, eye strain, constipation, bursting headaches

Hypericum—for cuts, grazes, bruising, lacerations, puncture wounds, cut lip, shooting pains, diarrhea and indigestion

Ledum—for cuts, bruises, insect stings, black eye, sore eye, bites, sprains and strains, particularly when they feel numb

Nux Vom.—for travel sickness, digestive problems, nausea with headache, overindulgence (after a birthday party, for example)

Phosphorus—for electrical burns or shock, nosebleeds, congestive headaches, burning pains, laryngitis with hoarseness, hemorrhaging

Pulsatilla—for thick, yellow-green and bland catarrh, tearfulness, digestive complaints (particularly those that are worse after eating), one-sided fevers, headaches, etc

Rhus Tox.—for red, swollen, itchy blisters, diaper rash, torn muscles, swollen joints, dislocated joints, cramp, muscle stiffness, arthritic or rheumatic pain which is helped by moving

Silica—for splinters, recurrent colds and infection, migraine, spots

Herbs

The best form of herbal remedies for children is a tincture, which can be used internally or externally as required. A tincture can be purchased at your local health food store or herbal supplier. Five to 15 drops, taken in a little water, is an appropriate dosage for children. Read the label when in doubt. Herbal tinctures can also be applied externally. Use them neat on cuts, bruises, bites and stings, and blend with a little olive oil for skin problems. See page 262 for more information on using herbs on children. Keep tinctures in a dark bottle, in a cool place.

Angelica—for coughs, travel sickness, fever, nervousness

Basil—for insect bites, vomiting, constipation, nervous complaints

Calendula—for cuts, bruises, grazes and minor skin problems

Catmint (catnip)—promotes perspiration in fevers, relaxes spasms and cramps, calms nerves, digestive problems, good general tonic, insomnia

Chamomile—fever, nervous conditions, sleep problems, swelling, sores, fatigue, digestive complaints

Echinacea—for fighting infection and warding off colds, flu and sore throats. Boosts the immune system while acting as a natural antibiotic. Use for boils, ulcers, measles, chicken pox, bacterial infections

Fennel—for indigestion, flatulence, colic

Garlic—for coughs and colds, thrush, wounds, bites, stings, infections, catarrh

Ginger—for indigestion and wind, circulatory disorders, travel sickness

Golden seal—general tonic, clears mucus from the body, mild laxative, chronic coughs

Hops—nervous pain and irritation, insomnia

Lavender—for stress (it promotes relaxation), insomnia, headaches, infection

Licorice—for digestive problems, as a tonic, catarrh, coughs, chronic sore throats, constipation (do not use in cases of high blood pressure or kidney disease)

Meadowsweet—for digestive problems, diarrhea and fever

Mint (ALL TYPES)—for headaches, insomnia, nervousness, coughs, migraine, flatulence, abdominal aches

Sage—for gastritis, diarrhea, throat problems, nervousness, wounds

Thyme—for coughs and colds, sore throat, catarrh, whooping cough, headaches, diarrhea, rheumatism, bruises

Valerian—for flatulence, nervous headache, insomnia, stress, tension

chapter ten

Natural Therapies for Children

....

Awhole new world of health care has opened up over the last decade and our children will represent one of the first generations to benefit from the cornucopia of treatments now available. Many parents have now tried a complementary therapy of some form; in fact, recent research shows that over 30 percent of us have seen a natural health practitioner and purchased natural remedies for home use. What is most exciting, however, is the breathtaking array of therapies now available to treat some of the most stubborn health conditions affecting both us and our children. Best of all, these therapies work with our children's natural energy levels, to prevent and treat health problems with few side effects, helping them to become stronger and more able to resist illness in the future.

In the last chapter, we discussed the importance of illness, and explained the concept of the vital force. It's important to bear these in mind when considering therapies for your children. Natural medicine has a fundamentally different approach to health, and you cannot expect to see instant cures or symptomatic relief. Certainly, some treatments will be quick and effective (sometimes within a few minutes of taking a remedy), but longer term, more chronic conditions will take more time to heal. This means you have to adapt your expectations, making long-term health a priority over short-term relief of symptoms. Natural therapies also work on a preventive basis, building up immunity and energy levels so that your child not only overcomes whatever health condition is troubling him now but also will also be more likely to deal with illness more effectively and efficiently in future.

Natural practitioners address each case on an individual basis. On the basis of a full physical and emotional assessment, you will be given treatment that works to balance your body's vital force, or energy. When you visit a natural health practitioner you will be expected to give all the details about your child and his health (see page 236) in order for your therapist to make an informed decision about treatment.

You will also need to go into some detail about your own health, and that of other members of your family. Remember that symptoms will not be treated, rather, their root cause will be investigated and dealt with. They do, however, impart important information about your child, and you can expect to discuss them in some detail. This can be offputting for parents used to spending a few moments in a doctor's office. Discussing the nature of a bowel movement, or the color of your child's nasal discharge, may represent a unique experience for you!

But remember, when you go natural, you are working with your child's body and her emotions in order to give her the best possible health care. Natural medicine provides a balance that simply does not exist in conventional medical treatment. Because your child—as a person, not just an "ill body"—is examined so fully, the treatment she receives will be tailored for her individual, specific needs, taking into consideration every aspect of her emotional, physical and spiritual health. Sufferers of serious conditions, such as cancer, have been helped enormously through natural medical treatment. Although the cancer itself may not be addressed, the body is encouraged to work more effectively, so the healing process will be more efficient. Even more importantly, the emotional effects of the condition will be treated, and your child's sense of well-being can be improved immeasurably. I have seen countless cases where a child's long-term health problems have been addressed by a natural health practitioner, and in almost every one of those cases, parents have remarked upon the positive change in emotional health and happiness in their child that resulted.

Complementing the conventional

Natural medicine is not a replacement for conventional medicine, but a complement to it. Modern medicine undoubtedly offers many miracles, and many lives are saved each year by conventional treatments. In emergencies, it can mean the difference between life and death, but even conventional practitioners themselves are aware of the shortcomings of the orthodox approach to chronic illnesses, such as asthma, eczema, chronic fatigue, excess catarrh, recurrent tonsillitis and ear infections, and even the inexplicable low-grade infections that seem to wipe children out for weeks at a time. These are the cases where natural medicine can make a real difference to your child's health, and there is no doubt that complementary therapies can heal on a level that conventional medicine never reaches.

Natural medicine is also important for acute (short-lived) illnesses, and it works on a much deeper level than conventional medication. You can expect your child to experience renewed energy and vigor, and a stronger immune system when he is treated with natural remedies. Most of us are aware of the side effects of many medications offered to children. After a course of antibiotics, for example, many children are exhausted and run-down. Long-term use of steroids for asthma can cause kidney damage, thinning of the skin and a variety of other health problems. Natural therapies are designed to work with the body, and general health is improved rather than reduced by their use.

But parents need to be on the lookout for serious disease, and to call in medical professionals if they have any concerns or doubts about their children's health, or the natural treatment they are being offered. As parents, we are in the unique position of being able to offer the best of both worlds—a natural approach to overall health, and a conventional medical service that can treat conditions needing urgent attention. Going natural doesn't mean swapping one discipline for another—it involves judging which approach is best for your child's individual circumstances. Don't be tempted to dump long-term medication in favor of a natural quick fix. Change will be gradual and you may need to continue with drug therapy for some time. All good therapists will help you to make decisions based on your child's needs, and none will suggest discounting conventional medicine altogether.

Natural therapies are gaining recognition across the world, and many doctors now study complementary theory as part of conventional training, if only to advise curious parents on what there is to offer. You won't offend your doctor if you choose to treat your child with other treatments. Doctors are, first and foremost, healers and will want your child to become well, whatever means are required to get her there. A *Journal of the American Medical Association* report[1] suggests a 47.3 percent increase in total visits to alternative medicine practitioners, from 427 million in 1990 to 629 million in 1997, thereby exceeding total visits to all U.S. primary care physicians. AMEDNEWS.com (an online newspaper for physicians) cites[2] a recent survey by the American Academy of Pediatrics that reports that 93 percent of pediatricians were queried about such therapies by parents. Many natural treatments are covered by your health plan, particularly if they are recommended by a doctor.

The best way to ensure that your treatments are complementary is to tell your doctor about any natural treatments you are receiving, and tell your natural health practitioner about any conventional medication.

Judging the effectiveness of natural remedies

There is a great deal of contemporary research into the efficacy of natural therapies. There is no question that most of them do work, although modern science has had difficulty in justifying that on a scientific level. Natural healing, for instance, works for thousands and thousands of people each year, and in some cases terminal illnesses have been cured. There is no explanation for how this has happened, but we know that it has. Some therapies require more of a leap of faith—for instance, Bach flower remedies, or homeopathy, which are based on the concept of vibrational medicine. But don't be put off by the differences between orthodox medicine and these types of healing. There are many, many studies showing that they are effective, even if we cannot prove exactly how. The theories behind these types of therapies are too complicated to explain here, but I will focus on the main issues when looking at each therapy, to give you a general understanding of what is going on in your child's body when you take them on.

Other therapies are similar to Western conventional medicine, in that you seem to take medication for a specific complaint. Massage, osteopathy and chiropractic are enough like conventional physiotherapy to silence the skeptics, and acupuncture has now achieved mainstream appeal and approval, although, once again, its effects cannot be explained scientifically. Some people believe that natural medicine works because there is so much time spent in consultation with the practitioner, which is, in itself, therapeutic. But this doesn't explain the fact that most of the therapies listed in this book work on infants, babies and also people who are no longer able to think for themselves. Nor does it explain how remedies prepared and administered at home can be enormously successful in treating all types of illness—serious and minor.

Choosing a therapy

There is a huge variety of treatments on offer, and you may find that some are more successful than others. One of the best ways to choose is to find the one that appeals to you most. If your child is a needle-phobic, acupuncture may not be appropriate. If she hates having her feet touched, then skip reflexology. Some of the general therapies, such as Ayurveda, traditional Chinese medicine and homeopathy are a good place to start, because they offer treatments for a wide range of physical and emotional complaints. However, specific problems following birth, for example, may be best dealt with by a cranial osteopath; or if your child's problems seem to be largely emotional, then try flower essences first. You can always complement therapies with home remedies, using aromatherapy oils, flower essences or homeopathic remedies for acute problems. Just make sure you tell your therapist about anything else you are trying or using, and try to stick to one major discipline at a time. Nutrition and massage are parts of many therapies, and can be used alongside all of the therapies discussed.

Read through the therapies described below, and have a look at the conditions that they are known to treat successfully. Or go straight to chapter 11, where you will find a list of common ailments, for a selection of natural treatments that can be undertaken at home, and details of the most appropriate therapies.

Choosing a practitioner

The success of alternative therapies can be enormously dependent on a good practitioner/patient relationship, and your choice of a therapist is as important as the choice of therapy. You and your child will need to feel comfortable talking to your practitioner, and if you feel embarrassed or ill at ease, you will be less likely to get across all of the essential information. A good therapist will naturally draw out the important information, and you and your child will go away feeling reassured and comfortable.

Take your time, check the therapist's qualifications, ask for recommendations from friends, your doctor or another therapist, and do not commit yourself until you are sure you will have a rapport. Also, make sure that the practitioner has experience treating children. Although all of the therapies listed in this book are appropriate for children, many treatments have to be adapted to work properly. As all parents know, children respond best to "child-friendly" adults, so an experienced therapist used to working with adults may be able to provide effective treatment, but your child will not come away with a sense of well-being and confidence, which can help the healing process too.

The consultation

The consultation is the most important part of any natural therapy session. This is the first session with a therapist, and the one in which the most information is exchanged. The first session usually lasts longer than any subsequent sessions because your therapist will aim to find out all about you and your child before any diagnosis can be made.

▶ Tips for preparing for a consultation

Your therapist will ask you about the following matters relating to your child. Be ready to discuss:

- your child's physical condition, including past and present illnesses, any medication he is taking, what his birth was like, whether or not he was immunized, any symptoms and interesting aspects (such as whether pain is sharp or dull, or whether a cough is worse at night or after being in fresh air)

- your child's diet, including cravings, appetite, any weight problems, habits, obvious dislikes and reactions to foods

- your child's sleeping patterns

- school and home life, whether there are any obvious stresses, sibling rivalry, parental tension, poor concentration, difficulty making friends, driving himself too hard or giving up too easily, undertaking too many extra activities

- your child's exercise patterns

- your child's emotional state—is there anything making him unhappy? Has he recently moved house, fallen out with a friend, lost someone important, failed an important exam? Is he grumpy in the morning, or irritable at particular times of day? Does he withdraw when he's unhappy, or does he become aggressive? Is he competitive or uninspired? Is he dreamy or outspoken?

- any other treatment he may be undergoing, both conventional and complementary, including any home treatments you may be offering

- what you hope to get from treatment.

Older children will be able to answer questions for themselves, and some therapists may ask that you leave the room in order for your child to speak freely. No therapist will judge you on the basis of whatever your child has to say, so don't be alarmed if your therapist wants him on his own. The most important aspect of the consultation is to get across every tiny bit of information you can summon up, no matter how trivial it may seem at the time. This presents a clear picture for the therapist, who will be able to offer treatment based on all the important facts, whether they seem relevant to you or not.

Many therapists use a variety of diagnostic techniques alongside the information you provide. For example, a Chinese therapist will use personal touch and observation, including:

- pulse-taking (there is more than one pulse in Chinese medicine)

- abdominal touch

- posture, movement and skin texture diagnosis

- tongue diagnosis

- possibly urine analysis.

Other therapists may use some of the following techniques.

- **Dowsing**—a pendulum is held over the body's "energy centers" or chakras to indicate strengths and weaknesses in the energy system. It may also be used to give yes/no answers (by swinging clockwise or counterclockwise) to specific questions about the person's health status and requirements.

- **Radionics**—using instruments to measure different aspects of a your child's energy state from a "witness" (a hair clipping or drop of blood) to provide a diagnosis of overall health.

- **Aura reading**—many healers appear to be able to "read" people's auras or energy fields by clairvoyance, touch or instinct. Most healers "scan" the energy field with their hands, sensing areas of heat, cold, pain, tingling and so on that indicate problems. Some therapists actually see and interpret the colors of the aura, and can pick up the effects of past traumas and potential future problems.

- **Kirlian photography**—developed by a Russian engineer, Kirlian photographs show the energy radiations emitted by living things, including plants and animals. A healthy person emits strong radiations while weak radiations are said to show imbalances that need to be treated.

- **Muscle-testing**—or applied kinesiology.

- **Iridology**—the iris of the eye represents a map of the glands, organs and systems of the whole human body. Problems show up on the iris as spots, flecks, white or dark streaks, and texture and color indicate a person's general state of health.

- **Reflexology**—is based on the theory that "reflex" points on the hands and feet represent different parts of the body and can be treated externally by a variety of palpations. For more see page 287.

- **Hair analysis**—a chemical analysis of hair is often used to reveal nutritional deficiencies in the body, particularly of minerals.

- **X rays.**

Don't be surprised if none of these is used, or if you are presented with something completely different. All therapies have their own methods of diagnosing health imbalances, and the majority are not intrusive. If you feel uncomfortable with any of the diagnostic techniques offered, suggest giving them a miss, or choose a therapy that is completely noninvasive (homeopathy, for example).

How to judge the results

Many parents do not seek out natural therapies until they have become thoroughly disillusioned by the conventional medical system and, by then, many long-standing conditions have become quite deeply entrenched. Some might be new parents, who want to use only natural treatments on their children, and they will find that they heal much more quickly than older children with chronic health conditions. The best course of action is to use natural medicine from the very beginning of any health condition, not when it has begun to affect your child's quality of life. Furthermore, use therapies preventatively, so that when a health crisis does arise, your child will respond better and more quickly to treatments of any sort.

It is normal for treatments to take some time. These are not miracle cures, but gentle and effective means of encouraging your child's body to work for itself. For example, it is normally believed that it takes as long to treat eczema as the length of time your child has suffered from the condition.

Many therapies initiate a process of detoxification, which means that toxins are forced out of the body. When this happens, your child may experience some symptoms like headaches, dizziness, bad skin, rashes, mild diarrhea, nausea and discharge. This is normal, and such symptoms should never be so uncomfortable as to be unbearable. You may find that her symptoms become worse or change as treatment progresses (a healing crisis). This is also normal, and it shows that your child's body is hard at work. If symptoms become alarming or your feel concerned for any reason, contact your child's practitioner immediately.

If your child experiences no change in her condition, or she is feeling much worse, chances are the treatment is not working and you should go back to your therapist. Always give a therapist a second chance; diagnosis is extremely complicated and you may, unknowingly, have omitted a major piece of information that changes the whole treatment picture. If several attempts to effect a cure fail completely, you may think about trying a different therapy, or a different therapist. Remember that it will take time, and your therapist can be only as good as the information you have given.

The therapies

Acupuncture

Many parents will be surprised to see acupuncture suggested for children, but it can have a dramatic effect on overall health. Most children are not naturally frightened by needles, and will be curious to see what happens. Acupuncture is not painful, and, in the hands of a good therapist, it can be a pleasurable experience, treating many chronic and acute health conditions.

Giles Davies, a London acupuncturist, treats children (his own included) regularly, and he has found that most children respond much more quickly than adults and seem to enjoy the treatment. Some of the children he treats prefer not to watch, and he finds that playing soft music and talking throughout treatment helps to overcome any fears that children might have. Always go for a therapist with experience in treating children.

What is it?

Acupuncture works by balancing the body's energy to encourage it to heal itself. It can be used to treat a wide range of conditions, including disorders where conventional medicine has not been able to cure or to even find a cause for the condition.

Chinese medical practitioners believe that a vital force, called "chi," flows through our body in channels, or meridians. When this vital force, or energy, becomes blocked or stagnant, disease and disharmony result. Acupuncture works by stimulating or relaxing points along the meridians to unblock energy and to encourage its flow.

Traditional Chinese medicine theorizes that the more than 2,000 acupuncture points on the human body connect with 12 main and 8 secondary pathways, called meridians. Chinese medicine practitioners believe these meridians conduct chi

Acupressure

Many acupuncturists will use finger pressure on points along the meridians instead of needles or moxa (an herb burnt at the site of accupuncture points). The principles are the same, but it is a gentler approach.

between the surface of the body and internal organs. Chi regulates spiritual, emotional, mental and physical balance. Chi is influenced by the opposing forces of yin and yang. According to traditional Chinese medicine, when yin and yang are balanced they work together with the natural flow of chi to help the body achieve and maintain health. Acupuncture is believed to balance yin and yang, keep the normal flow of energy unblocked, and restore health to the body and mind. Traditional Chinese medicine practices (including acupuncture, herbs, diet, massage, and meditative physical exercises) all are intended to improve the flow of chi.

Western scientists have found meridians hard to identify because meridians do not directly correspond to nerve or blood circulation pathways. Some researchers believe that meridians are located throughout the body's connective tissue.

What happens during treatment

The first consultation will last for up to 90 minutes, and your child's therapist will take great trouble to make an accurate diagnosis, since the success of the treatment depends upon it. He will ask you questions about your child's health, lifestyle, medical history, symptoms, sleep patterns, sensations of hot and cold, any dizziness, eating habits, bowel movements, emotional problems, relationships and many other factors.

He will note your child's general appearance, in particular facial color. He will then look at your child's eyes and tongue. He will listen to your child's breathing patterns, speech and the tone of her voice. Next he will use his sense of smell to decide where your child is imbalanced. Finally, he will take pulse readings on each wrist—and there are six basic Chinese pulses, three on each wrist. He will then decide on a course of treatment to restore your child's energy and ensure that she experiences optimum health.

Your child will have to lie on a table or couch and undress so that the acupuncturist can reach the relevant points on her body. In some cases only the socks need to be removed! The needles will be inserted into the skin, and manipulated to calm or stimulate a specific point. He will use up to eight needles, which will be left in for about 30 minutes, or removed very quickly. Your acupuncturist may also suggest some Chinese herbal treatment, or dietary or lifestyle changes to go alongside treatment.

You may carry on having treatment for as long as it is necessary to treat your child's condition. Chronic conditions like asthma and eczema take a little longer

THE WORLD HEALTH ORGANISATION recognizes the use of acupuncture in the treatment of a wide range of medical problems, including abdominal pain, allergies, constipation, diarrhea, indigestion, anxiety, depression, insomnia, nervousness, neurosis, cataracts, gingivitis, poor vision, tinnitus, toothache, athletic performance, chronic fatigue, immune system tonification, stress reduction, arthritis (including juvenile), back pain, muscle cramping, muscle pain/weakness, neck pain, headaches, migraines, bladder dysfunction, asthma, bronchitis, common cold, sinusitis, tonsillitis, childhood illnesses, flu.

Conditions like cancer, ME, irritable bowel syndrome and allergies, which have not been satisfactorily explained or treated by conventional medicine have been, in some cases, cured by acupuncture.

than acute conditions like flu—which has been lifted by acupuncture almost immediately in some cases. You should, however, see some improvement after three or four treatments. Many people return to their acupuncturists every two to three months for a "rebalancing" session after their initial illness has been cured. Acupuncture can also work preventatively, to improve whole health.

The needles are typically inserted ⅛ inch to ½ inch (0.3 to 1 cm) deep, but some procedures require the needles to be inserted as deep as 1 inch (2.5 cm). The acupuncture points are then stimulated either by gentle twirling, by heat, or by stimulation with a weak electrical current. Acupuncture points also can be stimulated by pressure, ultrasound, and certain wavelengths of light. Occasionally herbs are burnt at acupuncture points, and this technique is called moxibustion.

People experience acupuncture needling differently. Your child should feel only a tingling sensation as the needles are inserted; some feel absolutely no pain at all. Once the needles are in place, there is no pain felt. Acupuncture needles are very thin and solid and are made from stainless steel. The point is smooth (not hollow with cutting edges like a hypodermic needle) and insertion through the skin is not as painful as injections or blood sampling. The risk of bruising and skin irritation is less than when using a hollow needle. Because all acupuncturists carefully sterilize the needles using the same techniques as for surgical instruments, or use disposable needles, there is no risk of infection from the treatments.

As energy is redirected in the body, internal chemicals and hormones are stimulated and healing begins to take place. Occasionally the original symptoms worsen for a few days, or other general changes in appetite, sleep, bowel or urination patterns, or emotional state may be triggered. These should not cause concern, as they are simply indications that the acupuncture is starting to work. With the sessions, it is quite common for your child to have a sensation of deep relaxation or even mild disorientation immediately following the treatment. These pass within a short time, and never require anything more than a bit of rest to overcome.

Aromatherapy

Few therapies are as immediately pleasurable and effective as aromatherapy, and many children (boys included!) respond well to a variety of oils. There are several studies[3] showing the efficacy of aromatherapy on babies and toddlers and it can be a wonderful addition to a nighttime routine, or an afternoon baby massage (see Massage, page 274). Older children struggling through exams, or finding the transition between childhood and adolescence difficult, can also benefit from regular aromatherapeutic massage or baths.

What is aromatherapy?

Aromatherapy uses essential oils, which are the "life force" of aromatic flowers, herbs, plants, trees or spices, for therapeutic purposes. The word "aromatherapy" literally means "treatment using scents," and the therapy has evolved as a branch of herbal medicine. Unlike the herbs used in herbal medicine, essential oils are not taken internally (except in very rare cases), but are inhaled or diluted and applied to the skin. Each oil has its own natural fragrance and a gentle, healing action.

How it works

No one knows exactly how different scents can have such a dramatic effect on health, but studies show they do work. It is believed that receptors in the nose convert smells into electrical impulses, which are transmitted to the limbic system of the brain. Smells reaching the limbic system can directly affect moods and emotions, and improve mental alertness and concentration.

Essential oils enter the body by inhalation and by absorption through the pores of the skin. Once in the body they work in three ways: pharmacologically, physiologically and psychologically. The chemical constituents of the oils are carried in the bloodstream to all areas of the body where they react with body chemistry in a way that is similar to drugs. Certain oils also have an affinity with particular areas of the body, and their properties have a balancing, sedating, stimulating or other effect on body systems. It can take between 20 minutes and several hours for oils to be absorbed into the body, but on average it takes about 90 minutes. After several hours the oils leave the body. Most are exhaled, others are eliminated in urine, feces and perspiration.

Understanding essential oils

Essential oils are extracted from the leaves, flowers, fruit, wood, bark and roots of plants and trees. They are natural chemical compounds, more complex and safer than pharmaceutical drugs, but slower acting so they are best used as a preventive or complementary treatment.

About 150 essential oils have been extracted for use in aromatherapy. Each essential oil has a unique fragrance and more than 100 different chemical components, which work together to heal mind and body. All the oils are antiseptic and may have numerous other actions (anti-inflammatory, pain relieving, decongestant, antispasmodic, antibacterial or antidepressant, to name just a few). Every oil also has a dominant characteristic, so it is classified as stimulating, relaxing or refreshing, for example. Some oils are specialist oils that can adapt to treat whatever is required in the body at that time. For example, lavender oil can either relax or invigorate, depending on the body's needs. These types of oils are called "adaptogenic."

How to use essential oils

There are lots of ways to use essential oils at home, and some are more appropriate for children than others. A drop in the bath is probably the best way, but remember that smaller children need far less of these oils than adults, and too much can be toxic (see below). The main ways to use the oils are as follows:

Massage

Dilute the essential oil in a vegetable carrier oil such grapeseed, sweet almond, olive or sunflower oil. Use two drops of essential oil in five tablespoons (100 ml) for babies, and four drops in the same quantity for children over the age of three. Always dilute the oils for massage, as they can cause rashes and an uncomfortable reaction if used neat.

Steam inhalations

Add three to four drops of oil to a bowl of boiling water. Older children can be encouraged to bend over the bowl, with their head covered with a towel. Ask them to breathe deeply for a few minutes. Hot water and children don't mix, so this is not an appropriate treatment for children under the age of about ten. Steam inhalations for younger children can be used by running hot water in the bathroom sink, adding the oils to the water, and then closing the door until the bathroom fills with steam.

Vaporizers can be electric or a ceramic ring that is heated by a light bulb, but most are ceramic pots warmed by a small candle. Add water and six to eight drops of oil to the vaporizer. Alternatively, add the oil to a bowl of water and place by a radiator.

Baths

Children need only one or two drops of essential oils in the bath. Make sure you swish the water around with your hand to ensure that the drop disperses. If you use oils in your child's bath, try to keep the water away from his eyes.

Creams, lotions and shampoos

Add one or two drops of essential oil to creams, lotions and shampoos and massage into the skin or scalp. Using tea tree oil in shampoo or conditioner, for example, can help to prevent head lice. Once again, keep away from your child's eyes. Add a drop of chamomile oil to aqueous or calendula cream for eczema or itchy skin, or a drop of lavender in a gentle moisturizer to ease a fractious baby off to sleep. For a baby, one or two drops of essential oil in five tablespoons (100 ml) cream, shampoo or lotion is about right. For an older child, you can use up to four drops of essential oil.

Gargles and mouthwashes

Dilute one to two drops of essential oil (tea tree, clove or lavender) in a glass of warm water and swish around the mouth or use as a gargle. This is only for children who are old enough to know not to swallow! No aromatherapy oils should be used orally without the advice of a practitioner.

Neat

A few essential oils such as lavender, tea tree oil and sandalwood can be applied undiluted to the skin (in the case of chicken pox, for example, or cuts or burns). Most oils should not be used neat, and for that reason bottles should be kept well away from children.

Hot and cold compresses

Add one to two drops of essential oil to a bowl of hot or cold water. Soak a folded clean cotton cloth in the water, wring it out and apply over the affected area. Children should use only hand-hot water, no matter what the ailment.

Safety notes

Aromatherapy is compatible with conventional medicine and most other forms of holistic treatment. However, if your child is taking medication, consult your doctor. Some oils are not compatible with homeopathic treatment. Aromatherapy is safe to use at home for minor or short-term problems, providing you follow certain guidelines.

▶ Top safety tips

- Do not take essential oils internally.

- Do not put essential oils in or near your child's eyes.

- Keep all oil bottles away from your children.

- Do not apply oils undiluted to the skin, unless recommended in this book, or by a qualified practitioner.

Consult a qualified practitioner for advice and treatment if your child:

- has allergies of any kind (particularly to plants)

- has epilepsy or another chronic health condition
- has chronic or serious health problems or if a problem becomes severe or persistent

Putting aromatherapy into practice

There are many conditions that will benefit from aromatherapy. Babies, small children, adolescents and parents can all use the oils safely, provided you follow the above instructions for use. Need some ideas? Try these top tips.

Stop the snuffling

If your child has a cold that is keeping him awake at night, place a few drops of eucalyptus oil in a bowl of hot water on the bedroom radiator and close the door. Eucalyptus oil is a decongestant and the steam will help to open blocked airways. Add a drop of lavender oil to the bowl as well, to ease your child off to sleep and to disinfect the environment.

Colicky babies

Add two or three drops of roman chamomile oil to five tablespoons (100 ml) of a warmed light carrier oil (grapeseed is a good one) and massage your baby about an hour before symptoms normally set in (often in the evening). Concentrate on the abdominal area and the back and shoulders. Chamomile oil is digestive and relaxing, and can help to reduce the symptoms of colic.

Head lice about?

Add one drop of tea tree oil to your child's conditioner and leave on the hair for five or ten minutes. Comb through and rinse thoroughly. This will help to prevent head lice from settling on the hair follicles, and will kill eggs that are there (see page 366). Do this two or three times a week as a preventive measure (not every day). Tea tree oil is antiparasitic

Stressful times

Exam time? A big game coming up? Or just problems in the playground or at home? A drop or two of lavender oil in the bath every evening will help to relax and rejuvenate, reducing the physical and emotional symptoms of stress. If your child is having trouble sleeping, it will help to ease her off to sleep. Lavender oil also works to counter stress hormones, leaving your child feeling fresher and more relaxed.

Groggy mornings

If your children have trouble getting up and going in the morning, place a few drops of rosemary oil in a water-filled pan on the stove. Bring to the boil and let the kitchen fill with invigorating steam. It's a great pick-me-up and gives your child a good start to the day.

The best oils for children

- **Benzoin:** a pulmonary antiseptic that can be used to help expel mucus and relieve respiratory congestion. Not suitable for babies under age one.

- **Bergamot:** an uplifting oil for physical or emotional fatigue. It is indicated for some types of eczema, and can help to heal pimples, boils and wounds. Not suitable for babies.

- **Roman or German chamomile:** an anti-inflammatory oil that helps to calm, soothe and control skin problems and allergies. It has pain-relieving qualities, making it ideal for teething, headaches and growing pains. Chamomile is antispasmodic and a sedative and is widely used for sleep disorders, colic, hyperactivity, anxiety, stress, indigestion and flatulence. Safe for children of all ages.

- **Eucalyptus:** an antiseptic, antibiotic, analgesic, anti-inflammatory, antiviral and stimulating oil that is great for reducing fevers in babies and children. Helps to take the itch out of chicken pox spots, helps to clear mucus and ease congestion in the respiratory tract. Use as an antiseptic for cuts and grazes. Safe for children of all ages.

- **Geranium:** an antiseptic, antidepressant, astringent, fortifying, refreshing and uplifting oil that is used to help a wide variety of ailments, including skin problems, wound healing, fatigue, symptoms of stress and mild depression. It can also be used as an insect repellent. Safe for children of all ages.

- **Lavender:** the prince of aromatherapy oils! It is a gentle oil with a huge range of properties, including antiseptic, antibiotic, analgesic, antidepressant, antiviral, antifungal, antispasmodic, healing and sedating. It is used for skin problems, such as eczema, diaper rash, spots, burns and cuts; it relaxes, relieves headaches, migraine and growing pains, and can help to soothe a child off to sleep. It's also used to calm, relieve pain, treat thrush and encourage the healing process. Safe for children of all ages.

- **Tangerine:** a gentle oil that is refreshing, antiseptic, tonic, digestive and mildly relaxing. It's ideal for tummy upsets, nerves, constipation, indigestion and colic. Safe for children of all ages.

- **Rose:** an expensive, luxurious oil with a wide range of effects, including antiseptic, antibiotic, antidepressant, anti-inflammatory, and tonic. It's used for depression, grief, sadness, shyness and as an everyday antiseptic. It's great for skin conditions, including diaper rash, and helps digestive complaints. Safe for children of all ages.

- **Tea tree:** an antibiotic, antiseptic, antifungal, antiviral and disinfectant oil that can be used for many conditions affecting children, including skin infections, head lice, boils, warts, thrush, athlete's foot, recurrent infections, wound healing and for boosting the immune system.

Caution:

The following oils should never be used on babies or children unsupervised: basil; clary sage; hyssop; juniper; myrrh; sage.

Art and Music Therapies

Art therapy

Art therapy is a form of emotional or "psycho" therapy that allows for emotional expression and healing through nonverbal means. Unlike most adults, young children cannot express themselves verbally, and as they become older they are often shy and self-conscious about expressing emotion. Art therapy is designed to help children break through self-expression barriers, using simple art materials.

By providing a safe and nonthreatening environment, art therapists invite your child to express his feelings through a variety of art media. Every child is encouraged to explore and interpret his own art, which is a form of empowerment, according to art therapists.

Artwork can be spontaneous, but it may also be directed by your child's therapist. Through the creative process, it is believed that children can often approach difficult issues and convey a message much more clearly and safely than with words. The art product serves as a record of these events, upon which your child can later reflect and eventually understand with greater clarity.

Art therapies are believed to help children:

- express feelings too difficult to talk about

- increase self-esteem and confidence

- develop healthy coping skills

- identify feelings and blocks to emotional expression and growth

- provide an avenue for communication

- make verbal expression more accessible

Art therapy at home

You can easily encourage your child to express himself creatively, and it simply involves offering plenty of good supplies and lots of praise. Disturbed adolescents often find art therapy one of the most acceptable therapies in which to explore their problems. Ask your child to paint or draw various emotions, such as anger, happiness, fear or excitement. Never discourage any attempts, or try to read anything into his efforts. Ask him to explain if he feels like it, but don't push the matter. The fact that he is using art to express emotion is what you are aiming for. Alternatively, use art in a variety of situations: when your child is upset, angry, confused, withdrawn or sad. Notice the difference between the types of work he produces in different emotional states. Use clay, paper, pens, paint, glue, scissors (at an appropriate age)— anything that will encourage the creative process.

If you are concerned about your child's emotional health on any level, do try these therapies at home, but consider involving your child in an art therapy group, with a trained practitioner who will be able to guide and interpret according to specific therapeutic criteria.

Music therapy

Music therapy involves using music and musical play to promote, maintain, and restore mental, physical, emotional and spiritual health. Music has nonverbal, creative, structural and emotional qualities. A trained therapist will use these to facilitate contact, interaction, self-awareness, learning, self-expression, communication and personal development.

According to the American Music Therapy Association, based in Silver Spring, Maryland, some of the elements of structured music therapy include

- vocal and instrumental improvisation

- singing and instrument playing

- music listening

- lyric discussion

- imagery and music

- rhythmic movement

- songwriting and composition

Seeing a music therapist

During the initial sessions a music therapy assessment is completed and specific therapeutic goals are established. The therapist then develops a treatment plan with short-term objectives as steps to achieve the long-term goals. Evaluation of the treatment effectiveness is an ongoing part of the treatment plan.

What can music therapy treat?

According to research, music therapy treats a wide range of health and emotional conditions in people of all ages, regardless of disability or musical background. Some of the most relevant applications include treating autism and other developmental disabilities, insomnia, digestive upsets (particularly those caused by stress), emotional traumas, hearing impairments, mental health, neonatal care, oncology, pain control, physical disabilities, speech and language impairments, adolescent problems, visual impairments.

How does it work?

The American Music Therapy Association has had unprecedented success using this type of therapy with children and suggests it works in the following ways:

- Singing is used to help children (and adults) with speech impairments improve their articulation, rhythm and breath control. In a group setting, children develop a greater awareness of others by singing together.

- Playing instruments can improve gross and fine motor coordination in individuals with motor impairments. Playing instruments in a group helps a child with behavioral problems to learn how to control disruptive impulses by working within a group structure. Learning a piece of music and performing it develops musical skills and helps a person build self-reliance, self-esteem and self-discipline.

- Rhythmic movement is used to facilitate and improve an individual's range of motion, joint mobility/agility/strength, balance, coordination, gait consistency, respiration patterns and muscular relaxation. The rhythmic component of music helps to increase motivation, interest and enjoyment, and acts as a nonverbal persuasion to involve individuals socially.

- Listening to music has many therapeutic applications. It helps develop cognitive skills such as attention and memory. It facilitates the process of coming to terms with difficult issues by providing a creative environment for self-expression. Music evokes memories and associations. Actively listening to music in a relaxed and receptive state stimulates thoughts, images and feelings that can be further examined and discussed, either with the therapist alone or within a supportive group setting.

Using music therapy at home

Encourage music in children of all ages—dancing, playing instruments, singing, listening to all types of music from the latest Disney hits to opera and classical music. Get them to talk about the music and how it makes them feel. Use it as an emotional outlet and never discourage their tastes, even if they seem obscure! Music has been proved to have a wide variety of therapeutic benefits, including lulling children off to sleep (lullabies were invented for a reason!) and improving mood.

If you want to use music to help treat health problems, particularly if they are chronic or congenital, contact a registered music therapist, who will undertake an appropriate program. But don't just leave it to the experts—fill your children's lives with music as much as you can.

Buteyko method

Children as young as four or five years old have successfully learned the Buteyko method, which is a therapy indicated for asthma (in particular) and other health conditions, including allergies, sleep apnea, hay fever and even digestive problems. It is highly recommended that you take a course alongside your child, or visit a Buteyko therapist, as the therapy itself involves changing breathing habits.

What is it?

The basic premise is that a number of illnesses are caused by hyperventilation or "overbreathing." Symptoms of hyperventilation include chest tightness, feelings of breathlessness, blocked nose, frequently breathing through the mouth, irritable upper airways, overproduction of mucus, poor sleep patterns, nightmares, chronic tiredness, irritable coughing, frequent yawning and/or sighing, phlegm, dizziness, "spaced out" feeling, indigestion, clammy hands and erratic heartbeat.

Dr. Konstantin Buteyko was a Russian doctor who over the years studied hundreds of patients and developed the theory that much ill health is the result of the body's defense mechanisms trying to compensate for a lack of carbon dioxide. Overbreathing, he argued, was not just a symptom, but a cause of illnesses ranging from cardiac problems to breathing disorders.

He showed that many of us breathe too deeply, and his observations suggest that a higher proportion of carbon dioxide, traditionally regarded as a waste product of breathing, is essential if the body is to function properly.

Putting it into practice

- The basic exercise is called the Control Pause, which is the length of time that your child can hold her breath after breathing out, and not feel the need to breathe again. An ideal control pause is 60 seconds; a control pause of 15 or below shows serious and chronic asthma.

- Children can be taught the control pause, or they can use another method of measuring time—taking steps. Ask your child to pretend that she is underwater. Ask her to blow out all the air in her lungs. Without drawing in any breath, ask her to walk around the room at a slow pace. Count the number of steps she takes.

Ideally, your child should be able to take 120 steps, which is the equivalent, of a Control Pause of 50 to 60 seconds; 120 steps means that she is unlikely to suffer from asthma. Don't worry unduly if she is well below 120; it will gradually build up over time.

- When your child cannot hold her breath any longer, she should start to breathe shallowly. Tell her to resist the temptation to gulp when she releases her nose. Join in with her if you think it would be helpful.

- Once she has completed her steps, she should continue to breathe shallowly with her mouth shut. Any child who began this exercise with a blocked nose will probably find that it is becoming less congested.

- Ask your child to sit still and breathe gently—like a small mouse—for three or four minutes. To check that she is doing this correctly, put a finger under her nose to feel the air flow. It should feel very, very light. Teach your child to do this at the first sign of any asthma problem.

Children also need to be encouraged to breathe through their noses at all times. Unless they are eating, talking or drinking, they need to keep their mouths shut. Buteyko therapists suggest taping their mouths shut (not as draconian as it sounds; micropore tape is used and it can be easily removed by children of all ages), particularly at night.

Practice this exercise two or three times a day, noting down the control pause figure, or the number of steps. Encourage your child to exercise—running and playing in the backyard, for example—with her mouth closed. Over time, her breathing habits will change completely, and with higher concentrations of carbon dioxide in the blood (in ratio to oxygen), she should experience a significant decline in asthma symptoms, as well as enhanced concentration and mood.

Cranial osteopathy

Osteopathy is one of the most conventionally accepted complementary therapies, treating a wide range of health conditions in people of all ages. While general osteopathy is commonly and successfully used to treat children, it is cranial osteopathy that has most recently attracted a great deal of attention. I'll focus on this type of osteopathy here, mainly because of the dramatic impact it can have on your child's health. Studies show that 80 percent of children with learning difficulties, including autism and dyslexia, suffered a traumatic birth. Taking that one step further, osteopaths point to research showing that some 80 percent of all children suffer trauma at birth, which can affect immunity, overall health, development and even language skills.[4] By reversing the damage caused at birth, osteopaths—cranial osteopaths in particular—can cure chronic health conditions, improve well-being and sleeping habits, and make a big difference to your child's health on every level.

What is cranial osteopathy?

The philosophy of osteopathic medicine is based on the theory that the human body constitutes an ecologically and biologically unified whole. All body systems are united through the neuroendocrine and circulatory systems. Therefore, when looking at disease and other health problems, osteopaths address the whole body, not just symptoms.

The name "osteopathy" stems from the Latin words *osteon* and *pathos*, which translates to "suffering of the bone." This name has caused some confusion, for it suggests that osteopaths treat only conditions involving bones. However, the name was chosen because Dr. Andrew Still, the American founder of osteopathy, recognized that a well-balanced, properly functioning body relies on both the muscular and skeletal systems being healthy and well.

Cranial osteopathy was developed in the 1930s, by American osteopath Dr. William Garner Sutherland, a disciple of Dr. Still. His training taught him that the bones of the skull that are separate at birth grew together into a fixed structure and so could not move, but he noticed that the bones of the skull retained some potential for movement even in adulthood. If they could move, they could also be susceptible to dysfunction. Dr. Still had taught his students that cerebrospinal fluid (the clear watery fluid surrounding the brain and spinal cord) was "the highest known element in the human body." Dr. Sutherland discovered that the fluid had detectable rhythms which he called "the breath of life," as the rhythms appeared to be influenced by the rate and depth of breathing. By gently manipulating the skull he found he could alter the rhythm of this fluid flow and suggested that it might stimulate the body's self-healing ability and help to heal conditions that appeared unrelated to the cranium.

Dr. Sutherland found out that manipulation could bring about a range of reactions that varied from physiological to emotional changes. He concluded that good physical and mental health depends not only on the bones of the skull being in the right position, but also on the ability of the sutures to allow for slight movement. Through research it was discovered that this movement was not confined to the head, but that it could be felt throughout the body.

Dr. Sutherland spent 30 years studying this self-regulating movement, which he called the primary respiratory mechanisms (PRM). This mechanism is characterized by light movement of the bones in the skull and sacrum, the membrane system (visceral) and the central nervous system's cerebrospinal fluid. More recently research has proven that the cranial sutures are indeed like the other joints in the body and that the head actually has a moving structure. At the request of the American Academy of Osteopathy, the PRM has been measured by NASA physicists and numerous papers have been published to prove its existence.

Birth trauma

Viola Frymann, an American osteopathic doctor who trained with Sutherland, studied over 1,500 babies through eight years. All were examined within the first five days of birth and many were seen within 24 hours of birth. This study revealed the startling fact that approximately 10 percent of the newborn babies had perfect, freely mobile cranial mechanisms. Another 10 percent had had such severe trauma to the head that the diagnosis was obvious even to untrained observers. But the most fascinating result of this study was the fact that the remaining 80 percent all had some strain patterns in the cranial mechanism.

During labor and delivery, structures of the baby's body may become significantly compressed, resulting in a general decrease in function. The symptoms associated with these birth-related structural problems vary with the degree of distortion and between individual children.

According to osteopathy, health involves

- proper drainage of venous blood and lymphatic fluid

- proper supply of arterial blood

- proper flow in the nerves

- proper breathing of body tissues

Decreased health occurs when the body structure is compromised, affecting all of these areas. Any trauma, such as a difficult birth, may cause a strain to the tissues from twisting, overstretching or compression. If the trauma is small, the body may be able to heal by itself. If it is moderate to large or the recuperative capacity is too compromised, it cannot fix itself. Then the nervous system will contain these distortions, in an attempt to negotiate balance. If the forces are too great, the nervous system cannot fully compensate and the imbalances will appear extreme.

For example, according to cranial osteopaths, one common cause of colic is trauma during birth to the occipital area (back of the head). The occipital bone is composed of four parts at birth, and nerves that pass between these parts may be compressed from the forces of labor on the head. In addition, there are also other important nerves and veins that travel between these parts and the adjacent area (temporal bones). With the compression of the occipital area, and the possible change in the shape and relationship of parts of the head, pressure may be placed on these structures, altering the way in which they work and causing further symptoms.

There are many factors that can cause birth trauma, including a long labor, false labor, failure of the mother's cervix to dilate, the use of drugs to increase contraction intensity, vacuum extraction, forceps, incorrect positioning in the birth canal and even fetal distress.

Most common problems involve

- impaired suckling

- impaired swallowing

- irritability of the stomach and colon

- frequent spitting up or vomiting

- colic

- sleeplessness [5]

- learning disabilities

- behavioral problems

- mechanical problems, such as scoliosis

A cranial osteopath will gently "listen" with his hands to detect little areas of tension and built-up pressure that may be having a disturbing effect on a child.

How does it work?

Cranial osteopathy is a specialist technique used to manipulate the bones of the skull with a touch so light that many people claim they can barely feel it.

The human skull is made up of some 26 bones that are not fixed but can move slightly. Inside the skull the brain is surrounded by cerebrospinal fluid. The fluid is secreted in the brain and from there flows out of the skull and down the spine, enveloping the spinal cord and the base of the spinal nerves. Practitioners believe that cerebrospinal fluid is pumped through the spinal canal by means of a rhythmic pulsation, which has its own rhythm, unrelated to the heartbeat or the breathing mechanism.

When the bones of the skull move normally the cranial rhythm remains balanced, but any disturbance to the cranial bones can disturb the normal motion of the bones and consequently alter the cranial rhythm. This affects the functioning of other parts of the body.

A trained osteopath can feel the rhythm of the cranial pulse anywhere in the body, but principally at the skull and the sacrum. By holding and exerting very gentle pressure on the skull the practitioner can feel the rhythm of the cranial pulse and detect irregularities. The technical approach used involves extremely gentle, but specifically applied, adjustments to the movement of body tissues. Cranial osteopathy is both gentle and noninvasive, making it a very safe method of diagnosis and treatment for even newborn babies.

During treatment your child will usually feel only a very light pressure from the practitioner's hands, and many of the techniques require a very gentle touch indeed. The osteopath's hands may be placed on the head, spine or sacrum, as well as on an arm or leg or over an organ such as the liver.

Your child will be lying down for most techniques, although in some cases, sitting is advised. Your child will feel deeply relaxed during the treatment, and immediately afterward.

There are many conditions that have been successfully treated by cranial osteopathy, including asthma, coordination difficulties, dental problems, digestive problems, dyslexia, glue ear (see page 353), hyperactivity, colic, sleeping problems, migraines and headaches, digestive disorders (including colic), speech problems, and also scoliosis (abnormal curvature of the spine).

Flower remedies

This delightful therapy is misleadingly simple, but the results can be dramatic. Children are often more expressive than adults, wearing their hearts on their sleeves and their tempers on the tip of the tongue. For that reason, negative emotions—the basic tool for assessing appropriate remedies—are often easily recognized and treated.

Flower essences, or flower remedies, as they are more commonly known, are used therapeutically to harmonize the body, mind and the spirit. The bottled flower essences are said to contain vibrations of the sun's energy, absorbed by the flowers' petals when immersed in sun-warmed water. The remedies use the vibrational essence of the flowers to balance the negative emotions that lead to and are symptoms of disease. They are a simple, natural method of establishing personal equilibrium and harmony.

How they work

Flower remedies do not work in any biochemical way, and because no physical part of the plant remains in the remedy, its properties and actions cannot be detected or analyzed as if it were a drug or herbal preparation. Therapists believe the remedies contain the energy or "memory" of the plant from which it was made and work in a way that is similar to homeopathic remedies—on a vibrational basis (see page 267).

Some of the remedies are known as "type remedies." Your child's type remedy is effectively the remedy that is most compatible with your child's personality or basic character, and it can be taken when the negative side of his character threatens the positive. The difficulty with the type remedy lies in analyzing your character and deciding which remedy matches it best. For example, if you have a perfectionist child who works hard at school, and seems happy and proud of his work, his insistence upon perfection would be considered a positive side of his character. If, however, he becomes obsessive about his work, becomes aggressive and difficult to please, and demands too much of other people, then the negative side of this characteristic has taken over, and the appropriate essence would right the balance.

Flower remedies are ideal for home use, being simply made and used. They are made in water, preserved with alcohol and employ the ability of flowers to change and enhance mood, and to balance the negative emotions which contribute to disease. Some parents are concerned about using a remedy preserved in brandy or another alcohol, but only a drop is required and this would have no effect on your child's health. If you don't want to offer an alcohol-based treatment orally, rub a few drops into your child's pulse points and even put a few drops in the bath. The effects may be slower, but the remedies will still work.

Understanding negative emotions

Negative emotions depress the mind and immune system, repress activity and contribute to ill health. Some of the most common negative emotions include fear, uncertainty, loneliness, oversensitivity to influences and ideas, despondency, overconcern for the welfare of others and despair. There are many others, and you will recognize some of them when your children become ill. Just before physical symptoms set in, you may notice tearfulness, irrational fears (of being alone, for example), depression or anxiety. These are all negative emotional states that can be addressed using flower essences.

Flower essences work to right the negative emotion, improving well-being on an emotional level that transmits to good physical health. They can be used to prevent and treat illness by working on an emotional level.

A word about Dr. Bach

Until recently, the name Dr. Edward Bach was almost synonymous with flower remedies. His set of 38 remedies became the inspiration for the worldwide development of hundreds of different remedies. Dr. Bach's remedies are still the cornerstone of flower essence therapy, and they remain some of the simplest to use, and the most widely available. They are an excellent starting point for any parent who wants to experiment with flower essence therapy, and they come with literature explaining exactly how they work and in what situations.

While working in the London Homeopathic Hospital, just after the First World War, Dr. Bach noticed that people with similar attitudes often had similar complaints. He concluded that mood and a negative attitude predisposed toward ill health. He believed that illness was a manifestation of a deeper disharmony. Over five years he identified seven main negative states and made the "12 healers" or flower remedies to address them. Over the next few years he dedicated himself to finding natural remedies from the countryside and at his death had made 38 separate remedies.

Bach Flower Remedies are mainly made from the trees and flowers Dr. Bach studied on his travels. Apart from vine and olive, most are native to the U.K., although they are widely available in flower essence form around the world. On the basis of his work, remedies have been developed in other countries—in particular the U.S. and Australia. Over the last 20 years, dozens of new remedies have been explored, making the range wider and more exciting than ever before. Flower essences, flower remedies and bush flower essences are all common names for these gentle remedies, which shouldn't be confused with essential oils. All flower essences address the emotional self, unlocking repressions, liberating negativity and encouraging positive well-being.

The Bach remedies

The 38 Bach flower remedies support every conceivable personality, attitude and negative state of mind. They were developed as a complete system and, before his death, Bach gave instructions that no more remedies were to be added to the set. His aim was to keep the system as simple as possible, and although some therapists may find the system restrictive, the remedies were devised for self-help, and most users find their simplicity appealing.

Bach classified all emotional problems into seven major groups: fear; uncertainty and indecision; insufficient interest in present circumstances; loneliness; oversensitivity; despondency or despair; and overcare for the welfare of others. Through their subtle vibrational energy, the remedies work to heal every negative aspect of these seven types of emotional illness, thereby restoring mental harmony and preventing physical illness from taking hold.

Using the remedies

Flower remedies can complement other types of therapies such as herbalism, homeopathy or aromatherapy, or be used alone. Flower essences are simple and effective and can be used to:

- support in times of crisis

- treat the emotional symptoms produced by illness

- address a particular recurring emotional or behavioral pattern

- help prevent illness by identifying negative emotional states that are the precursors to ill health

Remedies act quickly, and there should be an improvement within days, although it make take months to fully address a long-standing pattern.

The flower remedies or essences bought in a store are sold in stock bottles. These should not be used straight from the bottle, but mixed to make a personal remedy. Sometimes a single flower remedy is needed, but in most cases two or more are combined.

Successful treatment depends on accurate diagnosis. Get to know the different essences available and then aim to match the remedies to your child.

Personal remedies

Every flower essence has specific properties, and you will need to discover which is the most effective for your child. Often a blend is the most effective, and your choice of remedies will depend upon your child's overwhelming emotional characteristics at the time.

You'll need:

- 1 oz (30 ml) glass amber dropper bottle

- 1 oz (30 ml) spring water or ⅓ oz (10 ml) brandy and ⅔ oz (20 ml) spring water

Decide on the remedies that are most applicable. Many parents find that a number of remedies appear to be suitable. Choose four or five that seem most appropriate and try these first. After a month or so, you may want to try a different combination.

Put four drops of each remedy into a clean dropper bottle and fill with clean spring water. The remedies should be used within a week or so and kept in the refrigerator. If you want to keep the personal blend for longer, you can add ⅓ oz (10 ml) of brandy before filling with spring water, but many parents may not like the idea of adding more alcohol.

The standard dose is to take four drops, under the tongue, four times a day. In stressful or traumatic situations, add two drops to a glass of water and sip as required.

For babies or anyone who has been seriously injured, or is intolerant of alcohol, rub the drops into pulse points (on the wrists and the neck), or add to the bath water.

Safety notes

Like homeopathic remedies, people of all ages will benefit from these essences and they are appropriate for even the youngest babies. They will not interfere with any other form of treatment, and they can even be used successfully on animals and plants!

Starting with Dr. Bach's system

A good way to begin using flower essences is to understand the types of negative emotions they address. Dr. Bach's system is straightforward and covers the vast majority of negative emotions.

Agrimony	For those who hide their feelings behind humor and put on a brave face.
Aspen	For fear of the unknown. Vague, unsettling fears that cannot be explained.
Beech	For the perfectionist who tends to be intolerant of other people's methods and experience.
Centaury	For those who find it impossible to say no to others' demands and thus exhaust themselves by doing too much.
Cerato	For those who lack confidence in themselves and are constantly seeking the advice of others.
Cherry Plum	For the fear of losing the mind and having irrational thoughts or behavior.
Chestnut Bud	For those who find it hard to learn from life and keep making the same mistakes.
Chicory	For the self-obsessed, mothering type who is overprotective and possessive.
Clematis	For the absent-minded daydreamer who needs to be awake and have the mind focused on the here and now.
Crab Apple	For those who feel unclean or polluted on any level. Physical, emotional or spiritual. For those who need a purification ritual.
Elm	For those who suffer temporary feelings of inadequacy brought on by their high expectations of themselves.

Gentian	For despondency and those who are easily discouraged and set back in life. Pessimism.
Gorse	For those who suffer hopelessness and despair after a long struggle and who are stuck in a negative pattern.
Heather	For those who like to be the center of things and talk constantly about themselves. Poor listeners.
Holly	For those who develop a victim mentality and suffer bouts of anger, jealously and envy.
Honeysuckle	For those who suffer from nostalgia or who dwell in the past to escape a painful future.
Hornbeam	For those who are stuck in a rut and exhausted so that work that used to be fulfilling is now tiresome.
Impatiens	For impatience and irritability. For those who are always in a rush and are too busy to slow down.
Larch	For those who feel worthless and who are suffering from lack of confidence or low self-esteem.
Mimulus	For the fear of known things. For the strength to face fears that can be named, for example the fear of flying.
Mustard	For depression and those who feel they are under a dark gloomy cloud, for no apparent reason.
Oak	For the fighter who never gives in and is exhausting themselves by being too narrow minded in the same old fight.
Olive	For those who are exhausted on all levels. Fatigued and drained of further optimism and spirit.
Pine	For those who suffer self-reproach and guilt. For those who say sorry even when things are not their fault.
Red Chestnut	For those who are over-anxious for the welfare of family or friends.
Rock Rose	For those who feel helpless and experience terror or panic. There may or may not be a reason but the feeling is real.
Rock Water	For perfectionists who are hard on themselves and demand perfection in all things.
Scleranthus	For those who suffer from indecision and who cannot make up their mind.
Star of Bethlehem	For shocks of all kinds, accidents, bad news, sudden startling noise and trauma.
Sweet Chestnut	For utter despair and hopelessness, for when there seems no way out.

Vervain	For overstraining and stress. For perfectionists, hard on themselves and overstrained by trying to meet their own exacting ideals.
Vine	For the overstrong and dominating leader who may tend toward tyranny. For bullying.
Walnut	For change. For breaking links so that life may develop in another direction.
Water Violet	For people who are aloof, self-reliant and self-contained. To relax the reserved and enable sharing.
White Chestnut	For tiresome mental chatter and the overactive mind, full of persistent and unwanted patterns of thought.
Wild Oat	For those who need help in deciding on the path and purpose of their life.
Wild Rose	For those who drift through life resigned to accept any eventuality. Fatalists.
Willow	For those who feel they have been treated unfairly. For pessimism and self-pity.

Rescue Remedy (also called Five-Flower Essence) is made from equal amounts of these five essences:

- **Cherry Plum** for feelings of desperation.

- **Rock Rose** to ease terror, fear or panic.

- **Impatiens** to soothe irritability and tension.

- **Clematis** to counteract the tendency to drift away from the present.

- **Star of Bethlehem** to address the mental and physical symptoms of shock.

▶ *Other good essences*

Not in the Bach range, these flower essences are, however, also extremely useful, and widely available (particularly by mail order):

- **Aloe Vera** for energy and revitalization.

- **Black-Eyed Susan** for awareness of hidden emotions (when your child is always sweet, for example, but clearly hiding hidden anger or fears).

- **Strelitzia Essence** for indecision (particularly important in adolescence, which is a time of great decision-making and change) and to assist in finding the right path.

- **Adolescence Essence** is specifically designed to assist teenagers in the transformative process. It is a combination of the following seven South African essences, each of which can also be used individually when it seems appropriate: cape almond, dune calendula, loquat, maple, mountain cabbage tree, plumbago and wild pear.

- **Ixia Essence** strengthens self-confidence and is indicated for shyness, timidity or introversion.

- **Oreganum** allows your child to be at ease with himself, without the need to pretend to be what his peers expect him to be.

- **Wattle** for unexpressed emotions.

- **Dog Rose** for grief that is being denied or not verbalized.

- **English Hawthorn** for broken-heartedness, intense grief or remorse.

- **Cancer Bush** for inner turmoil and torment.

- **Peach** for the effects of past trauma or even for a melancholic state of mind.

- **Loquat Essence**, when your child complains of being bored, or doesn't want to get out of bed.

- **Freesia** is a wonderful essence for apathy.

- **Cucumber** for lack of vitality and interest in life, for a sense of being defeated, and pessimism.

- **Australian Tea Tree** or **Jacaranda** are useful for procrastination.

- **Maple Essence** is for those who burn the candle at both ends, possibly depleting their physical resources. It is particularly recommended for periods of physical growth and brings about a sense of balance and harmony.

- **Zimbabwe Creeper** brings a sense of moderation for children who drive themselves too hard to achieve, for whom no success is enough, or who feel they have to do it all by themselves.

- **Belladonna Essence** is for the desire to blame and punish and for uncontrollable temper; **Wild Pear** is for bitterness, resentment, holding grudges and the inability to forgive; and **Fuchsia** is applicable when the anger is suppressed and emotional expression inhibited.

There are many, many other flower remedies. Look in your local health store, or order over the Internet (see page 444), according to your child's unique characteristics. There are special pre-blended remedies for things like exam stress, bowel problems, impatience, and even several designed for parents (try Parent Essence, a South African blend).

Putting flower essences into practice

The blend you choose for your child will be unique to her personality and character. For that reason, it is difficult to give blanket suggestions. There are, however, some tried-and-tested remedies for certain situations and types of children.

▶ *Top tried-and-tested flower remedies*

- If your child is afraid of anything "known"—in other words, something tangible, such as the dark, cats, school, her best friend's mother—use Mimulus. This is also a good remedy for stage fright before the school play or exam nerves.

- In the case of any shock, injury, trauma, bereavement or emotional or physical disturbance, use Rescue Remedy. Rescue Remedy rebalances the body after any upset. Rescue Remedy speeds healing after accidents, operations and dental surgery. It's great when you have a hysterical child or baby on your hands. Take a few drops yourself.

- Use Rescue Remedy Cream after sunburn, cuts, bruises or damage from accidents. It is also good for any type of skin trauma, including allergic rashes, eczema and insect bites and stings.

- If your child has been chronically ill, seems to have little energy or enthusiasm for anything, and seems to be slow to heal, try Olive, which works to alleviate feelings of utter fatigue.

- If your child has started a new school, changed teachers, gone through a parental divorce, lost a loved one, entered adolescence or experienced significant change of any type, offer Walnut.

- For an impatient child, who cannot seem to accept life's pace, his own short-comings or those of others, and who seems to be set back by his own inability to wait, try Impatiens. It's also a good remedy for parents at the end of their tether—and temper.

Herbalism

Western herbalism takes a different approach from practitioners trained in the East (China, Japan or India, for example), but it has strong roots in the Western folk tradition, and in much early medicine. Herbs are very good remedies for children, and can complement a broad range of other therapies.

Herbalism embraces the use of plants, particularly herbs, for healing. Like many other complementary therapies, it is based on a holistic approach to health, and treatment will be undertaken after an assessment of your child's individual symptoms, as well as lifestyle factors and overall health, on a physical, emotional and spiritual level. For many parents herbalism is an easy therapy to apply and use, and it appears, on the surface, to be closest to our conventional medical system. Like drugs, many herbs have a specific effect on symptoms or a part of the body. The difference is, however, that they do much more than work on a physical level.

How it works

Herbal medicine is designed to be gentle, stimulating the body to return to health by strengthening its systems as well as attacking the cause of the illness itself. Probably the most important principle of herbal medicine is that extracts are taken from the whole plant (or the whole of a part of the plant, like the leaves or the roots), not isolated or synthesized to perform specific functions. While this may seem an odd thing to point out, it is relevant. Many common drugs are based on herbal medicine. The difference is that scientists have often isolated the active ingredient and used this as the basis of the medicine. In some cases, they synthesize it (make it synthetically), which takes it one step further from nature. As most of us know, many drugs have side effects, even those with a natural, herbal base. However, herbs are used in their natural form, and the problems caused by using single ingredients do not exist. In fact, most herbs have very few side effects whatsoever.

Furthermore, professional advice and treatment is always tailored to individual needs and because of this there is far less chance of having an adverse reaction to treatment. The aim of herbalism is to help the body to heal itself, and to restore balanced health, not just to relieve the symptoms of the disorder being treated.

Using herbs

Herbal medication is designed to help the whole body, and to stimulate its responses in order to cure disease. One or many herbs may be administered in the following forms, depending on your child's symptoms and all of the information that you have provided to your herbalist. Herbs can also be used successfully at home, but it's important to remember that they are powerful healing agents and can be toxic in high doses (see below).

It's important to remember that the fresher, or more recently picked the herb, the stronger its active properties. Dried herbs are more readily available and are about one-third as strong as the fresh product—and in some cases actually must be used.

Tinctures

Powdered, fresh or dried herbs are placed in an airtight container with alcohol and left for a period of time. Alcohol extracts the valuable or essential parts of the plant and preserves them for the longest possible time. Children would take about five drops of a tincture, but you should always read the label as dosages differ between products. If you are using herbal tinctures for a baby, use only one drop, and only on the advice of a registered herbalist.

Decoctions

The roots, twigs, berries, seeds and barks of a plant are used and, much like an infusion (see below), they are boiled in water to extract the plants' ingredients. The liquid is strained and taken with organic honey or brown sugar to make it palatable. Decoctions should be refrigerated and will last about three days. Don't be surprised if your child rejects a herbal decoction. Blending a little in some fruit juice may help the medicine go down.

Infusions

Effectively another word for tea, an infusion uses dried herbs or in some instances fresh, which are steeped in boiled water for about ten minutes. Infusions are most suitable for plants from which the leaves and flowers are used, since their properties are more easily extracted by gentle boiling. Always cool an infusion before offering it to a young child.

Tisanes

Tisanes are mild infusions, usually prepackaged and sold in the form of a teabag, which can be boiled for a much shorter period of time than an infusion. Chamomile or peppermint tea available at the supermarket would be considered a tisane. Once again, serve warm, not hot, to young children.

Powders

Herbs in this form can be added to food or drinks, or put into capsules for easier consumption and convenience. You can make your own powder by crushing dried plant parts with a mortar and pestle, or chop them finely in a food processor or coffee grinder. This is a good way to get herbs into small children who don't like the idea of a pill, or the taste of herbal teas or tinctures.

Syrups

Many herbs sold for children are available in syrup form and flavored with ingredients that will appeal to children. Read the label before giving your child any syrup. Syrups not intended for children can be dangerous for them.

Pills

Herbal remedies rarely take this form, since it is more difficult to mix more than one herb and to control the quantities. Some of the more common remedies will be available from professional herbalists or health food stores, and there are many that are designed specifically for children. Always read the label to check suitability for children.

Compresses and poultices

Compresses and poultices are for external use, and can be extremely effective, since the active parts of the herb are able to reach the affected area without being altered in any way by the digestive tract.

A poultice is made up of a plant that has been crushed and then applied whole to the affected areas. You can also boil crushed plant parts for a few minutes to make a pulp, which will act as a poultice, or use a powdered herb and mix with boiling water. Because they are most often applied with heat and use fresh parts of the plant, they are more potent than compresses. Poultices are particularly useful for conditions like bruises, wounds and abscesses, helping to soothe and to draw out impurities. Always cool a poultice slightly before placing on any part of a child's body. Adults can stand much higher extremes of temperature, and anything too hot could burn your child.

Compresses are usually made from infusions or decoctions used to soak a linen or muslin cloth. The cloth is then placed on the affected area, where it can be held in place by a bandage or plastic wrap. Compresses can be hot (in the case of children, only hand hot) or cold and are generally milder than poultices.

Ointments and creams

For external use, herbal ointments and creams are often prescribed. You can make your own by blending tinctures with coconut oil (which solidifies), aqueous cream or even another gentle herbal cream like calendula. Creams and ointments should also be kept in the refrigerator to maintain freshness and effectiveness.

Essential oils

Often used in other therapies, like aromatherapy (see page 242), the essential oils of a plant are those that contain its "essence," or some of its most active principles. Essential oils are useful for making tinctures and ointments, and for massage.

Baths

Many herbs can be added to the bath (a handful under running water) for external symptoms, such as skin conditions. This can be messy, but it's very effective.

Putting herbalism into practice

Herbalism is not a miracle cure and, like any other therapy, works best for specific conditions. Having said that, almost anyone can benefit from the prudent use of herbs as a form of restorative and preventive medicine. Herbs are a rich source of vitamins and minerals, aside from having healing properties, and can be an important part of your child's daily diet, eaten fresh, or perhaps drunk as a tisane. An herbal tonic is useful, for example, in the winter months, when fresh fruit and green vegetables are not such a regular part of our diets. Or something like echinacea or garlic can be taken regularly to improve the general efficiency of the immune system. One study showed that natural killer cells were up to 155 percent more effective when garlic was supplemented in the diet.[6]

Some of the most common conditions that respond to herbal treatment include hay fever, colds and respiratory disorders, digestive disorders (like constipation and diarrhea), cardiovascular disease, headaches, anxiety, depression, chronic infections, skin problems and anemia.

There are literally hundreds of herbs and herbal products now widely available, and it makes sense to educate yourself about any herb that you propose to use. Make sure it is suitable for children, and always follow the dosage instructions. There are many herbal treatments that work extremely well in children.

▶ *Top herbal remedies for children*

- If your child has difficulty falling asleep or unwinding, try a warm mug of chamomile tea before bedtime. Sweeten with a little cold-pressed organic honey to taste, and make it part of a good bedtime routine for as long as the problem persists. Babies can have a teaspoon of cooled chamomile tea before bedtime. This will not interfere with breastfeeding.

- For travel sickness, try ginger, which can be chewed as a preventative before a journey, or added to cookies. Ginger is a natural digestive and eases nausea.

- If your child is suffering from conjunctivitis, combine chamomile, eyebright (euphrasia) and marigold (calendula) in some warm water. Soak cotton balls and use them to clean the eyes, from the center to the outside, using a new ball for each eye. Place clean, soaked cotton balls over your child's eyes while he is sleeping. Don't worry if they fall off!

- For indigestion, offer a cup of cooled fennel tea after eating, or serve it iced, with a little honey and lemon.

- For mild sunburn, bathe the skin with cold water to reduce the heat and then use one of the following herbal ointments: calendula, chickweed, aloe vera (gel) or comfrey juice.

- If your child suffers from periodic cold sores when she is run down, you will need to address the condition externally and internally. On the inside, offer herbs that boost the immune system (such as echinacea, astragalus or garlic) and herbs that help your child's body to detoxify (such as nettles or dandelion root). On the outside, dilute a tincture of echinacea or St. John's wort mixed with calendula (called hyperical) and apply daily to speed up the healing of the blisters and discourage secondary infection.

- For hay fever, offer echinacea to boost immunity and euphrasia for symptoms such as running eyes. These herbs can be blended together and offered, a few drops at a time, several times daily.

Is it safe?

Other than purchasing herbal teas or products specially designed for children (for some good sources, see page 444), it would be wise to consult a registered medical herbalist before offering your children herbal treatment. The majority of herbs are safe for most people, but there are also many contraindications—especially in children, and particularly so if they suffer from a long-term, chronic or serious health condition (epilepsy, for example). Herbs are natural, but they are very powerful. There is some evidence that they can affect the uptake and efficiency of some conventional drugs, so make sure you tell your herbalist about any medication your child is taking, and tell your doctor about any herbal products. If you are interested in reading more about the actions of a particular herb, visit one of the medical herbalism websites (see page 444), or invest in a good materia medica.

Homeopathy

I can think of few therapies that are more appropriate for children than homeopathy. It's a gentle therapy, with no danger of toxicity or side effects, and it can be used alongside many other complementary therapies to provide relief from a wide range of health conditions affecting your child's emotional and physical health. Since converting completely to homeopathy several years ago, my family has not required a single trip to a conventional doctor and although we do still succumb to the occasional bug, we are all stronger, fitter and happier than we have been in years.

What is homeopathy?

Homeopathy is a system of medicine that supports the body's own healing mechanism, using specially prepared remedies. It is "energy" medicine, in that it works with the body's vital force (see page 203) to encourage healing and to ensure that all body systems are working at optimum level. Homeopathic remedies use plants, minerals and even some animal products as a base. They are prepared through a process known as "potentization" to bring out their subtle healing properties.

We know from modern physics that our seemingly solid bodies are just dense fields of energy. A disturbance in our energy field can give rise to disease, and a potent form of energy can rebalance us. Homeopathy uses "potentized" remedies to rebalance the body's subtle energy system. Once this is back in balance, the immune system and all the other interconnected systems in the body start functioning better.

The term "homeopathy" comes from the Greek, meaning "similar suffering." It reflects the key principle behind the homeopathic method—that a substance can cure the symptoms in an ill person that it is capable of causing in a healthy person.

Homeopathic remedies

A homeopathic remedy is an extremely pure, natural substance that has been diluted many times. In large quantities these substances would cause the same symptoms the patient is trying to cure. In small, diluted doses, the substance is not only safe and free from side effects but also will trigger the body to heal itself.

Many scientists have claimed that a study of the remedies themselves has proved that there is little or even no trace of the original substance in the pill. This is the basis of the scientific assertion that homeopathy effects cure through positive thinking alone. Don't be fooled by these claims. Homeopathy is an extremely subtle medicine, based on the concept of "vibrational medicine." Because the remedies are so diluted, they often contain only a vibration of the original substance, and it is this vibration that works on the body's natural energy field. It's rather like a radio signal rather than an overt substance, but it is that subtle signal that effects a cure.

Homeopathic remedies are classified into three levels of potencies: X, C and M refer to 10, 100 and 1,000, respectively, in terms of the amount of dilution. The more a tincture is diluted, the more potent it becomes. So, while a C is more dilute than an X, the C is more powerful. M-classified remedies are extremely potent, and are normally prescribed by homeopathic practitioners on a constitutional basis.

To make the 6C potency (properly called the 6 centesimal potency) of Nat. Mur. (salt), for example, one part of salt is added to 99 parts of milk sugar or alcohol and succussed (vigorously shaken), and this process is repeated 6 times. A 30C potency has gone through the same process 30 times. Although a 30 potency has been diluted more than the 6 potency, the succussion has made it more powerful. The number on the label tells you just how many dilutions the remedy has been through.

Why use homeopathy?

No homeopathic remedies are tested on animals. Because they've all been tested on healthy people, we know their effect on the human body. In acute illness, homeopathy:

- treats acute symptoms safely and effectively

- has no side effects

- works with the immune system rather than against it

- improves resistance to infection

- shortens recovery time after illness—often preventing complications

Choosing a remedy

If you plan to use homeopathic remedies for your children, you'll need to learn to take into account many factors apart from overt symptoms. Choosing the correct remedy involves "matching" the symptom picture of the remedy as closely as you can to your child's symptoms. Symptom pictures, or descriptions of symptoms, take into account the condition of the whole child, not just one symptom. If two remedies seem to be very close and it is difficult to decide between them, pick the one that best matches your child's most prevalent symptom.

Here is an example. Your child has a cold and a runny nose. In conventional medicine, the diagnosis would be simply a cold, with various symptoms. In homeopathy, however, you need to look much further:

- What is your child's emotional state? Is he tearful, anxious or irritable?

- What color is the discharge?

- Does the discharge burn or is it bland?

- What makes the symptoms worse—going outside, for example, or heat?

- Is he worse after eating? At night?

- Is he hungry, thirsty or off his food?

Then, look at the remedies that seem most appropriate:

- If your child is clingy and tearful, with a thick yellowish nasal discharge that doesn't burn or sting and he seems to be thirstless, then Pulsatilla is probably the right choice.

- If your child is anxious with a burning discharge and very thirsty for small sips of cold water, then Arsenicum might be indicated.

There are obviously many more remedy choices, but the trick is to find the remedy that best matches all of the features of your child's overall picture.

Choosing a potency

Homeopaths prescribe potencies based on a wide range of factors, including how long your child has had the condition, what his energy and the energy of the condition are like, how well the remedy fits the symptom picture, and whether they believe the overriding factors are emotional, mental or physical:

- 6C dilutions are best for physical conditions, and you can confidently self-prescribe these for acute conditions.

- 30C dilutions are prescribed for physical conditions that have a good emotional symptom picture. Again, these are safe to use for self-prescription.

- 200C is prescribed when there are strong physical and emotional factors present.

- 1M and above is prescribed when the condition has a strong emotional base.

Don't play around with the higher potencies, particularly those that have a dramatic effect on mental or emotional health.

How to take a remedy

- Remedies come in pill form or as granules (for young children). Try to buy the loosely packed pills for older children. They dissolve more quickly. Tinctures and creams are also available.

- One pill (or a few granules) is enough for one dose—taking more than one does not increase the effect. Encourage your child to dissolve the pill under her tongue, or to suck it slowly. Crush pills in paper for small children or babies, but try to avoid touching it with your own hands. If you don't have time to crush the pill, place it between your child's bottom lip and his gum. If she spits it out, don't worry. She'll probably have taken in enough to have an effect.

- Children can also have a pill dissolved in a small quantity of water, but again, don't touch the remedy with your own hands.

- Your child should not eat, drink, or clean her teeth (or smoke) for at least 15 minutes before or afterward. Some homeopaths believe that strong substances can antidote the remedies.

- Store the remedies in their original containers away from direct light, heat and strong-smelling substances.

- Don't panic if your child takes more than one pill—the effects will be no greater than if she had just taken one. Swallowing the contents of a whole bottle may cause a little diarrhea (the pills are normally made with milk sugar), but it will pass.

Is it safe?

Homeopathy is one of the safest of all the natural therapies, and it is suitable for people of all ages—babies and the elderly included. There are, however, guidelines that make the remedies more effective, and help to prevent bringing out undesirable emotional or physical symptoms.

▶ *Tips for taking homeopathic remedies safely*

- Don't attempt to treat your child at home if he has a serious health problem.

- Don't self-diagnose instead of seeing a doctor or a homeopath.

- Never take your child off conventional medication without advice.

- Don't take a number of different remedies at the same time (unless prescribed by a registered homeopath). Stick to one, and if it doesn't work, change to another (see below). Multiple remedies are appropriate if you purchase an over-the-counter blended preparation, but it's best not to take a hit-and-miss approach yourself.

- Don't keep taking a remedy if it is not working. This can aggravate symptoms in the long term.

- Don't take high potencies (200 and over) unless prescribed by a registered homeopath.

- Homeopathy is compatible with osteopathy, counseling, meditation and dietary management. While homeopathy is safe to use when taking conventional medicines, it may not be as effective as when used alone.

How to tell if a remedy is working

For acute conditions, you can expect a quick reaction, where physical and mental symptoms improve (within half-an-hour or less). Chronic conditions may take some time to react to treatment, but you should notice a change of some sort—on an emotional level perhaps—within a few days. Homeopathy is a gentle therapy, and you won't see miracle cures. Be patient—the results are worth waiting for:

- Within a day or so, your child should experience an enhanced sense of well-being—with improved mood and energy levels.

- Sometimes physical symptoms get worse when the mental state improves. According to the laws of homeopathy, and depending on the potency of the remedy, the mental symptoms improve first, then the emotional symptoms and finally the physical symptoms.

- Sometimes your child will start to feel better and then get stuck. If the symptoms are the same, continue taking the remedy. If they are different, you will need to switch remedies according to the new symptoms. Homeopathy is a little like peeling an onion. The remedies work on the top layer, and when that's dealt with, another one emerges. In cases of chronic emotional or physical health, your child may require a long-term course of different remedies as each new layer presents itself. Even acute ailments can have dramatically different symptom pictures that emerge one by one. Try to be objective and look carefully at changes as they occur.

- If your child's symptoms do not improve, or she feels much worse, the wrong remedy may have been selected. Try again. If physical symptoms improve, but your child feels worse emotionally, there may be a "constitutional" (fundamental) imbalance, which will require the attention of a registered homeopath.

- Continue offering the remedy for a few days after it is working. The tendency is to stop when the symptoms are abating, when longer-term treatment may be required.

- If a remedy has no effect whatsoever, try a different one.

Seeing a professional

Homeopaths treat the same range of complaints as doctors. A skilled homeopath can treat psychological problems (depression, anxiety, even shyness or phobias) or serious chronic illnesses like multiple sclerosis and, in some cases, cancer. Deep-seated problems, such as allergies (eczema, hay fever and asthma) and repeated infections often respond very well to homeopathic treatment, but you will need to put your child in the hands of an experienced practitioner.

Homeopaths differentiate between acute illnesses—usually short illnesses that blow up quickly and blow over quickly as well—and more serious (chronic, or long-term) "constitutional" problems. In constitutional treatment a single homeopathic remedy is often chosen to address the physical, mental and emotional symptoms. Classical homeopaths, who practice according to traditional techniques, usually give just one high potency dose of a remedy and carefully watch your child's response. If it's the correct remedy, this high-potency stimulates your child's energy, improving his mood and sense of well-being, before balancing out his body systems, including the immune system, hormones, circulation and digestion. Specific physical symptoms are then addressed by the body's own self-healing mechanisms.

Constitutional treatment may involve monthly sessions over several months— or even years, depending on how long your child has been suffering from health problems.

▶ When to seek advice from a registered homeopath

- If your attempts to treat your children don't work. If you have tried two or three remedies, with no effect, it's time to get some help.

The laws of cure

While it may seem unnecessary to absorb the theory behind complementary therapies when you intend to use them for simple, at-home treatments, in the case of homeopathy, an understanding of the basic laws of cure will help you to assess whether the treatment you are offering at home, or getting from a homeopath, is working. For cure to be taking place:

- The disease should go from within to without (in other words, organs will be treated before skin problems).

- From organs of greater importance to lesser importance (in the case of a child with asthma and eczema, for example, the lungs will respond first, and the skin probably last, because the lungs are a more crucial organ).

- From above to below (facial skin would clear first, and the skin on the feet last, in a child with whole-body eczema).

- Symptoms should disappear in reverse order to their original appearance. This is one of the reasons why homeopaths take such a careful case history. They will be able to see old conditions "coming out" as part of the treatment, and they can assess whether the symptoms that appeared last are the first to go. If your child suddenly develops hay fever, but has suffered from eczema all his life, the hay fever should be the first to go. If it happens the other way around, chances are the wrong remedy has been chosen.

- If your child is very run-down and suffering from general, low-grade symptoms (tired, irritable or tearful; not fighting off infections, for example). A constitutional remedy is probably required.

- If your child seems very out of balance—either emotional or physically, or both. Again, constitutional treatment is necessary.

- If your child suffers from serious health problems of any nature.

Putting homeopathy into practice

There are literally thousands of homeopathic remedies, and the wide range of symptoms they address can be daunting for a first-time home practitioner. There are, however, some very commonly used remedies for a variety of health conditions, and you may want to experiment with some of these first, until you feel more confident prescribing. Children respond very well to homeopathic remedies, probably because they have fewer "layers" to peel before the root cause becomes apparent.

▶ *Top homeopathic remedies for children*

1. For a crying, irritable, inconsolable baby who needs to be carried everywhere, try Chamomilla. This remedy is also indicated for teething.

2. For a tearful child with green nasal discharge and no apparent thirst, try Pulsatilla. This is a great remedy for the heart-breaking, "I want my mommy" tears of a toddler.

3. For a condition that comes on suddenly, after exposure to cold air, for example, try Aconite. It's a good first-try remedy for colds or earaches that appear from nowhere.

4. For fever, with a red face, try Belladonna. It's also useful for any pains that seem to be hot, red or throbbing.

5. For tummy bugs, with diarrhea or vomiting that seems to be burning, and a great thirst for sips of cold water, try Arsenicum. It's ideal for traveler's tummy.

6. Remember ABC when treating a sick child. It stands for Aconite, Belladonna and Chamomilla. Many children's acute health conditions (fevers, coughs, colds, earaches, etc.) that come on suddenly respond to these remedies, taken in ABC order. Leave about 20 minutes between each remedy.

7. Croup often responds to Spongia, taken at 30C for two or three doses.

8. For falls, bruises or injuries of any kind, take Arnica. In fact, keep a bottle on hand at all times.

9. Strained muscles and joints will respond to Rhus Tox. This is also a first-line treatment for chicken pox.

The best-selling flu remedy in France is a homeopathic medicine. Anas barbariae 200C, commonly marketed under the trade name Oscillococcinum, is also popular in the U.S. and is effective primarily at the first signs of influenza. A study with 478 patients suffering from influenza showed that almost twice as many people who took the homeopathic remedy got over the flu after 48 hours, as compared to those given a placebo. [7]

Massage

The therapeutic effects of massage are well documented, and although skeptics insist that any health benefits derived from treatment are the result of an improved sense of well-being, rather than any biological response by the body, there is no doubt that massage works on many levels to improve overall health. Even ticklish children enjoy a soothing massage, and this is one therapy that you can undertake at home in a variety of situations. A professional massage may be a luxury for a young child, but older children who are under stress of any type, or suffer from chronic health conditions, will undoubtedly benefit.

How does massage work?

Massage is one of the oldest, simplest forms of therapy and is a system of stroking, pressing and kneading different areas of the body to relieve pain, relax, stimulate and tone the body. Massage does much more than make your child feel good; it also works on the soft tissues (the muscles, tendons and ligaments) to improve muscle tone. Although massage largely affects those muscles just under the skin, it is believed that it also reaches the deeper layers of muscles and possibly even the organs themselves. Massage also stimulates blood circulation and assists the lymphatic system (which runs parallel to the circulatory system), improving elimination of toxic waste throughout the body.

Here are some of the proven physical effects:

- Massage is known to increase the circulation of blood and flow of lymph. The direct mechanical effect of rhythmically applied manual pressure and movement used in massage can dramatically increase the rate of blood flow. Also, the stimulation of nerve receptors causes the blood vessels (by relaxation) to dilate, which also encourages blood flow.

- For the whole body to be healthy, the individual cells must be healthy. These cells are dependent on an abundant supply of blood and lymph because these fluids supply nutrients and oxygen, and carry away wastes and toxins.

- It causes changes in the blood. The oxygen capacity of the blood can increase by 10 to 15 percent after massage.

- Massage can help loosen contracted, shortened muscles and can stimulate weak, flaccid muscles. This muscle balancing can help posture and promote more efficient movement. Massage does not directly increase muscle strength, but it can speed recovery from the fatigue that occurs after exercise. Massage also provides a gentle stretching action to both the muscles and connective tissues that surround and support the muscles and many other parts of the body, which helps keep these tissues elastic.

- Massage increases the body's secretions and excretions. There is a proven increase in the production of gastric juices, saliva and urine. There is also increased excretion of nitrogen, inorganic phosphorus and sodium chloride (salt). This suggests that the metabolic rate (the utilization of absorbed material by the body's cells) increases.

- Massage balances the nervous system by soothing or stimulating it, depending on what your child needs at the time of the massage.

- Massage directly improves the function of the sebaceous (oil) and sweat glands, which keep the skin lubricated, clean and cooled. Tough, inflexible skin can become softer and more supple.

- By indirectly or directly stimulating nerves that supply internal organs, blood vessels of the organs dilate and allow greater blood supply to these organs.

When massage is not a good idea

There are some conditions that can be exacerbated by massage, and it should never be undertaken in these situations:

- areas of local infection (e.g., shingles, ringworm, athlete's foot)

- bruising (never work directly over a bruised area)

- eczema (weeping)

- fever or high temperatures

- full stomach—always allow at least an hour between eating a meal and massage

---

Keeping up touch

The importance of touch for babies is now recognized, but as children grow older, physical contact often declines. Children become busy, there are siblings to consider, and then the old pride and self-consciousness slide into action, and your children may not want to be seen touching, kissing, hugging (in some cases even speaking) to you in front of their peers. Despite all this, growing children need touch. Being held is a sign of love and reassurance, and children sometimes need a way to express their emotions physically as well. Incorporating massage into your daily life can be a link for both children and adults. They can "touch" you, under the guise of a quick stress-relieving shoulder massage (my two boys are experts already), and you can touch them to do the same. There is no question of unnecessary or embarrassing affection. This is work! By adolescence, many children are receiving little or no touch from their parents, or, indeed, from anyone, until they begin exploring in the context of a sexual relationship. Remember that all children need to touch and to be touched. Don't be alarmed by any sexual connotations. Massaging an adolescent is a way to keep in physical contact without any pseudosexual elements intruding. Even if it's just a shoulder or foot rub, massage can keep open the channels of communication between you and your children as they get older.

- heart conditions

- nausea

- open cuts or sores

- recent major operation

- swelling or inflammation

- tumors or undiagnosed swellings

When to see a professional

It's certainly possible to practice massage at home on your children, and there are a variety of books and courses available teaching the basics of the therapy. There are a number of different strokes that help to produce the therapeutic benefits, and it is important to learn these to produce significant health changes. An amateur massage at home will, however, work on several levels, including enhancing well-being, which will affect your child's physical and emotional health. There are times when a professional should be called in, including cases of chronic illness (colic, insomnia, colds, ear infections, asthma, nonweeping eczema, juvenile arthritis, diabetes and others).

Basic baby massage

Babies and children usually enjoy being massaged, but they will often keep still only for a short length of time. You don't need to learn any special strokes to massage your baby—just explore her body with gentle rhythmic or stroking movements, and she'll soon let you know what feels good. Massaging your baby is an excellent way of settling her, and of establishing a close physical relationship. She will feel loved and cared for, and you may find that you bond more easily and more deeply if you spend a little time exploring her body on a regular basis. Touch is very therapeutic, and you will both benefit from close, loving contact.

Studies at the Touch Research Institute, located in Miami, Florida, have also found that premature babies massaged three times a day for as few as five days consistently fare better than equally frail babies who don't get massages. Full-term infants and older babies also benefit from them. The International Association of Infant Massage in the U.K., estimates that 10,000 American parents took infant-massage training last year. New converts say it helps their babies sleep better, relieves colic and helps hyperactive children relax. In fact, new research shows that premature infants are more alert, sleep better and gain weight more quickly when they are massaged regularly. [8]

If your baby is small enough, you can sit on the floor and massage her on your lap. Otherwise, spread a towel on the floor or on any safe, raised surface. Make sure that the room is warm, and free of drafts. If your child objects, wait until she is feeling calmer. Try massaging before a feed, or as part of the bedtime routine. You may want to consider using a drop of aromatherapy oil to enhance the effect (see page 246 for suitable oils). Always use a gentle massage oil, such as grapeseed, olive oil or apricot kernel oil, to help your hands glide over her body. It's a good idea to gently heat the oil first. Be careful when you are finished—your baby will be slippery!

Front of the body

- Starting with your baby on her back, gently stroke her face, starting in the middle of the forehead and working out to the temples.

- Stroke across the cheeks from the nose to the ears and then from the cheeks down to the chin.

- Gently stroke across the eyebrows, and back around under the eye.

- Make gentle circles around the temples.

- Stroke up the front of the body and out along the arms.

- Make clockwise circles around the navel using both hands.

- Do gentle wringing strokes across the abdomen and up the body. [9]

- Lift arms one at a time and stroke the length of the arm from the shoulder to the hand.

- Use one hand to squeeze the arm, starting from the shoulder and moving down the arm.

- Massage the hand and squeeze and rotate each of the fingers in turn.

- Repeat for the other arm.

- Gently wring or squeeze up the leg.

- Stroke down the leg using a light, feathering stroke.

Back of the body

- Turn the child onto her front and gently stroke her back.

- Stroke up and over the back and along the arms.

- Gently knead shoulders.

- Make a gentle wringing stroke up over the body.

- If your child is a baby, massage her bottom using gentle kneading or pinching strokes.

What can massage treat?

Studies show that massage can be used to treat many common health conditions, particularly the following:

- arthritis (including juvenile)

- asthma

- carpal tunnel syndrome

- chronic and acute pain

- circulatory problems

- gastrointestinal disorders (including spastic colon, colic and constipation)

- headache

- immune function disorders

- insomnia

- premature infants

- sports injuries

- stress (which is significant; experts believe that 80 percent of all health conditions are caused or made worse by stress)

- Smooth down the spine using alternating hands, starting at the base of the neck and working down to the base of the spine.

- Use gliding strokes down the legs.

- Bend the knee up and work on the foot.

- Work around the anklebone with fingertips.

- Sandwich foot between heels of hand and massage, moving both hands in a circular motion.

- Squeeze the heel with one hand and massage up the sole of the foot using your thumbs.

- Massage each toe, gently squeezing, rotating and pulling each in turn.

- Sandwich foot between hands and hold firmly for a few seconds.

- Stroke from one foot up the leg, across the sacrum (base of the spine) and back down the other leg.

- Use light strokes down the body, starting from the top of head right down to the feet.

Nutritional therapies

We've discussed the importance of nutrition in chapters 1 and 2, and you will, by now, have a good idea how the elements of nutrition can impact health. Nutritional therapy is an umbrella term for a wide variety of therapies that use nutrition as their base, and the majority of complementary therapies do offer some nutritional advice as part of the healing program. Nutritional therapies are, however, more than healthy eating. They can involve using supplements and foods for specific health conditions, and they work to rectify small or large imbalances in the body. Children need good nutrition, and in many cases they need supplements. However, under no circumstances should you ever undertake a nutritional program using large doses of any supplement without the advice and guidance of a registered nutritional therapist. Many therapists will help to work on individual health complaints, and address food allergies and intolerance. This is a safe therapy, but only in the hands of an experienced professional.

What are nutritional therapies?

Everyone should try to eat a good, well-balanced diet, rich in fresh, whole, organic foods, in order to get the optimum levels of vitamins, minerals and other elements of nutrition. However, body chemistry is very complicated, and each nutrient works both on its own and in combination with other elements in the body. Furthermore, each individual has different requirements, and what may balance and work therapeutically for one person may unbalance and cause problems in another.

Nutritional therapy is a sophisticated system of health care that depends on an increasingly broad-based knowledge of biochemistry, physiology and chemistry to use the tools available within nutrition to address the health needs of the individual. There are three basic diagnoses that are made by the nutritional therapist, and they are allergy (or intolerance), nutritional deficiencies (often subclinical) and toxic overload.

All children should take a good "insurance-level" vitamin and mineral pill, to ensure that they are getting adequate levels of the nutrients they need. Some vitamins and minerals are safe in large quantities and will not upset the balance of the body when taken in "mega doses"; however, you will need a good understanding of how they work in the body before you attempt to take large doses to achieve health.

If you are looking for a general improvement in your child's health rather than addressing a particular ailment, you can probably treat your child at home safely, without upsetting the fine balance of his body. However, if you wish to use supplements for a health condition, you are advised to see a registered practitioner, who can run a series of tests to ascertain any nutritional deficiencies and prescribe supplements that are required for your child's individual needs.

Nutritional therapists are often medical doctors who have trained specifically in nutrition. The practitioners of other complementary therapies such as naturopathy, homeopathy and herbalism, may also be trained in nutritional therapy and offer it as part of the treatment.

A consultation normally takes up to an hour, during which the therapist takes a full case history. Many practitioners suggest analyzing hair, urine, sweat, blood, muscle testing and perhaps a questionnaire to pinpoint specific deficiencies. Further therapy will be based on your child's physical symptoms. From this information a diet plan will be produced for your child, individual to his needs, and any supplementation prescribed. Exercise and herbal treatment may be incorporated into the treatment. The number of sessions required depends on how quickly your child responds to treatment, how long he has suffered from symptoms or illness and how carefully you manage to incorporate the lifestyle and dietary changes suggested.

Combining treatments

Vitamins, minerals and other elements of nutrition are, in essence, simply parts of food, and in most cases they are safe to take with other medication and with complementary treatments (although you must always check with your therapist for possible contraindications). Some therapies, such as herbalism, use herbs and other plant products for nutritional as well as medicinal purposes, and you should tell your practitioner if you are taking supplements, as the action can be duplicated and you could end up taking too much of one thing.

How long will it take to work?

Marginal deficiencies will often be righted in a short period of time, and you should begin to see effects within a few weeks. Righting deficiency should not take long, and you should not expect to have to take extra supplements, or large doses of any vitamins and minerals, for much longer than several months. However, there are cases where your child's lifestyle, eating habits, and body chemistry and metabolism will increase his need for nutrients. Some children with chronic health problems may need to take a series of different supplements on an ongoing basis. Generally speaking, however, if you do not begin to see results within two to three weeks of beginning supplementation, chances are it is not doing any good.

Children's needs are much lower than an adults', so supplements should be given with great care. Read the label to ensure that the product is safe for children, and follow it carefully.

Is a healthy diet enough?

The answer should be yes, but unfortunately it isn't. Ideally, a balanced, healthy diet contains foods that are high in all of the nutrients we need. However, vitamins are easily destroyed by canning, processing, refining and even cooking. Minerals are not necessarily present in foods—the quality of the soil and the geological conditions of the area in which they were grown play an important part in determining the mineral content of food. Even a balanced diet may be lacking in essential minerals or trace elements because of the soil in which it was grown. There's pretty strong evidence that intensive farming robs soil of its nutrient content (although many farmers make a considerable effort to put some back), which means that our food is, naturally, lower in minerals than it should be.

Secondly, and perhaps most importantly, our modern, overscheduled lives place demands on our bodies that cause them to require extra nutrients. Pollution, noise, stress, food additives and many other factors combine to put stress on the body. Stress of any kind—whether it is emotional or physical—increases our need for nutrients.

The answer to this perplexing state of affairs is not to give up on the idea of healthy eating, for it has many, many roles other than supplying vitamins and minerals. Food is important, so don't think that you can swap it for a packet of foil-wrapped, bubble-packed nutrients. Children in particular need a wide variety of healthy foods in order to grow and develop into strong, healthy adults.

This does, however, raise the question of supplementation. There is no question that supplementation has become necessary from a fairly early age, unless you can afford to eat exclusively organic foods (see page 39). Breastfed babies have no need for vitamin drops, and bottle-fed babies are unlikely to either, but when table food becomes the norm, it's time to consider supplements as an essential part of a healthy diet.

● Top tips for taking supplements

- As we discussed on page 13, you can supplement your child's intake of essential fatty acids in the form of cod liver oil and flaxseed oil. A good source of omega-3 EFAs is fish oils, such as, salmon oil or Norwegian liver oil. Evening primrose oil contains the highest amount of gamma-linolenic acid (GLA) of any food substance and is helpful for prevention of hardening of the arteries, heart disease, multiple sclerosis, high blood pressure, hyperactivity, skin problems, some arthritis (including juvenile) and liver problems.

- All children will benefit from a multivitamin and mineral pill. Look for "slow-release" pills if you can find them. Take the pills according to manufacturers' instructions, and always with food to make sure they are properly assimilated.

- Chewable pills can damage children's teeth if they are eaten between meals. Sugar-free is always best, or if they are unpalatable, look for pills sweetened with a small amount of fruit sugar.

- For small children, powders and drops are available. Mix them in with food or a little juice. Don't be alarmed by resulting brightly colored urine—this is normal.

- For children with recurrent infections (colds, coughs and ear infections), make sure they get extra vitamin C, which helps to boost the immune system. Many experts recommend extra vitamin C as a matter of course, to help ward off illness. Between 100 and 1,000 mg is the usual dosage, depending on the child's age. A two-year-old, for example, might have an extra 100 mg. If there is any diarrhea after taking the pills, reduce the dose by half.

- Similarly, if anyone in the house smokes, extra vitamin C is necessary. Adult smokers lose about 25 mg of vitamin C for every cigarette smoked. While passive smoking loss is substantially less, there is undoubtedly some loss above and beyond what children in a smokeless home would experience. Use the same dosages mentioned above. The same goes for children living in areas of high pollution.

- With iron-deficiency anemia on the increase (see page 302), it may be necessary to supplement iron. Most good vitamin and mineral pills contain iron, and you should never consider supplementing anything beyond this without the advice of your doctor.

- Stress reduces many nutrients in our bodies—in particular, the B vitamins. It may seem ludicrous to suggest that children suffer debilitating stress, but there are many cases where this is so. If your child finds exams, a house move, school, homework, friendships, relationships or almost anything else difficult to cope with, or if she is undergoing a particularly traumatic time, such as a parental divorce or bereavement, she may well need some extra vitamins. B vitamins work together, so don't try supplementing any one at a time, unless recommended by a nutritionist. Once again, a good multivitamin or mineral pill should adequately cover the B vitamins, but for children over the age of six, 10 to 25 mg a day is the usual level at which to supplement.

- Children who are unable to eat or drink dairy produce because of allergies, or because they simply don't like them, should be able to get enough calcium from vegetable and fruit sources. However, if you have a picky eater on your hands, you might need to consider supplementation of calcium. One good source is the new "calcium-enhanced" orange juices, which contain a whole day's supply in one glass. If the juice is out, talk to your doctor about special supplements, or visit a nutritional therapist (see page 438).

- Antioxidant nutrients, including vitamin A, beta-carotene, vitamins C and E, and the minerals selenium and zinc, help to protect the body from the formation of free radicals that can cause damage to cells, impairing the immune system and leading to various degenerative diseases such as heart disease and cancer. Free radicals in the body may be formed by exposure to radiation and toxic chemicals, such as those found in cigarette smoke, overexposure to the sun's rays or various metabolic processes, such as the process of breaking down stored fat molecules for use as an energy source.

- Acidophilus is a source of friendly intestinal bacteria (flora). Healthy bacteria plays an important role in our bodies, and unless it is continually supplied with some form of lactic acid or lactose (such as acidophilus) it can die, causing a host of health problems. Many doctors and health practitioners recommend taking acidophilus alongside oral antibiotics, which can cause diarrhea, destroy the healthy flora of the intestines and lead to fungal infections. Acidophilus may also help to ensure vaginal health. It can aid in the treatment of skin problems, can aid absorption of nutrients in food and can relieve and prevent constipation and flatulence. The best source is natural, unflavored "live yogurt." Acidophilus is not toxic and can be taken daily, with food, in unlimited amounts. Many practitioners recommend taking it as a daily supplement. It is safe for children, and is available in chewable, vanilla-flavored pills. Keep the pills in the refrigerator.

- Bee propolis, a resinous substance collected from various plants by bees, is an excellent aid against bacterial infections. It is believed to stimulate white blood cells that destroy bacteria. Studies show that it is good for inflammation of the mucous membranes of the mouth and short, dry coughs, halitosis, tonsillitis, mouth ulcers, acne and for boosting immunity. [10]

- Garlic has been shown to cleanse the blood and help to create and maintain healthy bacteria (flora) in the gut, help to bring down fever, act as an antiseptic with antibiotic and antifungal actions, tone the heart and circulatory system, boost the immune system, help to reduce high blood pressure, treat infections of the stomach and respiratory system, and act as an antioxidant and decongestant. Garlic is widely used in cooking, but heat destroys its medicinal effects, so it is best to use it only slightly cooked, or raw, or to take it in supplement form.

- Amino acids are organic compounds that comprise the "building blocks" of proteins. Experts suggest that amino acids should not be supplemented without the supervision of a trained practitioner.

- Algae are plants that grow in water. Spirulina, one of the most common types, are blue-green bacteria or algae, which are rich in GLA (see page 283) and a wide variety of nutrients, including beta carotene. Recently, there have been a number of cases of algae contamination because some algae is grown outdoors in open lakes. Some symptoms of contamination have included hair loss. Deep-sea algae products are believed less likely to be contaminated, and therefore safer. Seaweeds are another form of "algae," and are believed to have antiviral activity, and some studies have concluded that they act as a preventative for cancer. Seaweeds may help to reduce the effects of carcinogenics, including radioactive material, and are therefore useful for reducing the damage done by chemo- and radiotherapy. Seaweeds are believed to be natural antacids, and are often used in the treatment of intestinal disorders.

- Coenzyme Q10 (CoQ10) is a vitamin-like substance found in all cells of the body. It is biologically important since it forms part of the system across which electrons flow in the cells in the process of energy production. When it is deficient, the cell cannot function effectively and the rate at which the muscle cells work is adversely affected. Coenzyme Q10 is also known as ubiquinone or vitamin Q, and it is concentrated in the human body in certain organs, especially the liver and the heart. Coenzyme Q10 stimulates both the immune system and overall immunity, and may help in the treatment of obesity. Clinical studies suggest it enhances immunity, improves the heart-muscle metabolism, is anti-aging, necessary for healthy functioning of the nervous system and the brain cells, boosts energy levels and is used in the treatment of gum disease. Co-enzyme Q10 is found in organ meats, spinach, polyunsaturated vegetable oils, and cold-water fish, such as tuna and sardines.

- Polyphenols, which are also known as polyphenolic flavonoids, are powerful antioxidants related to tannins, and found in green tea and red grapes. Flavonoids, also known as bioflavonoids, are colorful antioxidants found in plants, and are responsible for the colors of fruits. There are 12 basic classes of flavonoids, and apart from their antioxidant qualities, they are known to help strengthen capillary walls and may be useful in the treatment of heavy menstrual bleeding. Some flavonoids are anti-inflammatories, helping to form prostaglandins. Bioflavonoids were originally called vitamin P, and are also known as flavones. They accompany vitamin C in natural foods, and their primary job is to protect the capillaries, to keep them strong and to prevent bleeding. Many of the medicinally active substances of herbs are bioflavonoids. Best sources include citrus fruits, apricots, cherries, green peppers, broccoli, and lemons. The central white core of citrus fruits is the richest source. Bioflavonoids are not toxic, and should be taken with vitamin C for best effect.

Is my child deficient?

Some obvious and not-so-obvious symptoms rear their heads when there is vitamin or mineral deficiency. Do any of the following fit your child's health patterns?

Problem	Possible deficiency
Chronic constipation (not linked to fiber intake)	B-complex vitamins
Chronic diarrhea (not linked to fiber intake or illness)	niacin (B3) and vitamin K
Eye problems	vitamin A
Fatigue	zinc, iron, vitamins A, B, C, D
Hair problems	vitamins B12, B2, B6, E and selenium
Recurrent infections	vitamins A and C, calcium, iron potassium
Muscle cramps	B vitamins, vitamin D
Nervousness or anxiety	B6, B12, B3, magnesium, vitamin C
Skin problems	vitamins A, B-complex, E, copper, biotin

If you have concerns about deficiency, try a multivitamin and mineral pill first. Check the label to ensure that the appropriate elements are there. Some pills contain only a few vitamins. Others contain the whole range. Go for the latter. Give it a couple of weeks and if symptoms don't clear up, consider a trip to a nutritional therapist.

There are many, many more supplements that are commonly used for children, and many herbal products are used alongside. The best advice is to see a registered practitioner, who will advise you on the best therapeutic supplements for your child, according to his individual needs.

Reflexology

This is a gentle and effective therapy for children, and most of them enjoy the experience of having their feet, and sometimes their hands, massaged. The effects can be dramatic, but longer-term health problems can take some time to treat effectively.

Reflexology involves stimulating, massaging and applying pressure to points on the hands and feet that correspond to various systems and organs throughout the body to stimulate the body's own healing system. These points are called "reflex points," and each point corresponds to a different body part or function.

Reflexologists believe that applying pressure to these reflex points can improve the health of the body and mind. Depending on the points chosen, reflexology can be used to ease tension, reduce inflammation, relieve congestion, improve circulation and eliminate toxins from the body. Like many other complementary therapists, reflexologists do not claim to cure anything, rather they aim to stimulate the body to heal itself. They do this by working on the physical body to stimulate healing at the physical, mental and emotional levels.

Pressure applied to nerve endings can influence all the body systems, including the circulation and lymphatic systems. Improvements in circulation and the lymphatic system result in improved body functioning because nutrients and oxygen are transported more efficiently around the body and toxins are eliminated with greater ease. Energy pathways are opened up so that the body is able to work more effectively, and harmony or "homeostasis" is restored.

How does reflexology work?

Reflexologists believe that the body is divided into ten vertical zones or channels, five on the left and five on the right. Each zone runs from the head right down to the reflex areas on the hands and feet, and from the front through to the back of the body. All the body parts within any one zone are linked by the nerve pathways and are mirrored in the corresponding reflex zone on the hands and feet. By applying pressure to a reflex point or area, the therapist can stimulate or rebalance the energy in the related zone.

Each zone is a channel for energy (or chi), and stimulating or working any zone in the foot by applying pressure with the thumbs and fingers affects the entire zone throughout the body. For example, working a zone on the foot along which the kidneys lie will release vital energy that may be blocked somewhere else in that zone,

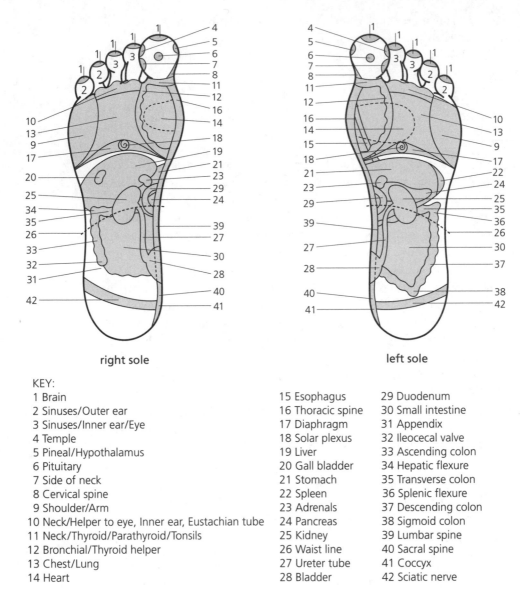

right sole

left sole

KEY:
1 Brain
2 Sinuses/Outer ear
3 Sinuses/Inner ear/Eye
4 Temple
5 Pineal/Hypothalamus
6 Pituitary
7 Side of neck
8 Cervical spine
9 Shoulder/Arm
10 Neck/Helper to eye, Inner ear, Eustachian tube
11 Neck/Thyroid/Parathyroid/Tonsils
12 Bronchial/Thyroid helper
13 Chest/Lung
14 Heart

15 Esophagus
16 Thoracic spine
17 Diaphragm
18 Solar plexus
19 Liver
20 Gall bladder
21 Stomach
22 Spleen
23 Adrenals
24 Pancreas
25 Kidney
26 Waist line
27 Ureter tube
28 Bladder

29 Duodenum
30 Small intestine
31 Appendix
32 Ileocecal valve
33 Ascending colon
34 Hepatic flexure
35 Transverse colon
36 Splenic flexure
37 Descending colon
38 Sigmoid colon
39 Lumbar spine
40 Sacral spine
41 Coccyx
42 Sciatic nerve

such as in the eyes. Working the kidney reflex area on the foot will therefore revitalize and balance the entire zone and improve functioning of the organ.

What does it treat?

Reflexology is an excellent whole-body system, and can be used both to prevent illness and to encourage the body to heal. It is particularly useful for stress and related disorders, emotional disorders, digestive problems, circulatory disorders, menstrual problems, insomnia, fatigue, and most chronic and acute illnesses.

Are there any side effects?

Because the body is being encouraged to heal itself, some symptoms can be "thrown up." In most cases, this is nothing to worry about—it simply represents a "healing crisis," whereby some symptoms appear to become worse before they get better. Most children will not experience any symptoms, but you should be aware that the following can occur:

- coldlike symptoms like a running nose, as catarrh and sinus congestion is cleared

- a cough, as mucus is cleared from the lungs and respiratory passages

- more frequent emptying of the bladder

- more frequent emptying of the bowels

- flatulence

- headache

- increased sweating

- skin rash—some skin conditions may get worse before they get better

- yawning

- tiredness

- increased energy

Trying it at home

A full treatment will involve working all of the areas on the right foot and then all of the areas on the left foot—starting with the toes and working each section of the sole of the foot and then the sides and top of the foot. Chronic conditions should be treated by a registered practitioner, but it is possible to treat acute conditions (such as colds, headaches, colic, backache, coughs, etc.) at home. If you don't have any success, get some professional help.

The main parts of the body are reflected in the following areas of the feet:

- the head and neck—within the toe areas

- the spine—down the inner border of both feet

- the chest—between the levels of the shoulder girdle and the diaphragm on both feet

- the abdomen—below the level of the diaphragm to just above the pad of the heel on both feet

- the pelvis—over the pad of the heel

- the limbs—on the outer side of the feet

- the reproductive glands—on the sides of the feet near and over the ankles

- the lymphatic system and breast—on the top the feet

▶ *Tips for home reflexology*

- So, if your child has a headache, try massaging the big toe on both feet, working upward with firm strokes.

- For colic or indigestion, use your thumb to press into the stomach, intestine, diaphragm and solar plexus areas on both feet.

- For colds, work the head area. Then work with your thumb on the affected areas such as the nose, throat and chest. If your child has a temperature, work on the pituitary gland reflex.

- For constipation, start by stroking both feet and, beginning with the right foot, work thoroughly all over the small intestine area on both feet. Then rub your thumb along the colon, which runs across both feet. Finally, press firmly on the solar plexus area. Repeat on the left foot.

- For insomnia, work all over the foot, giving special attention to the head area. Press on the solar plexus and then press your thumb down the spine. Finish by gently stroking the top of your child's feet from the toes down toward the ankle.

Other suitable therapies for children

Hypnotherapy

Hypnotherapy has been very successful in treating many emotional and physical problems in children. From the age of about six (or as soon as they can understand what is being said), they can benefit from treatment. Younger children can be hypnotized or taught self-hypnosis (positive affirmations) for relaxation. In 1981 self-hypnosis was introduced into the national curriculum in Sweden. Hypnosis is a tool for reaching and dealing with problems of the mind and body, using a state of mental relaxation in which the patient is open to suggestion. In the hypnotized state, emotional problems can be addressed and resolved, and body functions can be improved to restore normal activity. There is evidence that hormonal problems, respiration, heart rate, circulation and digestive activity can be influenced by hypnosis, and many people find they can cut off completely from sensations of pain. Some of the ways that hypnotherapy works include:

- Hypnohealing, which is aimed at healing pathological disease. The therapist helps your child to uncover the cause of illness and through the use of visualization encourages her to release it.

- Cell command therapy or "cellular regeneration" is a similar technique, which is being used to slow down aging and associated degenerative diseases.

Hypnotherapy is especially useful in the treatment of behavioral and habitual difficulties, such as eating disorders, phobias, etc. Other conditions treated include arthritis (including juvenile), asthma, digestive troubles, eczema, insomnia, migraine, stress and many childhood problems, like colic, bedwetting and hyperactivity. It is very good for chronic pain, such as sciatica and headaches. Some cancers respond to treatment.

Traditional Chinese medicine

Traditional Chinese medicine (TCM) is a holistic system of medicine that embraces a wide range of therapies, including herbalism, acupuncture and acupressure (see page 239), diet, massage, exercise (including Qigong) and lifestyle factors. It can be enormously helpful for children suffering from chronic and acute health conditions, and for preventive health care. Many parents swear by the Chinese approach, which believes that health is not just the absence of symptoms but also the presence of a vital and dynamic state of well-being. Many conditions can be cured completely with appropriate treatment suggested by a registered TCM practitioner, including asthma, skin diseases, menstrual problems, neurological disorders, allergies, arthritis, depression, digestive disturbances (including colic) and migraine (including abdominal migraine,[11] common in children), colds, coughs, flu, sore throats, period pains (common in young girls), nausea and vomiting, nasal blockages, insomnia, constipation, aches and pains (growing pains included) and earaches.

Yoga

Yoga is good for children, encouraging flexibility, relaxation skills and breathing. Used therapeutically, yoga can help with muscle joint mobility, flexibility, breathing disorders, musculoskeletal pain, nervous system and endocrine disorders, digestive problems, fatigue, insomnia and stress-related conditions. Children aged 10 and 11 at Heathfield Primary School in Nottingham, in the U.K., are learning exercises, breathing and relaxation techniques prior to exams. Teachers and students have reported that it has helped them to cope with stress. In the U.S. and Canada, yoga for children has been introduced at a wide range of health clubs and fitness centers, with a view to encouraging healthy exercise habits, but also relieving stress and aiding overall health.

Traditional forms of yoga may be difficult for some children, requiring enormous self-discipline and concentration; however, there are now a variety of courses available that teach yoga in children's terms. For example, some encourage children to take on the movements and postures of animals, which are put into a sequence and linked with a jungle story. Another good form for children is called Oki-do yoga, a form of yoga with both dynamic and relaxing aspects that was introduced to the West in the 1970s. It was developed in Japan by Masahiro Oki, and he combines Indian yoga, Eastern healing methods and martial arts in a program that is brilliant for children.

Ayurvedic medicine

Ayurvedic medicine (Indian medicine) is fast gaining acceptance in the West, and, as a system of medicine addressing all aspects of health, it can be a good choice for children who are chronically ill or simply need a boost. Some of the elements of Ayurvedic medicine include:

- a type of aromatherapy

- breathing

- detoxification

- diet

- exercise

- herbs

- manipulation of vital energy points (called marma)

- meditation

- music therapy

- techniques aimed at emotional and psychological health

- yoga and meditation

The basic Ayurvedic belief is that everything within the universe, including ourselves, is composed of energy or "prana." By balancing that energy within, practitioners promote health on all levels. Ayurvedic practitioners believe that we comprise constantly changing energy. Ayurveda teaches us and our children how to encourage the balance of energy, which controls the functions of every cell in our bodies. That means our thoughts, feelings, actions, food, sleeping patterns, relationships, personal habits and fears—and everything else that is a part of us—affect our energy levels, the quality of that energy and, through that, our health itself.

Ayurvedic practitioners often work on the immune system, in order to balance the energies and keep it strong so that it is able to fight invaders and relieve chronic conditions. There are seven main constitutional types, and once your child's is established, he'll be given a set of guidelines to follow, which are an individually prepared plan for health, mind and spiritual maintenance. Every Ayurvedic program is completely different and tailored to the individual. There is no one treatment that works for an ailment in every person. The combination of energies that make up one person might lead to optimum health. In another person, that balance of energies may cause illness. Ayurvedic medicine can, in theory, address any type of health problem, and is particularly useful for shifting long-term or chronic conditions, such as allergies, digestive disorders, anxiety, depression, headaches, insomnia, respiratory problems, skin problems and stress.

There's more!

Other therapies that are appropriate for children include healing, chiropractic, Alexander Technique, color therapy (see page 159), shiatsu, naturopathy and relaxation and visualization. New therapies appear all the time, and one of the most pleasurable aspects of the wealth of therapies available means that you can experiment and explore. As long as you are convinced that your proposed therapist has experience with children, and is registered in her given field, showing evidence of training and an affiliation with a recognized body, you can try anything that might work. If you are ever in doubt, don't do it! The therapies listed above are all appropriate for children in the right hands, and many can be undertaken safely at home on a basic level. No parent should ever take risks with her child's health, no matter how ill that child is. Use the best of both worlds—complementary and conventional—to get the most appropriate treatment for your child.

Part Three
Natural Treatments for Common Ailments

Treating Common Health Issues

This chapter discusses the most common ailments that affect children, offering parents some alternatives to conventional drugs and intervention. In most cases, natural treatments can be taken alongside orthodox medication, or you may find that drugs will, after time, be unnecessary. Remember that natural medicine can be as powerful as any drug, and you will need to ensure that you get the dosage right, and that the remedies are appropriate for your child. If you are concerned about your child's health for any reason, see your doctor. With the benefit of a little knowledge you can make choices about how you treat your child, but it's never a good idea to play doctor unless you are experienced in natural health or medically trained.

All of the natural treatments suggested are given on the basis that your child is normally healthy, has a good diet, gets enough sleep and exercise, and is well cared for. The best medicine is always preventive, so make sure that you keep your child strong and healthy by addressing these aspects of his lifestyle. When illness strikes, help is at hand!

Giving medicine to children

Whether you choose natural medicine, over-the-counter (OTC) drugs or your child is taking prescription medication, it is important that you follow the dosage exactly. More is never better, as it can be toxic and even life-threatening. The same goes for natural medicines. Many remedies are gentle, working to encourage your child's body to heal itself. However, natural doesn't necessarily mean safe. These remedies are safe and appropriate when taken as required, in the recommended dosages.

Whatever you choose, make sure you consider the following:

- Always read the label.

- Make sure treatment is necessary before you even open the bottle.

What's more important is vigilance: giving the medicine at the right time at the right dose, avoiding interactions between drugs, watching out for tampering, and asking your child's doctor, therapist or the pharmacist about any concerns you may have. Before administering any drug or remedy, it is important for parents to understand why it has been prescribed and how it should be given to the child. A parent should ask a number of questions before accepting any remedy:

- What is it and what is it for?

- Will there be a problem with other drugs or remedies that my child is taking?

- How often and for how long does my child need to take it?

- What if my child misses a dose?

- What side effects does it have and how soon will it start working?

Check all bottles for signs of tampering in any OTC product (herbal, homeopathic or otherwise). The safety seal should be intact before opening. Also, be extra careful to read the label of OTC medicines. Labels are designed to provide valuable information and they should be read thoroughly before giving your child any medication. If you have questions about the label information, ask a therapist, your pharmacist or your physician.

Make sure the drug is safe for children. This information will be on the label. If the label doesn't contain a pediatric dose, don't assume it's safe for anyone under 12 years old. Children are more sensitive than adults to many drugs and remedies, and you should watch your child closely for any side effects.

And before using any self-prescribed drugs or remedies, consider whether they're truly necessary. Not every health condition requires medication or even remedies. Most will run their course in a few days with a little "tincture of time." Homeopathic remedies, flower essences and aromatherapy, among others, will gently encourage the healing action, but they are not drugs and should not be considered in the same light. Don't expect miracle cures or instantaneous symptom relief, and don't give up and run out to buy an OTC product if they don't work overnight. The whole basis of natural medicine is a gentle, long-lasting treatment that will stand your child in good stead in the future. What any parent hoping to go "natural" needs to remember is that the "pop a pill" culture has no place in natural medicine.

In this chapter you'll find a description of the health condition in question, a note of what your doctor might suggest, a list of some of the most appropriate natural therapies, some self-help measures and lots of natural remedies that are commonly used to treat the condition. Most of the remedies can be undertaken at home, but try them one at a time, and always read the label. It can be daunting to take responsibility for a child's health, but with experience, you will develop an instinct for your child's health, and know what to use and when. This chapter is designed to offer you the information you need to make choices. There are no set prescriptions and no rules set in stone. See what works best for your child, and watch her flourish.

ABSCESSES

Abscesses are pockets of pus that are normally the result of a bacterial infection. White blood cells are sent by the body's defense system to attack the bacteria by engulfing them, thereby creating the pus-filled swelling. They can be painful, with swelling and discomfort, and they may feel hot to the touch. If the abscess is big, there may also be fever, nausea and sweating.

Conventional treatment

Antibiotics will normally be offered, but because they cannot penetrate the lining of the abscess cavity, most abscesses will be surgically drained as well.

NATURAL TREATMENTS

- Homeopathic remedies can be very successful in treating abscesses. Try the following:
  - Hepar sulf., for an abscess that is tender, causing sharp pain
  - Belladonna, for early stages, where there is tenderness and throbbing pain
  - Silica, for a slow-forming abscess, with swelling, that doesn't appear to come to a head
- A warm compress with essential oil of chamomile, lemon, lavender or thyme will help to bring it out. Tea tree oil is a natural antiseptic and can be applied neat to abscesses.
- Echinacea, taken two or three times daily, will boost the immune system and help to purify the blood, as well as acting as a natural antibiotic.

Useful therapies

Herbalism, aromatherapy, homeopathy, Ayurveda and naturopathy.

SELF-HELP

- Take steps to boost your child's immune system, which will help to keep infection at bay (see page 207).
- Keep skin clean with regular baths. If your child is prone to abscesses, get some good advice from a registered therapist.

ACNE

Acne is a skin disorder most common among adolescents, and it causes enormous embarrassment and self-consciousness in some teens. It is caused by the hormonal changes at puberty that lead to an increase in the activity of the sebaceous (oil-producing) glands. The sebum produced is trapped beneath the skin, causing inflammation and eventually the characteristic raised red spots on the skin itself. There may also be blackheads. The face, chest and back are most usually affected, and in some cases scarring may occur. Sweating can aggravate acne, as do some oral contraceptives, face creams and cosmetics.

Conventional treatment

Topical treatments are most often used, including benzoyl peroxide, retinoic acid, antibiotic lotions and sulfur-containing creams. Ultraviolet light may also be used with oral antibiotics if the topical treatment fails. These can be given for up to six months at a time.

NATURAL TREATMENTS

- Offer your child acidophilus pills and take three times daily. Alongside, offer zinc gluconate (5 mg pills), taking one pill daily. If your child's skin improves, stop the pills for several weeks, returning to the program for two weeks and then stopping again. This should help to control the condition in most teens.
- Homeopathic treatment will be constitutional, but the following remedies may help. Try:
  - Silica, when there is scarring
  - Antimonium Tart., for pus-filled pimples
  - Sulfur, for chronic acne, with rough hard skin; best in a child who is prone to diarrhea
  - Kali. Brom., for itchy spots or unpleasant dreams
  - Hepar sulf., for large boil-like spots
  - Pulsatilla, when the acne is aggravated by rich, fatty foods, your child dislikes stuffy rooms, and is often tearful
- Gorse flower essence is useful if the acne has gone

on for some time. It will help your child feel less distressed and depressed by his condition.

- Boost your child's immune system (see page 207), which will help prevent infections and encourage healing.
- Rub vitamin E or evening primrose oil into spots (with clean hands) to encourage healing and help prevent scarring.

Useful therapies

Homeopathy, herbalism, nutritional therapy, Ayurveda, aromatherapy, acupuncture, traditional Chinese medicine.

SELF-HELP

- Try to ensure that your child feels good about himself, and take steps to boost his self-esteem and self-image. Skin conditions can have a dramatic effect on self-confidence, and he'll need constant reassurance.
- Although diet is no longer linked to acne, it is important for overall health. Ensure that your child gets plenty of fresh, whole foods for skin health.

ALLERGIES

An allergy is the immune system's abnormal response to contact with a specific substance. The system over-reacts when faced with foreign substances or organisms—allergens—and deals with them as if they were harmful, as it would with invading bacteria, for example. The result is an allergic reaction, also known as a histamine reaction (histamine being the substance produced in response to attack). Common allergens include foods (see page 344), grass pollens, spores, fabrics, drugs, household chemicals and stress. Some of the most common allergic responses are urticaria (see page 359), dermatitis (see page 337), asthma (see page 304) and hay fever/rhinitis (see page 355).

Symptoms vary between children, but some of the most common include sneezing and runny nose, wheezing, excess catarrh, urticaria and anaphylactic shock (see page 302).

Conventional treatment

Histamine reaction allergies will be treated with anti-histamines, topical nasal steroids, and cromolyn sodium—any of which can be used alone or in combination. Immunotherapy may also be suggested, which involves desensitizing allergy shots.

NATURAL TREATMENTS

In natural medicine, allergies are considered a fundamental imbalance within the body, and this will be best addressed by a trained practitioner who will tailor treatment to your child's constitution and symptoms. The best thing that you can do is to take steps to boost her immune system, remove as many toxins from your environment as possible (see page 142), which reduces stress on the body and its systems, and deal with symptoms naturally, helping your child to become strong enough to resist attacks rather than suppressing symptoms.

Alongside natural therapies, you can consider the following:

- Echinacea acts as a natural antibiotic while building the immune system. Other useful herbs include chamomile, elderflower, red clover and yarrow.
- Add a small amount of ginseng powder or syrup (children's strength) to drinks to overcome the tendency to allergic attacks, such as hay fever.
- Offer a little local honey in a cup of warm water with two tablespoons of apple cider vinegar to reduce the reaction to allergens. Particularly useful during hayfever seasons.
- During a sudden allergic reaction, offer Bach Rescue Remedy (see page 260).
- Homeopathic treatment has proved to be very successful in the treatment of allergies. Remedies will be prescribed according to your individual case, so it is best to see a registered practitioner to ensure that your prescription is exact. In the short term, however, Urtica will help with hives, Pulsatilla will help with thick catarrh (especially if your child is tearful) and itching eyes and Arsenicum will help with sneezing and itching eyes.
- Place a few drops of Roman chamomile in a vaporizer or on a light bulb to treat an allergic

Anaphylactic shock is a severe and life-threatening allergic reaction. The reaction occurs after an insect sting, a drug or a particular food. Entry of the allergen into the bloodstream provokes the release of massive amounts of histamine and other chemicals that have effects on body tissues. This causes the respiratory system to spasm, the tongue to swell, pain in the abdomen and sudden, severe lowering of blood pressure. It must be treated as a medical emergency. Summon emergency medical care immediately. The following homeopathic remedies can be given until help arrives:

- Aconite, when your child is restless and frightened
- Veratrum, when her skin is cold and mottled, with a cold sweat
- Arnica, for shock brought on by injury

reaction, including an asthma attack.

- Lavender oil, in a little light carrier oil, can be used in a gentle massage on the chest or the affected area to reduce spasm and boost immunity. For babies, use one or two drops of essential oil in five tablespoons of carrier oil; for older children use four drops of essential oil to five tablespoons of carrier oil.
- Evening primrose oil or blackcurrant seed oil are rich sources of essential fatty acids, which can prevent allergies in susceptible individuals.

Useful therapies

Nutritional therapy, Ayurveda, homeopathy, traditional Chinese medicine, herbalism, acupuncture, reflexology.

SELF-HELP

- Consider your child's diet carefully, and ensure that she is getting plenty of fresh, whole foods to keep her system balanced. You might want to consider whether her symptoms fit those of leaky gut syndrome (see page 264).

- There may be an emotional aspect to the problem as well; stress and anger, especially if the immune system is not functioning properly, are frequently contributing factors. In this case, flower essence therapy can help enormously, as can reducing stress in your child's life (see page 386).

ANEMIA

Anemia is an extremely common condition (in the U.S., millions suffer), characterized by a reduction in either the number of red blood cells, or the amount of hemoglobin in the blood. This results in a decrease in the amount of oxygen that the blood is able to carry. Some of the most common causes include drug use (even prescription drugs), infections, surgery, chronic inflammation, bone marrow disease and dietary deficiencies (especially iron, folic acid and vitamins B6 and B12). The most common cause is iron deficiency. Of those suffering from this type of anemia, 50 percent are children, and it is often considered a hidden disease in that its symptoms can go unrecognized. Watch out for

- Weakness and fatigue.
- Breathlessness on minimal exertion.
- Pale skin and lips.
- Headaches, dizziness and possibly fainting in severe cases.
- In pernicious anemia (caused by vitamin B12 deficiency) there may be nosebleeds, a sore tongue, and "pins and needles" in the hands and feet.

Conventional treatment

The normal treatment for iron-deficiency anemia is iron supplementation; B12 shots would be given in the case of pernicious anemia.

NATURAL TREATMENTS

- Homeopathic remedies include
  - Ferr. Phos., which helps the assimilation of iron from the diet
  - Nat. Mur., for anemia with constipation, headache and a tendency to cold sores

- Calc. Phos., for anemia during a growth spurt, accompanied by irritability
- Nettle tea is rich in iron and can be drunk daily (add a little honey if it is unpalatable).
- The herbs alfalfa, dandelion root, nettle, watercress and yellow dock are rich in iron, and safe for children of all ages. Add fresh to food, or take in tincture or pill form.

Useful therapies

Traditional Chinese medicine, homeopathy, herbalism, nutritional therapies.

SELF-HELP

- Omitting all sugars from the diet increases iron absorption. If your child is taking iron supplements (or extra iron in his diet), increase foods with vitamin C, which enhances absorption.
- Ensure that your child has a complete blood test to confirm that there is an iron deficiency before taking supplements. Iron supplements in excess can damage the liver, pancreas and immune cell activity, and have been linked to cancer. Iron is fine in moderation, when required, but extra iron will do no good unless it's needed.
- Watch oxalic acid, which inhibits iron absorption. It's found in foods such as almonds, cashews, chocolate, cocoa, kale, rhubarb, soft drinks, sorrel, spinach, chard and most nuts and beans.

ANXIETY

Most parents will have witnessed anxiety in their children at some stage or another, and it is actually a normal state of fear or apprehension in the face of threat or danger that causes adrenaline levels to rise. Anxiety can, however, become a chronic condition, characterized by a constant feeling of worry, and is often associated with depression. It can also become seriously acute, where your child suffers from panic attacks, or feels suddenly overwhelmed by fear and dread. Short-term symptoms include a dry mouth, sweating palms, a rapid pulse and palpitations. Longer term it can be debilitating, causing breathlessness, headaches, fatigue, abdominal pain and diarrhea, insomnia and loss of appetite. If your child seems constantly anxious and suffers from these types of symptoms, she will need some help from a registered practitioner.

Conventional treatment

Normally counseling or psychotherapy will be suggested; in extreme cases, drug treatment using psychotropic drugs.

NATURAL TREATMENTS

- Constitutional homeopathic treatment will be appropriate for chronic conditions, and there are a number of remedies that are useful for acute attacks, including
  - Aconite, for a panic attack that comes on suddenly
  - Arsenicum if your child feels insecure, restless, tired and tends to fight anxiety by being obsessively tidy or organize
  - Nat. Mur. may be useful if she dwells on morbid topics and hates fuss
  - Ignatia, if anxiety follows the loss of a loved one or a specific, distressing event
- Herbal remedies would be used to calm the nervous system and to relax your child. Skullcap and valerian are useful herbs, blended together for best effect. Offer as a tea when symptoms arise.
- Flower essences can be brilliant for anxiety: consider Elm for anxiety accompanying a feeling of being unable to cope, or Red Chestnut for anxiety over the welfare of others. Anxiety for no apparent reason might be treated with Aspen. Bach Rescue Remedy (see page 260) is useful during attacks.
- A relaxing blend of essential oils of lavender, geranium and bergamot in sweet almond oil or peach kernel oil may be used in the bath at times of great stress and anxiety.
- Ensure your child gets plenty of B vitamins, which work on the nervous system.

Useful therapies

Aromatherapy, reflexology, acupuncture, herbalism, homeopathy, yoga, hypnotherapy and flower essences.

SELF-HELP

- Open up the channels of communication with your child and help to encourage her to talk about anything that might be at the root of her anxiety. For example, if she becomes anxious after a problem at school, go through it with her and let her know that you are on her side. If she can offload any emotional factors, the physical symptoms will disappear.
- Make sure she gets enough sleep—both anxiety and depression are compounded by poor or inadequate sleep.
- Regular exercise—whether aerobic, or gentle, such as yoga—will help to disperse built-up adrenaline and help your child feel calmer.

Watch her diet. Food that is high in sugar can cause blood sugar swings, as can erratic eating. This can exacerbate feelings of anxiety. Stick to complex carbohydrates and small regular meals.

ASTHMA

Asthma is a condition in which the muscles of the bronchi (the air tubes of the lung) contract in spasm, obstructing the flow of air and making particularly breathing out very difficult. Asthma is becoming increasingly common, especially among children, and may be triggered by a number of factors, including allergens (such as house dust or pets), pollution, infection, emotional trauma or physical exertion. Asthma is divided into two categories: intrinsic for which there is no identifiable cause, and extrinsic, which is triggered by something, usually inhaled.

Asthma is one of the few diseases on the increase in the Western world, and although orthodox medicine can control all the worst symptoms, there is no sign of a cure being found. In the U.S., asthma is a major public health problem of increasing concern. Between 1980 and 1994, the prevalence of asthma increased 75 percent overall and 74 percent among children five to 14 years of age. Asthma now affects nearly five million people who are younger than 18 years of age. Asthma's effects on children and adolescents include the following:

- Asthma accounts for 14 million days of school missed annually
- Asthma is the third-ranking cause of hospitalization among those younger than 15 years of age
- The number of children dying from asthma increased almost threefold from 93 in 1979 to 266 in 1996
- The estimated cost of treating asthma in those younger than 18 years of age is $3.2 billion per year[1]

In many asthmatics, inflammation of the lining of the airways leads to increased sensitivity to a variety of environmental triggers that can cause narrowing of the airways, resulting in obstruction of airflow and breathing difficulty. In some children, the mucous glands in the airways produce excessively thick mucus, further obstructing airflow.

An asthma attack may be brief or last for several days. Typically, an attack begins within minutes after exposure to a triggering agent. Some children have only occasional or "seasonal" symptoms, while others have daily symptoms, including difficulty in breathing, an increase in pulse rate, wheezing (especially on the out breath), a persistent, dry cough (often at night) and tightness in the chest.

Conventional treatment

With two types of drugs: relieving drugs and preventing drugs.

- The relieving drugs such as salbutamol (Ventolin) and terbutaline (Bricanyl) act within minutes to open the airways and bring relief from symptoms, but wear off within a few hours and fail to deal with the underlying inflammation of the airways.
- Preventing drugs such as beclomethasone (Becotide), budesonide (Pulmicort) or sodium chromoglycate (Intal) tackle the root of the problem—the inflammation in the airways. They act slowly over several hours and their full effect may not be

apparent for several days. These drugs are used regularly, whether the child is well or ill, in order to keep the inflammation at bay and prevent long-term or permanent damage to the airways.

Leukotriene antagonists are a fairly new class of drugs, which block leukotrienes, 18 components of the immune system that cause constriction of the airways and excess production of mucus in allergic asthma. Leukotriene antagonists are usually taken orally and are prescribed for long-term prevention and exercise-induced asthma. They are not used for treatment of acute asthma attacks. Prescribed alone or in combination with steroids, these medications can reduce the need for inhaled steroids.

> **CAUTION**
> A prolonged attack of severe asthma that does not respond to simple remedies requires immediate medical attention.

NATURAL TREATMENTS

- Chronic asthma can be addressed by homeopathy, but it must be treated constitutionally. The following remedies can be used for mild attacks:
  - Ipecac, for wheezy children who cough until they vomit up a little mucus
  - Arsenicum, waking between midnight and 2 A.M. with difficult breathing
  - Bryonia, for asthma that comes on at the end of a cold, with a hard, dry cough
  - Nat. sulf., for asthma in damp weather; loose cough with yellowish mucus
  - Lachesis, for asthma that comes on in spring or autumn
- In traditional Chinese medicine, the cause of the illness is considered to be phlegm produced by weakness of the spleen and kidneys; almond and ephedra are two herbs that can be used to open lungs. Acupuncture will address weaknesses.
- Any of the herbs suggested for stress (see page 387) will help your child to relax, and decrease the incidence of attacks.

- The herb ginkgo biloba has been shown effective in many studies.
- A steam inhalation of chamomile, eucalyptus or lavender essential oils can be offered during an attack and immediately afterward to ease panic and help open airways.
- Bergamot, clary sage, neroli, chamomile and rose oils are antispasmodic, as well as relaxant, and they will be particularly useful for attacks brought on by stress.
- Children with asthma may be deficient in certain nutrients, such as vitamin B6, vitamin C, magnesium and selenium (see Appendix). Make sure they get plenty of these in their diet, or consider supplementing.

Useful therapies

Buteyko method, acupuncture, traditional Chinese medicine, homeopathy, herbalism, reflexology, aromatherapy.

SELF-HELP

- According to *Nutrition Health Review*, strong feelings of anger, anxiety and depression may be an important cause of asthma attacks. Ensuring emotional health can do a great deal to ease the condition.
- Include garlic and onions in your child's diet. These foods contain quercetin and mustard oils, which have been shown to inhibit an enzyme that helps the body to release inflammatory chemicals.
- Take steps to boost your child's immune system. Asthma is considered a largely allergic disorder (the airways are hypersensitive to certain stimuli, causing chronic inflammation), and a strong immune system is the basis for all treatment.
- Watch out for food intolerances (see page 344).

ATHLETE'S FOOT

Athlete's foot (or tinea pedis) is a fungal infection that attacks the warm, moist areas between the toes, most commonly between the fourth and fifth toes. It is highly infectious, spreading through close physical contact, notoriously at public swimming pools. Once acquired, athlete's foot is very persistent. It usually affects children with particularly sweaty feet, and those who fail to dry off properly after bathing.

Symptoms include discomfort and itching, followed by painful cracks in the skin, peeling skin and blisters.

Conventional treatment

Antifungal ointments will be offered, and antibiotic creams if the cracks become infected.

NATURAL TREATMENTS

- A foot bath with tea tree oil, eucalyptus, patchouli or lavender is effective as all the oils are soothing and antifungal. Also add to unscented skin lotion, such as aqueous cream or calendula and rub into the affected area.
- Echinacea tincture, which is antifungal, can be dabbed on the affected area as often as required.
- Apply a little live yogurt to the area daily, for its antifungal properties.
- Take acidophilus pills daily to help restore natural bacteria in the body to help fight fungal infections.

Useful therapies

Aromatherapy, herbalism, constitutional homeopathy, traditional Chinese medicine.

SELF-HELP

- Keep your child's feet clean and dry, and avoid swimming pools or other damp, moist places until cracking is healed. Buy cotton socks, but encourage your child to keep his feet bare as often as possible.
- Aim to boost your child's immune system, to help fight against fungal invaders.

ATTENTION DEFICIT DISORDER (ADD)

and

ATTENTION DEFICIT AND HYPERACTIVITY DISORDER (ADHD)

Watch out for this diagnosis. It has become increasingly common to label lively and uncooperative children—with or without emotional or learning difficulties—as hyperactive, or suffering from ADD. The terms ADD and ADHD developed after several years of misnomers for children who failed to conform to what were probably idealistic standards of learning and behavior.

In *The Limits of Biological Treatments for Psychological Distress* (eds. S. Fisher, R. Greenberg, 1989) Diane McGuinness says, "It is currently fashionable to treat approximately one-third of all elementary school boys as an abnormal population because they are fidgety, inattentive and unamenable to adult control." She insists that two decades of research have not provided any support for the validity of ADD and concludes that there is no convincing evidence that medications help learning or attention problems. She says that while the drug Ritalin may "reduce fidgety behavior," it does so in all children, regardless of diagnosis. She says, "The data consistently fails to support any benefits from stimulant medication," and cautions that stimulant medication is a drastic invasion of the body and nervous system. She also notes that the majority of children labeled as being ADD are, in fact, normal, healthy, energetic children.

ADD is not always a medically diagnosed condition; in fact, it is diagnosed when a child fits the description of 8 out of 14 items on a check list of characteristics, and has done for 6 months or more. Some of these characteristics include:
- loses things necessary to complete a task
- fidgets in his seat
- can't wait his turn
- blurts out answers
- shifts from one uncompleted activity to another
- has difficulty remaining seated
- interrupts or intrudes

It doesn't take a psychologist to assess the fact that the majority of these characteristics are common to most children, particularly those in stressful conditions.

Many experts now believe that ADD is nothing more than a buzzword. The fact that children are hyperactive or have difficulty concentrating is probably due more to the fact that Western diets are so poor, children are forced at an increasingly early age to sit still in a classroom or nursery with large numbers of other children watch too much television, get inadequate sleep and get little or no exercise. Place these restrictions on any adult, and the same behaviors could be expected. Also, the vast majority of children labeled ADD are boys, throwing into question our societal expectations of children who have natural activity, aggression and independence.

If you or anyone else suspects your child has ADD/ADHD it is essential that he be assessed by a child psychologist. Legitimate cases do exist, but too often the diagnosis is given without thorough assessment by a trained professional. Drugs may be necessary in the case of a clinical diagnosis, but medication should not be the only treatment. All aspects of the child must be assessed including socialization, parenting, school life, sleep, emotions and diet.

Conventional treatment

The solution has been to use drugs, particularly Ritalin, which has the effect of temporarily calming children (all children). But this practice is now under review. For example, Sweden has abolished Ritalin as dangerous and too easily abused. In March 2000, the U.S. government announced an effort to reverse the dramatic increase in prescriptions for psychotropic drugs such as Ritalin in preschoolers, and the National Institutes of Health (NIH) is conducting a nationwide study of the use of medication for attention-deficit/hyperactivity disorder in children under the age of seven. While Ritalin may be appropriate for a seriously hyperactive or unwell child, it should never be prescribed without the recommendation of a good child psychiatrist, who can assess the situation from a psychological as well as a behavioral and physical point of view.

SELF-HELP

So what do you do if your child is hyperactive or labeled as having ADD?

- Make your daily routine as simple and straightforward as possible. It will help to keep your child calmer and he will have more chance of remembering what comes next. Try to avoid rushing around, or eating on the run, which will make him feel unsettled.

- Be very specific when talking to your child. Explain everything, and don't expect too much.

- Several studies show that toxins in the environment may be a contributory factor. Take steps to keep your child's environment as pure as possible (see page 142). Have a hair analysis done to check for high levels of metals, such as lead. Do not use antacid pills, cough medicines, perfume, throat lozenges or commercial toothpaste (use a natural toothpaste instead).

- Avoid overstimulation. Playtime should be calm and reassuring, and no more than one or two other playmates should be involved. When things get out of hand, change the room or the venue (head off to the park, for example).

- Remember that hyperactivity is not bad behavior. There can be learning difficulties present, and your child may have some difficulty with coordination or controlling movement.

- Some studies show that children with a tendency toward hyperactivity benefit from increased parental attention—on a one-to-one basis. Many children are labeled "difficult," "hyperactive" or "hard work" when they first exhibit these symptoms and in some cases this can create a self-fulfilling prophecy. This type of negative labeling can harm a child emotionally, so it is important to offer positive reinforcement (see page 176) and to raise your child's self-esteem. There should be a period of quality time, in which positive behavior can be reinforced. Discipline should never be harsh, as your child is not usually willfully being naughty, but simply losing control. Removing your child from the scene of a tantrum or an outburst, or whatever behavior has got out of control, will help. Timeouts (see page 180), seem to help with some hyperactive children.

- Some children naturally have increased energy and physical requirements, and it is important for any child with these tendencies to get plenty of exercise. This can mean a break not offered to other children in a school environment. Talk to your child's teacher about allowing more breaks for physical release of tension (running around the playground, for example), which will help children to focus more in a school environment. If your child is extremely active, you may want to consider whether early schooling is a good idea. Many children are not able to handle the confines of the school environment until they are older, and it can exacerbate a problem if you start too early.

- Consider some of the natural therapies, such as cranial osteopathy, acupuncture (trials have shown it to be a useful alternative to standard medication), flower essences, herbalism, reflexology and homeopathy. If your child has been vaccinated, a postvaccination cleansing by a homeopath can make a dramatic difference—ADD did not exist before broadscale immunization.

- Dietary causes are now credibly linked with diagnoses of ADD and ADHD, and a food allergy (see page 344), toxic overload (see page 141), and nutritional deficiencies can be at the root of the problem. For example:

  - Researchers found that 74 percent of a group of 261 hyperactive children displayed abnormal glucose tolerance curves, suggesting a connection between hyperactive behavior and the consumption of sugar

  - Studies indicate that gamma-amino-butyric acid (GABA) decreases hyperactivity, as well as tendencies toward violence, epilepsy and learning difficulties

  - Behavior, learning and health problems were compared between boys with high and low intakes of essential fatty acids. More behavioral problems were found in those with lower omega-3 intakes, and more learning and health problems were found in those with lower omega-6 intakes.

  - Of 76 hyperactive children treated with a low-allergen diet, 62 improved and a normal range of behavior was achieved in 21 of these. Artificial colorings and preservatives were found to be the most common culprits.

  - A study of ten habitual juvenile offenders found they were very low in zinc, and had high hyperactivity scores. Some also had manganese and chromium deficiencies.

  - The hyperactivity ratings of 19 out of 26 children given a diet excluding wheat, corn, yeast, soy, citrus, egg, chocolate, peanuts and artificial colors and flavors, dropped from an average of 25 (high) to an average of 8 (low)

Consider making dietary changes. Strict elimination diets can be dangerous for children, so it's important that you alter their diet only under the guidance of a registered nutritionist. Suspect foods include all forms of refined sugar and any products that contain it; artificial colors, flavorings or preservatives; and foods that contain salicylates (including almonds, apples, apricots, cherries, currants, all berries, peaches, plums, prunes, tomatoes, cucumbers and oranges). Include plenty of other fruits and vegetables in your child's diet, plus breads, cereals and crackers that contain only rice and oats. If diet is the culprit, your child will not have to remain on a strict regime for the rest of his life. Many children outgrow the problem.

It is, of course, very difficult for parents to deal with a constantly active child, and you will need to get as much support as you can from friends, family and professionals. Get whatever help you need, including counseling, natural therapies, specially trained teaching for your child, and a support network of parents facing similar difficulties (see page 442).

AUTISM

Autism is a little understood brain disorder that affects approximately 4 out of every 10,000 people. It is usually diagnosed in early childhood (before the age of three) and characterized by a marked unresponsiveness to other people and the surrounding environment. There are no physical signs, but children exhibit marked differences in behavior from an early age. Most children appear indifferent to love and affection as babies, and as they grow older they often fail to form attachments in the way that most children do. Many autistic children exhibit unpredictable and unusual behavior, such as constant rocking, sitting for long periods of time in total silence or pounding their feet while sitting. There are learning difficulties present, but many autistic children are enormously bright, or at least within normal intelligence ranges. The cause is unknown, but many experts believe there may be a hereditary element, a neurological imbalance, or malfunction that makes an autistic child oversensitive to external stimuli. There may also be an immune basis.

A recent study showed that families of children with autism have an unusually high incidence of immune diseases, in particular rheumatoid arthritis. The results showed that in 46 percent of the families of autistic children two or more members had autoimmune disorders and 21 percent of autistic children had at least one parent suffering from such a disorder. This compared with 26 percent of normal children's families having such a disease and 4 percent of parents. This may lend credence to the idea that autism is linked to immunization. It may, however, not be the cause, and parents must be prepared for the fact that their child's autism is inexplicable.

Conventional treatment

Counseling and behavior therapy may be offered. In some cases phenothiazine antipsychotics are used (they are major tranquilizers), as well as fenfluramine and thioridazine.

NATURAL TREATMENTS

- Cranial osteopathy may be appropriate, as some experts believe that there may be head pain caused by overcompression of the skull during birth.
- Constitutional homeopathic treatment may aid children whose symptoms came on following immunization, and may be appropriate for mild

cases. But, there is no conclusive evidence that homeopathy will help children suffering from core autism, although it's worth a visit to a good homeopath to see if symptoms can be reduced in any way. For short-term relief try
  - Chamomilla, for a child who is irritable, restless and lashes out when approached, repeatedly bangs head and finds noise upsetting
  - Silica, for a child who retreats into a shell, sits on the floor and counts over and over, has head sweats at night and possibly sweaty feet
  - Hyoscyamus, for a child who is suspicious, muttering, goes into fits of laughter and plays with the genitals
- Nutritional therapy is indicated for behavioral autism, particularly magnesium, vitamin B6 and vitamin C. At present no studies indicate that core autism can be treated with diet, or indeed anything else. If your child suffers from behavioral autism, consider this:
  - In a trial administering vitamin B6 with magnesium to 44 autistic children, 15 showed a moderate clinical improvement and became worse when the supplements were discontinued
  - Questionnaires on the treatment of 4,000 autistic children revealed that among the biomedical treatments, the use of high-dosage vitamin B6 with magnesium was found to be six times more effective than fenfluramine and thioridazine
  - In one study, supplementation of autistic schoolchildren with 0.28 oz (8g) per 154lbs (70kg) body weight per day of vitamin C resulted in a reduction in the severity of symptoms
- Studies also show dramatic improvement in autistic children after chemical additives and allergenic foods (see page 344) were eliminated from the diet. A significant number have been found to have gastrointestinal disorders, including celiac disease and other food intolerances. A study by Dr. Michael Tettenborn, consultant pediatrician, showed that 28 out of 57 autistic children between the ages of 2 and 15 showed a "definite and sustained improvement" when they were given anti-fungal therapy and/or fed a diet low in yeast and milk products.

Fifteen got worse when taken off the treatment and six had "uncertain improvement" in their symptoms. Most of the school-age children are now in mainstream schools. The children who responded to treatment had several characteristics in common: most had developed autism after 16 months; many had poor socialization skills such as poor eye contact; there was often a history of altered bowel habits at the same time that autistic symptoms developed; many had been ill when symptoms developed and had been given antibiotics. They also shared a tendency to feel excessive thirst, a craving for milk or wheat products, nasal congestion, and had a very pale face with dark shadows under the eyes and abdominal distention.

- The herb ginkgo biloba is a powerful free radical destroyer that protects the brain. It also improves brain function by increasing circulation to the brain. It may interfere with drug treatment, but talk to a registered herbalist about use.

Useful therapies

Art therapy, music therapy, cranial osteopathy, homeopathy, nutritional therapies, herbalism and traditional Chinese medicine.

BALANITIS

Balanitis is inflammation and soreness of the foreskin of the penis. It is common in boys with a very tight-fitting foreskin, making it difficult for the urine to flow out easily. The foreskin often balloons when the child passes urine. Common symptoms include pain when urinating, inflammation and redness around the end of the penis and general discomfort.

Conventional treatment

Your doctor will probably first try a local antibiotic or anti inflammatory cream—eye ointment is commonly used for children. If this does not work, a course of antibiotics may be necessary. Circumcision may be required for recurrent balanitis.

NATURAL TREATMENTS

- Add saltwater to your child's bath, and gently bathe the area to encourage healing. If there is obvious infection, one or two drops of tea tree oil can be added to the bath water to help fight it off.
- Make sure your child has a good diet, rich in foods containing vitamin C, such as citrus fruit, broccoli and leafy green vegetables, which will help him to throw off the infection more quickly.
- The homeopathic remedy Mercurius 6C can be taken up to five times daily, for several days. If there is fever, offer Belladonna.

BEDWETTING

Bedwetting is not considered a problem until your child is at least five. Many children, boys in particular, are slow in getting the message that they should get up to use the toilet at night, but that is no reflection on the state of their health—mental or otherwise. If a child sleeps heavily it may take longer to achieve night dryness, but many children manage it by two or three years of age. Bedwetting in children who have already established a pattern of dry nights is usually caused by stress of some sort, like moving house, changing schools, family fighting. Children who have never been dry at night may suffer from immature nerves and muscles controlling bladder function. Other medical causes include diabetes, urinary infection, a structural abnormality, nutritional deficiencies and food allergies.

Conventional treatment

If there is no physical cause, a bed alarm may be suggested (a loud alarm rings when moisture hits the sheet). In rare cases antidepressant drugs may be offered.

NATURAL TREATMENTS

- Homeopathic treatment is appropriate, but should be constitutional. Try:
  - Equisetum, when the wetting occurs during dreams

- Belladonna, when it occurs early in the night
- Kreosotum, when wetting occurs during dreams in early night, and deep sleep
- Causticum, for wetting in first sleep, worse in clear weather or when your child has a cough
- Plantago, when all else fails
- Bedwetting is an ideal condition for flower essences, particularly if the condition seems to have an emotional cause (and even if not).
  - Try Wild Rose if he seems to drift through life
  - Walnut will help if the bedwetting is brought on by change, such as a new house, school or baby
  - Vervain may help if your child is stressed
  - Star of Bethlehem is recommended if bedwetting is related to a trauma or shock
  - Try Mimulus if the problem is linked to fear
- Offer St. John's wort in a cup of water and sweetened with honey, sipped throughout the day, to soothe an irritable bladder and encourage control of the bladder.
- If the bedwetting stems from an emotional upset or disturbance, the herbs vervain and lemon balm will relax and soothe.

Useful therapies

Any of the therapies suggested for stress, if the cause is believed to be emotional (see page 386), homeopathy, cranial osteopathy, traditional Chinese medicine, hypnotherapy, reflexology and flower essences.

SELF-HELP

- Try not to become angry, which can exacerbate the problem. Use a star chart and plenty of praise for dry nights, and ignore the situation if you find a wet bed. If your child is slightly older, you may suggest a sleepover at a friend's. Many children will not wet the bed under these circumstances, and it can break a long-term habit.
- Some children sleep very deeply and do not waken when the urge to pass urine is felt. You can, for a time, waken your child and take him to the toilet, in advance of the time when the bed is normally wet. This won't cure the condition, but it will prevent some wet nights until your child outgrows it.
- Keep evening drinks to a minimum, and make sure he urinates before bed.
- Don't be tempted to carry on using diapers—it can be belittling for older children, and younger children will continue to wet them as usual.

BOILS

A boil is a swollen, pus-filled area occurring on the site of an infected hair follicle. The staphylococcus bacteria is usually responsible, but other causes may include eczema, scabies, diabetes, poor personal hygiene or obesity. A boil begins as a painful red lump, then hardens and forms a yellow head. The most common areas for boils to appear are the back of the neck, groin and armpits. A boil on an eyelash is known as a stye (see page 388). A boil is characterized by a burning, throbbing sensation around the affected area, and enormous sensitivity when pus has formed.

Conventional treatment

Boils are often lanced, and topical and systemic antibiotics offered.

NATURAL TREATMENT

- Homeopathic remedies will help. Try:
  - Belladonna, for red, tender, new boils
  - Hepar sulf., for boils that are sensitive, and weep easily; this will also bring the boil to a head
  - Gunpowder, for weeping but not painful boils
- A warm compress with essential oil of chamomile, lemon, lavender or thyme will help to bring it out.
- Offer echinacea, two or three times daily, to boost the immune system and purify the blood. Drink infusions of thyme or red clover three times daily during attacks.
- Offer plenty of garlic if your child is prone to boils; garlic is cleansing and chronic boils indicate that she may have a high number of toxins in her body.

Useful therapies

Homeopathy, herbalism, aromatherapy, traditional Chinese medicine.

BRONCHITIS

Bronchitis is an inflammation of the lining of the bronchi (the air tubes of the lungs). Acute bronchitis in which mucus infected with bacteria is expelled from the lungs often follows a viral illness such as a cold or flu, or even childhood illnesses such as measles. Symptoms include a dry cough that becomes loose and moist, shortness of breath, fever, wheezing and occasionally chest pain.

Conventional treatment

Antibiotics are given only if there is a secondary bacterial infection, otherwise treatment is limited to broncho-dilator drugs and cough suppressants.

CAUTION

If there is blood in the sputum, your child turns blue around the lips or has an extremely high temperature, get emergency attention. If natural remedies do not work within two days, see your doctor.

NATURAL TREATMENTS

- Homeopathic remedies can be offered for acute bronchitis; chronic bronchitis must be treated constitutionally. Try:
  - Pulsatilla, for symptoms that are worse in stuffy rooms and dry cough at night, which loosen in the morning
  - Ipecac., for nausea, vomiting and a feeling of suffocation
  - Bryonia, for a dry, stabbing cough with headache and great thirst
  - Phosphorus, for tight, ticking cough; children who are pale, anxious and thirsty for cold water
  - Aconite, for sudden onset, with dry cough and chills
- Essential oils to help clear the congestion include eucalyptus and thyme, which can be inhaled in a steam bath or vaporizer as required.
- Ginger oil can be heavily diluted and rubbed into your child's chest for chronic bronchitis, to dispel mucus.

- Wild cherry bark extract can be added to any herbal drink to relieve coughing.
- Rub garlic oil into the chest to fight infection and encourage healing.
- Ginseng in hot water will help to eliminate infection and ease coughing.
- Honey and lemon in a little warm water can be sipped regularly to fight infection and ease coughs.

Useful therapies

Homeopathy, traditional Chinese medicine, acupuncture, herbalism, reflexology.

SELF-HELP

- Take steps to boost your child's immune system (see page 207).
- Try to stay calm, even if symptoms are alarming. They will become worse if your child is frightened.

CATARRH

Catarrh is the term used to describe the overproduction of thick phlegm by the mucous membranes of the air passages to the lungs, the larynx, the nose and sinuses. Inflammation of the membranes as a result of a cold or flu is the usual cause, but other triggers include passive smoking, inhalation of dust, chronic sinusitis, upper respiratory tract infection or allergy. A series of colds in close succession may lead to chronic catarrh, and it can follow other illnesses and immunization.

Conventional treatment

Nasal sprays, cough suppressants and, if there is secondary bacterial infection, antibiotics.

NATURAL TREATMENTS

Most natural therapies will need to be constitutional—that is, based on your child's individual constitution and environment. Many therapists believe that chronic catarrh is a symptom of general toxicity of the body, which can be addressed therapeutically.

- Onions are an excellent purgative, and can be offered raw or cooked as often as possible.
- Mustard powder can be added to a footbath to help decongest nasal passages and clear catarrh.
- Good, short-term homeopathic remedies include:
  - Arsenicum for thick, yellow discharge that makes the nose and the surrounding area sore
  - Pulsatilla, for yellow or green catarrh that is not painful; accompanied by weepiness
  - Nat. Mur., for catarrh like raw egg white, with a dry nose and loss of taste and smell
  - Calcarea, for yellow, smelly catarrh
  - Sulfur, when there are dry scabs inside the nose, causing bleeding, and nose stuffier indoors rather than outdoors
- Eucalyptus oil may be inhaled to ease symptoms, and lavender is useful by the bed to make it possible to sleep. Many oils, including chamomile and mint, are decongestant and expectorant. Rub into the chest and temples in a light carrier oil, or place several drops in a vaporizer and encourage your child to inhale.
- Herbs such as golden rod, elderflower and eyebright are anticatarrhal and astringent. When catarrh is accompanied by infection, supplement with echinacea and garlic.

Useful therapies

Reflexology, traditional Chinese Medicine, homeopathy, herbalism, acupuncture, nutritional therapies, cranial osteopathy, aromatherapy.

SELF-HELP

- Watch dietary causes. Chronic catarrh is one of the most common signs of food allergies (see page 344).
- Boost your child's immune system (see page 207), to prevent secondary infection and help to reduce overproduction of mucus.
- Ensure that your house is free of dust and that your child is not in contact with smoke.

CHICKEN POX

Chicken pox is an extremely contagious viral infection, which features headache, fever and general malaise, with spots starting usually on the trunk and spreading to most parts of the body, including the mouth, anus, vagina and ears. They appear as pimples, which soon fill with fluid to become little blisters. Eventually the spots dry up and form a scab, which may cause scars. These spots are very itchy and it is important that the child does not scratch, for scarring and bacterial infection can result. The incubation period is 10 to 14 days, and sufferers are contagious from just before the spots appear. Chicken pox is considered a cleansing illness, giving the body a chance to detoxify, so plenty of spots is a good sign, even if it is unsightly and uncomfortable for your child. One bout of chicken pox normally gives lifetime immunity against the illness, but the virus that causes chicken pox (varicella zoster) is the same virus that causes shingles in adults. The virus can lie dormant for years, then resurface as shingles.

Conventional treatment

Your doctor may suggest calamine lotion to ease the itching and acetaminophen to relieve the fever. In most cases, children will recover within about ten days. The Varicella vaccine is used to immunize against this condition.

NATURAL TREATMENTS

- A witch hazel compress can be applied directly to the spots, or a little added to the bath, to ease discomfort.
- Homeopathic remedies can be enormously effective. Try the following:
  - Variolinum can be taken once in cases where there is an epidemic of chicken pox, before your child acquires the illness, and symptoms should be less severe
  - Rhus Tox. can be taken for a few days after contact with an infected child, and then again as soon as the first spots appear
  - Aconite is useful in the early stages of the illness
  - Belladonna is useful for fever

- Add baking soda to the bath to ease itching.
- Flower essences can also help with negative emotional features of the condition:
  - Chicory, Hornbeam and Cherry Plum are usually suggested to help relieve some of the discomfort
  - Impatiens can ease irritability
  - Crab Apple may be diluted and applied directly to the spots to encourage healing
  - Olive will be useful for the convalescence period
- A few drops of Roman chamomile can be used in the bath to soothe
- Essential oil of lavender can be dabbed directly on spots to ease the itching and encourage healing. Lavender also has an antibacterial action, which will help prevent a secondary infection

Useful therapies

Aromatherapy, acupuncture, traditional Chinese medicine, homeopathy and herbalism.

SELF-HELP

- Keep your child's nails short and clean, and try to encourage her not to scratch the spots. Put mittens on a young child's hands if necessary.
- Offer freshly squeezed, diluted juices to encourage the cleansing process. When she is able to eat normally again, offer bland foods (bananas, fresh raw apple sauce or live yogurt) for a few days. Avoid processed or spicy foods for as long as possible.

> **CAUTION**
> When fever lasts for more than a couple of days, or there is an obvious chest infection accompanying the rash, see your doctor. Very rarely, chicken pox pneumonia can occur as a secondary infection.

CHRONIC FATIGUE SYNDROME (CFS) AND MYALGIC ENCEPHALITIS (ME)

These terms seem to be used interchangeably, and there is still little research into the causes of these conditions. Myalgic encephalitis (ME) is also known as postviral fatigue syndrome and chronic fatigue syndrome, and its cause is the subject of controversy: some think it is caused by a viral infection (possibly herpes, polio or Epstein–Barr), while others hold that it may be a psychological or neurological disorder, and others still a result of damage to the immune system. Symptoms may persist for years, aggravated by periods of stress or exertion—they include profound fatigue, fever, headache, nausea and dizziness, muscle pain, weight fluctuation, sleep disturbance, depression and even memory loss.

Interestingly, a recent study showed that the majority of children diagnosed with CFS first developed the illness during the autumn school term, and most came from the top two social classes, with half in private education. Only one in five came from a broken home. It is thought that the high stress environment of school (worse in private education), combined with the arrival of infectious illnesses brought on by the winter and the classroom environment can trigger the illness. In all, 76 percent of CFS cases started between September and December. Cases peak around exam time. Dr. Anita Sharma, who is researching CFS at the University of Birmingham in England, said many adults diagnosed with CFS often felt their symptoms had started after they had suffered some sort of infection, such as influenza, glandular fever or a stomach upset. She added that individuals who tended to be highly driven also seemed more likely to develop CFS. She speculated that a return to school in autumn might herald greater exposure to certain winter infections, which, together with increased work pressure, could comprise a greater risk. She said: "In addition, children are going from a relatively unregulated environment to a very structured one, and all the extracurricular activities are starting up again."

Conventional treatment

There is no cure for CFS or ME, and doctors recommend a period of rest with a little regular exercise. Occupational therapists can often provide a gradual rehabilitation with a graded exercise program and support from a team of practitioners. Occasionally antidepressants are offered.

NATURAL TREATMENTS

- First and foremost, take the new study as a warning. Before school starts, it's important to boost your child's immune system (see page 207) and to keep extracurricular activities to a minimum in the autumn term.
- Look at the Bach flower essences listed on page 258. If you have an enormously driven child, choose a remedy that will help to bring out the positive features of this trait. If he starts to become tired, offer olive, for deep fatigue. The idea is to prevent CFS or ME before they set in.
- If your child does become ill toward the end of the summer holidays, or early in the autumn term, ensure that he takes time to recover (see page 226) and don't rush him back to school.
- In traditional Chinese medicine, ME and CFS are believed to be caused by weakness of chi, deficient blood and damp heat, and herbal treatment would be given accordingly, probably in conjunction with acupuncture. Chinese angelica can restore energy and stimulate white blood cells and antibody formation.
- A good B-complex vitamin pill will help to ensure the health of the nervous system and give your child more energy.
- Some sufferers have food allergies (see page 344) that may exacerbate or even cause the condition; try an elimination diet to see if your child is allergic to anything; in particular, look at dairy produce and wheat.
- Chronic yeast infection may be at the root of the condition; try supplementation with acidophilus, and eating plenty of fresh live yogurt.
- Evening primrose oil, taken over three months, has proved useful in treating ME.
- Homeopathic treatment would be constitutional, based on your individual needs, but there have been many promising studies done into its effects. China may be taken every 12 hours, for 3 to 4 days, while waiting for constitutional treatment.
- Herbs that address the immune system, such as echinacea, are useful. Ginseng and ginkgo biloba will encourage energy.
- Rosemary and sage wines act as an excellent tonic when you are run-down and tired.
- Uplifting oils, such as rose and neroli, are useful to help with flagging spirits. Tea tree and niaouli will strengthen the immune system. Use any of these oils in massage, or in the bath.

Useful therapies

Acupuncture, homeopathy, traditional Chinese medicine, nutritional therapies and herbalism are the most useful; stress-relieving therapies such as yoga, reflexology and aromatherapy may help.

SELF-HELP

Emotional health is crucial to a full recovery (see Chapter 8) and you will need to offer plenty of support. A gradual exercise program is recommended.

COLD SORES

Cold sores are painful blisters caused by a herpes simplex infection and usually appear on the lips and nose. The virus is harbored by most people, but may cause problems when your child's immune system is compromised, dealing with other viral infections (such as a cold), or when he is rundown.

Conventional treatment

If cold sores are particularly troublesome, your doctor may prescribe idoxuridine paint or the antiviral drug acyclovir (in pill or cream form), or another antiviral agent.

NATURAL TREATMENTS

- Homeopathy will do a great deal to prevent recurring cold sores, but constitutional treatment will be required. The following remedies may help:

- Nat. Mur., for deep cracks in the lower lip, dry mouth and puffy, burning sores
- Rhus Tox., for mouth and chin sores, and ulcers at the corner of the mouth
- Sempervivum, for ulcers in the mouth, and bleeding gums; worse at night
- Capsicum, for cracks at the corners of the mouth, pale lips, rash on chin, blisters on tongue and bad breath

- St. John's wort tincture should stop a cold sore from appearing. Use at the first sign of tingling.
- Bergamot, eucalyptus and tea tree oils will help to treat the blisters, and should be applied at the first sign of a sore.
- Lavender oil will help to heal blisters that erupt.
- Cold sores tend to crop up when your child feels run-down, so it is important that he eat a healthy diet. Offer plenty of whole-grain cereals, fruit, legumes, nuts and seeds. Take a daily multivitamin and mineral pill—especially one containing high amounts of the antioxidant nutrients—to boost immune activity. Vitamin C stimulates immunity and is antiviral as well as anti-fungal. Zinc stimulates the immune system and is antiviral and antifungal.
- Acidophilus will encourage the healthy bacteria in your child's gut to help fight off infections and infestations.

Useful therapies

Any therapy that helps to reduce stress and boost immunity—try reflexology, homeopathy, traditional Chinese medicine, acupuncture, herbalism, aromatherapy and nutritional therapies.

SELF-HELP

Cold sores are infectious—wash hands carefully after applying any lotion, and give your child his own towel.

COLIC

Colic is characterized by a baby's apparently unending frantic crying, usually at around the same time of day or night. The legs are drawn up to the abdomen, and the baby appears to be in severe pain. Excessive crying causes the baby to swallow air, which can exacerbate the problem and lead to abdominal bloating. The cause is unknown, but may be caused by contractions of the colon, an allergy to something in the formula (if bottle-fed) or the mother's diet (if breastfed), or simply excessive air gulped in through repeated bouts of crying. There is some evidence that a difficult birth can lead to colic.

Conventional treatment

There are a variety of OTC antispasmodic drugs that might be suggested for your baby.

NATURAL TREATMENTS

- Because colic is exacerbated by tension, relaxing herbs are often suggested—used in the bath, or infused, cooled slightly and taken by bottle. Chamomile, lemon balm and lime flowers are most effective.
- A warm bath with an infusion of dill, fennel, marshmallow or lemon balm will soothe a colicky baby.
- The following homeopathic remedies will help:
  - Chamomilla is useful for babies who seem better when they are held
  - Pulsatilla is used for babies who are better in the fresh air, and when they are rocked
  - Cuprum Met. is used when the tummy rumbles, and the child curls her fingers and toes in discomfort
- Rock Rose flower essence is excellent for distress and fright, and Bach Rescue Remedy (see page 260) can be used to calm and help to reduce any spasm.
- A gentle massage of the abdominal area with one or a blend of essential oils of chamomile, dill, lavender or rose, will help to ease symptoms and calm a distressed baby.
- Try a drop of lavender or chamomile oil in a warm bath, just before evening feeds.

Useful therapies

Massage, cranial osteopathy, acupuncture, herbalism, aromatherapy, homeopathy, nutritional therapy (to address any potential allergies).

SELF-HELP

If you are breastfeeding, avoid dairy produce for a few days to see if this helps. Other foods that should be avoided are very spicy foods, citrus foods, gassy foods (beans, onions, cabbage, etc.) and sugar.

COMMON COLD

The common cold is an infection of the upper respiratory tract that may be caused by any one of up to 200 strains of virus. These are spread either by inhaling droplets coughed or sneezed by others, or more probably by direct hand-to-hand contact.

When infection occurs, the walls of the respiratory tract swell and produce excess mucus, giving rise to the typical cold symptoms of stuffy or runny nose, throat discomfort, malaise and occasional coughing. Colds can produce fevers of up to (102°F) 39°C in infants and children (such a high fever in an adult would indicate flu; but children do become hotter faster). The incubation period is from one to three days, after which symptoms occur, and most colds run their course in three to ten days.

In conventional medicine, colds are treated with rest and fluids, in addition to antihistamines, decongestants and cough medicines as needed. Aspirin is recommended only when symptoms are severe, because it increases viral shedding and makes the sufferer more contagious. Vaccines are of little use in prevention because so many kinds of viruses are involved. Research suggests that interferon (a protein produced by animal cells when they are invaded by viruses, released into the bloodstream or intercellular fluid to induce healthy cells to manufacture an enzyme that counters the infection) could prevent the spread of colds and may prove useful to persons at high risk for complications. In 1988, a drug called R61837 was found useful in preventing colds in persons exposed to some of the main cold viruses affecting the nose.

Small children are more susceptible than adults to the viruses causing colds and flu because their immune systems are immature. Don't be surprised if your child seems to contract every cold he comes into contact with. Symptoms of a cold include a running nose, headache and sometimes a cough. There may be a mild fever and a feeling of general malaise.

Conventional treatment

Your doctor may suggest you take steps to lower your child's temperature (see page 341) and advocate acetaminophen. Antibiotics will be prescribed only for a secondary infection.

NATURAL TREATMENTS

- If your child gets recurrent colds, it would be a good idea to get some constitutional homeopathic treatment. In the short term, however, the following remedies should help:
  - Aconite the first stages of a cold, particularly if it seems to have come on suddenly, after your child has been outside, for example
  - Belladonna, for colds with a high temperature, and great thirst
  - Nat. Mur, for watery colds, particularly if accompanied by cold sores
  - Kali. Mur. for catarrhal colds
  - Ferr. Phos. for hot colds
  - Arsenicum, for watery colds, particularly if your child is prone to frequent colds
  - Euphrasia, for colds affecting the eyes
  - Pulsatilla if your child is clingy and irritable, and when there is thick yellow discharge
  - Bryonia for an irritable child who is thirsty and wants to be left alone
  - Mercurius for a child with an earache, and swollen lymph nodes in the neck
- Bach Rescue Remedy (see page 260) will soothe any distress—rub the cream into the chest area to calm.
- Olive flower essence will help with fatigue.
- Goldenseal and elecampane are useful for chronic colds to clear mucus from the lungs and nasal passages.
- Elderflowers, drunk as an infusion, will reduce catarrh and help to decongest. Peppermint is another decongestant and will also work to reduce a fever.
- Chamomile will soothe an irritable child and

help him to sleep. Chamomile also has antiseptic action, to help rid the body of infection, and it works to reduce fever and feverish symptoms.

- Herbs to strengthen the immune system, including echinacea, can be taken throughout a cold, and afterward to stimulate healing and prevent subsequent infection.
- Place your child's head over a steaming bowl of water with a few drops of essential oil of cinnamon. Place a towel over her head to make a tent, and let her sit there for four or five minutes to ease congestion. If she is younger, use the bathroom steam method (see page 243).
- Try a few drops of lavender or tea tree oil in a warm bath to encourage healing and help open up the airways.
- Blackcurrant tea is excellent for catarrh and infections.
- Offer plenty of fresh garlic and onions to reduce catarrh and cleanse the blood. Garlic is also antibiotic and boosts the immune system.

Useful therapies

Homeopathy, acupuncture, traditional Chinese medicine, reflexology, nutritional therapies, herbalism.

SELF-HELP

Following a cold, take steps to boost your child's immune system (see page 207).

CONJUNCTIVITIS

Conjunctivitis is an inflammation of the conjunctiva (the mucous membrane that covers the outer layer of the eyeball and lines the eyelids). It's fairly common in young children, who tend to rub their eyes and touch their faces more often than adults. Conjunctivitis is generally caused by either viral or bacterial infection, or by an allergic reaction to substances such as pollen. Infectious conjunctivitis is contagious, so keep your child's hands clean and keep her towel and pillow away from other family members. The major symptom of bacterial conjunctivitis is a yellow discharge that hardens during sleep causing stickiness in and around the eyes. Viral conjunctivitis produces only minimal discharge, and in allergic conditions there may be swollen, puffy eyelids, but no discharge. In all cases, the eyeball may become extremely red—hence the name "pink eye."

Conventional treatment

Suspected infections are treated with eyedrops or ointment containing an antibiotic drug. Viral conjunctivitis tends to get better without treatment. Allergic conjunctivitis may be treated with antihistamine eyedrops, and occasionally eyedrops containing a corticosteroid drug.

NATURAL TREATMENTS

- Homeopathic treatment should be constitutional, particularly if your child is prone to conjunctivitis, but in the meantime, for acute, occasional attacks, try:
  - Euphrasia, for burning, itching eyes—one or two drops of Euphrasia tincture to bathe the eyes
  - Pulsatilla, for mucus collecting in corner of eyes
  - Hepar sulf., to draw out infection
- Boil fennel seeds to make an eyewash for conjunctivitis and sore, inflamed eyes.
- Honey water can be used to cleanse the eye; it acts to destroy any infection, soothes and encourages healing.
- Infusions of the following herbs can be taken internally to ease the condition: echinacea (boosts the immune system and acts as a natural antibiotic), eyebright, goldenseal and sage.
- Infusions of chamomile, elderflower, eyebright and goldenseal can be applied externally—some of these herbs can also be bought as a tincture and used to make a soothing eyewash.

Useful therapies

Homeopathy, herbalism, nutritional therapies, traditional Chinese medicine.

SELF-HELP

- Put a little olive oil on your child's eyelids and eyelashes at night, to make it easier to remove crusting the following morning.
- Clean eyes with a cotton ball dipped in a herbal substance (elderflower or eyebright, for example) and sweep from inside of the eye to outside. Use a clean ball for each eye. Never use hot water on the eyes.
- If the itching is extreme, put cucumber slices on shut eyelids and ask your child to sit as still as possible! If she can't do that, freshly squeezed cucumber juice can be used to soothe *shut* eyes.

CONSTIPATION

Constipation is common in children at various stages as they are more susceptible to dietary changes (such as during weaning). Some doctors define constipation as the failure to have a bowel movement every day, while others suggest that one every four or five days is acceptable, providing it is not hard or painful to pass. Some children do have irregular bowel motions and this is not a cause for alarm. However, it is important to remember that the longer the stool remains in the body, the more chance there is for toxins to be absorbed. This can cause liver problems in the long term, among other things. The best thing to aim for is regularity, which is possible for most children with a healthy diet (see chapter 1). Chronic constipation can be a sign of underlying health problems, including Hirschsprung's disease or hypothyroidism. It can also be the result of undue attention paid to toilet training. If you are concerned, see your doctor.

Conventional treatment

Laxatives may be suggested (lactalose syrup, for example), but the emphasis will be on increasing fiber in the diet.

NATURAL TREATMENTS

- In homeopathy, constipation is regarded as a constitutional problem, but the following remedies can help with occasional symptoms:

- Lycopodium, when there is flatulence but no need to open bowels for long periods of time and hard stools, passed with pain
- Nux Vom., for constipation that alternates with diarrhea
- Opium, when there is no desire to pass stool
- Silica, when there is a burning sensation after a bowel movement
- Causticum, for a stitchlike pain accompanying a bowel movement
- Bryonia, for large, hard, dry stools, with congestion in the abdomen causing distention, and a burning feeling in the rectum
- Alumina, for no desire to open bowels until rectum is full; stool may be covered in mucus
- Laxative herbs, which can be drunk as herbal infusions up to three times daily, include licorice, marshmallow root or senna.
- Massage a drop of marjoram or fennel oil, diluted in grapeseed oil, into the abdomen, to relieve constipation.
- Acidophilus will encourage the health of the intestines, and make bowel movements more normal.
- Chronic constipation may respond to an increased intake of B-complex vitamins, particularly if it follows a course of antibiotics. Vitamin B1 is most effective.

Useful therapies

Nutritional therapies, homeopathy, aromatherapy, reflexology, traditional Chinese medicine.

SELF-HELP

- Some foods, particularly milk and milk products, tend to delay things in the large intestine, causing constipation. Giving up milk should be the first step if your child is constipated. Give it two weeks, and, if symptoms continue, you'll know that dairy produce is not the culprit.
- Increase fiber (see page 18) and encourage your child to drink plenty of water throughout the day.
- Prunes and dried apricots (soaked to plump them up) can be added to foods to encourage bowel movements.

Coughs

There are many types of coughs, some of which accompany a cold. Others are caused by chemicals, other infections, like ear and tonsil infections, excess catarrh, inflammation of the airways and many other things. If the condition is caused by a virus, there is little that can be done, other than to keep your child warm and dry, and drinking plenty of fluids, until he throws off the illness.

Coughs are necessary to expel foreign bodies and mucus from the trachea and airways of the lungs. Coughing is a symptom rather than an illness, and can indicate sinusitis, croup, bronchitis, pneumonia, flu and other viruses, the early stages of measles, asthma, whooping cough, or an excess of catarrh from the nose or sinuses, usually due to irritation or infection.

A dry cough may be caused by mucus from infections or colds, chemicals in the atmosphere, a foreign object or nervousness that constricts the throat. A loose, wetter cough is caused by inflammation of the bronchial tubes produced by an infection or allergy. A constant nighttime cough, or one that recurs with each cold, and is hard to get rid of, may indicate asthma.

Conventional treatment

If there is reason to suggest a bacterial infection, antibiotics may be prescribed. Some doctors may advocate a cough suppressant, but this is not advised unless the cough is nonproductive and exhausting. Acetaminophen may bring down any fever, and reduce the discomfort.

Natural treatments

- Cayenne pepper can be added to your child's food (a few grains) to stimulate the body's immune defenses and clear the wet secretions from the lungs.
- If the cough is accompanied by a fever, try infusions of chamomile, catmint, hyssop and yarrow.
- Comfrey and coltsfoot are useful expectorants to help expel the mucus from the lungs and airways; use about ten drops of each tincture, mix with some warmed honey and serve by the teaspoonful as necessary.

- Elecampane and thyme can be infused and used to treat a wet cough.
- When the mucus is tough to shift, try strong infusions of ginger and fennel or thyme.
- Elecampane root tea, sweetened with honey and ginger, will help to reduce inflammation and reduce mucus.
- The following homeopathic remedies may be appropriate, although chronic coughs should always be treated constitutionally:
  - Belladonna, for when the cough is accompanied by a fever, and your child has bright red cheeks and neck
  - Pulsatilla, for a thick yellow discharge and when your child is clingy and tearful
  - Ant Tart., for a cough that causes the chest to rattle, and makes breathing painful
  - Bryonia, for a painful, dry cough, made worse with movement
  - Spongia, for croup (see below), and for a loud, crowing cough
  - Drosera, for a tickling cough, worse for lying down
  - Aconite, if the symptoms come on suddenly
  - Chamomilla, to soothe a child who is inconsolable, but better for being held
- Use Bach Rescue Remedy (see page 260) when your child experiences distress, or panics because breathing is difficult. It will also help your child to sleep. A few drops can be taken internally, or applied to pulse points, and Rescue Remedy cream (see page 260) can be rubbed into the chest.
- Olive flower essence is good for a child who is overwhelmed by fatigue.
- Vervain will help for the stress of a cough—particularly a chronic cough.
- Use lavender, eucalyptus or thyme in a vaporizer. A few drops of essential oil of thyme, pine, cinnamon, clove or eucalyptus can also be used in combination or singly in a foot bath to ease congestion.
- Add a few drops of eucalyptus and sandalwood to a carrier oil, or some petrolen jelly, and rub into the chest and upper back.

- If your child is over the age of 12 months, offer plenty of organic, cold-pressed and preferably pasteurized honey, which has antibacterial action and will also soothe a sore throat.
- Blackcurrant tea will ease the pain of a sore throat, and help to reduce catarrh.

Useful therapies

Buteyko method, aromatherapy, herbalism, traditional Chinese medicine, acupuncture, homeopathy, reflexology, nutritional therapies (for chronic coughs).

SELF-HELP

Plenty of fluids and bedrest will make it easier for your child to recover from a cough. Offer only fluids for the first couple of days, and then just light meals, avoiding dairy produce altogether until the catarrh has been coughed up.

> **CAUTION**
> If a cough is accompanied by a high fever, and your child has difficulty breathing, see your doctor immediately.

CRADLE CAP

Cradle cap is characterized by a thick, encrusted layer of skin on your baby's scalp. There will be yellow scales, which form in patches, especially on the top of the head. In severe cases, cradle cap can last for up to three years. Like dandruff, cradle cap is a condition in which the seborrhoeic glands are overactive, and it is often associated with seborrhoeic dermatitis, a skin condition in which there are red, scaly areas on the forehead and eyebrows, among other places.

Conventional treatment

If the skin becomes inflamed or seems infected, a mild ointment containing an antibiotic drug and corticosteroids will be prescribed until the condition improves. Occasionally a shampoo, such as cetrimide, may be suggested.

NATURAL TREATMENTS

- Rinse the scalp after washing with an infusion of meadowsweet, which acts as an anti inflammatory and will reduce any itching.
- Massage the scalp with calendula ointment.
- The homeopathic remedy Lycopodium is useful if the skin is dry but uninfected. See a homeopath for constitutional treatment.
- Rock Rose is useful if the itching causes distress. Rescue Remedy cream (see page 260) may be massaged into the scalp to reduce symptoms.
- Add two drops of Rescue Remedy to the rinse water, and use after a shampoo.
- Massage a drop of lavender or lemon oil, mixed in a light carrier oil, into the scalp before bedtime. Rinse gently each morning.
- Olive oil can be massaged into the scalp each evening, and then gently shampooed away in the morning.

Useful therapies

Homeopathy, herbalism, aromatherapy, traditional Chinese medicine.

SELF-HELP

Overwashing will make the condition much worse. Gently brush away loosened crusts with a soft brush.

> **CAUTION**
> Try not to loosen crusts that have not pulled away on their own—bleeding and infection may result.

CROUP

The characteristic cough of croup is a definite loud bark or whistle, caused by inflammation of the vocal cords. Croup occurs when the larynx (voice-box) becomes inflamed and swollen. It can be the result of a bacterial or viral infection, or even simply a cold. Because the larynx swells and blocks the passage of air, breathing can be very difficult, which can panic a child.

Conventional treatment

Your doctor will recommend steam inhalations (filling the bathroom with steam is useful) and, if the cause is bacterial, a course of antibiotics. Acetaminophen, which has anti inflammatory action, may also be recommended.

NATURAL TREATMENTS

- Lobelia and black cohosh will reduce spasm, soften the phlegm and clear the lungs.
- Wild cherry syrup can reduce spasm and help deal with phlegm.
- Try infusing lavender flowers or chamomile in a bowl of hot water, placing your child's head over it to calm and help breathing.
- Infuse some chamomile, catmint or wild cherry, and give your child small sips before bedtime and during an attack.
- A footbath with some thyme or eucalyptus oil should help.
- Homeopathic treatments can be amazingly effective. Try:
  - Spongia, taken every 20 minutes during an attack. Aconite can be taken alongside
  - Phosphorus, for croup when there is a thirst for cold drinks (which may be vomited up)
  - Drosera, for a deep, hoarse-sounding cough, with gasping and retching
- Bach Rescue Remedy (see page 260) will help to calm the child and make breathing easier. Alternatively, rub a little Rescue Remedy cream into the chest and upper back.
- Rock Rose will help if your child is frightened, and Olive can be taken after an attack if your child is exhausted.
- Essential oils of eucalyptus, lavender, pine, chamomile, cinnamon and thyme can be added together, or separately, to a vaporizer or a footbath.
- A few drops of eucalyptus or lavender can be placed on a hanky by the child's crib or bed to ease breathing and encourage the child to relax.
- Rub a few drops of lavender oil mixed with olive oil into your child's chest and upper back.
- If your child is over 12 months old, offer a hand- hot honey and lemon drink to ease the symptoms. Honey has strong antibacterial properties and will be useful if the cause of the croup is bacterial infection.

Useful therapies

Traditional Chinese medicine, homeopathy, aromatherapy, acupuncture, herbalism.

SELF-HELP

- Put your child in a bathroom with the door shut and the hot taps running, or fill a bowl with boiling water and gently place your child's head over it, covered by a towel. Steam will open the airways and reduce symptoms.
- Raise the upper end of the crib or bed so that breathing is easier.

> **CAUTION**
> If your child does not respond to treatment, call your doctor immediately. If he or she becomes blue around the mouth, this condition should be treated as a medical emergency.

CRYING

Babies cry for different reasons, and although we are told that the average baby cries for about four hours a day, there are few that conform. If your baby cries inconsolably for hours, she may have colic (see page 316), be hungry or uncomfortable, or she may require constant physical comfort. She may have diaper rash (see page 325), a problem with formula milk, or, if you are breastfeeding her, with something that you have eaten.

Many babies cry because they are tired. Lack of sleep causes irritability just as it does in older children and adults, and makes it even more difficult to fall asleep. Babies are also very sensitive to their environment, and if you are feeling angry or tense for any reason, she may sense it and cry even harder. As your baby becomes more settled—usually around the six-week to three-month mark—her crying will change and you will be able to distinguish between the cries that indicate her different needs.

SELF-HELP

- Many babies respond to being held and rocked, although you may find, frustratingly, that something that worked one day may not work the next. If your baby does require constant comfort, you may want to carry her next to your body in a sling, as you get on with things around the house. Many babies like to have their heads near your chest, in order to hear your heartbeat.
- Rhythmical sounds soothe many babies, and you can buy a recording of a mother's heartbeat as your baby would have heard it in the womb, which can be very effective. Low music may also help, and many babies will settle instantly at the sound of the vacuum cleaner.
- If your baby is eased off to sleep by rocking, bring stroller inside, and settle yourself in a position where you can comfortably rock the cradle with a free hand or foot.
- Many babies like to feel securely wrapped, and you can make her feel more comfortable by swaddling her—that is, wrapping her quite tightly in a blanket—before settling her down. Other babies may feel too constrained by swaddling.
- Some need to suck to get to sleep, or to settle, which is why they feed almost constantly when they are upset. Sucking will not stop a hungry baby from crying, unless she gets milk from it, but it will certainly soothe a crying baby who is not hungry. Your baby might benefit from a pacifier, which can always be used as a last resort, or you can help her to find her thumb or fingers, which she might want to suck to quiet herself.
- Make sure she is not hungry—calm her down before a feed by giving her a light massage with a soothing oil, perhaps blended from a drop of lavender or Roman chamomile oil in some baby oil, and talk to her gently as you feed her.
- If she is frightened of the bath, avoid giving her a whole-body bath, and concentrate on "topping and tailing"(face, neck and behind ears, diaper region and feet), which will be adequate until she is old enough to cope better.
- If you are tense, and find it difficult to cope with her crying, take a few drops of Bach Rescue Remedy (see page 260) on your tongue, which normally provides nearly instant relief. Take time for yourself, perhaps giving her to your partner while you have a soothing bath with lavender oil, or drink a cup of chamomile tea. If you are feeling exhausted, see page 136. Most importantly, try not to be anxious. Babies have amazing antennae and will respond to your distress in kind.
- Flower essences are also gentle enough for babies, and if your baby is distressed and fearful, she may respond to mimulus, or try chicory if she needs constant attention and reassurance.
- You may find that if you set up a routine that makes her feel secure (page 119), she will calm down and feel more comfortable in the day.
- If crying begins after feeding, after switching from breastmilk to formula or a change in formula, talk to your doctor or midwife. There may be problems with the formula she is taking.
- Try the homeopathic remedy Chamomilla if she seems inconsolable and wants to be held constantly. For older children who are regularly tearful, try Pulsatilla.

DEPRESSION

Depression is a prolonged feeling of unhappiness and despondency, often magnified by a major life event such as bereavement or parental divorce. Many children and adolescents suffer from depression, which can also be the result of fluctuating hormones or undue stress. It can also follow a viral illness, such as glandular fever (see page 352).

If your child is depressed, try to remember that it is an illness and they won't just "snap out of it." It's important to be patient and to spend as much time as you can boosting self-esteem (see page 174) and helping your child to feel good about himself, even in the depths of despair.

Some common signs of depression include poor

concentration, irritability, loss of self-esteem, insomnia and early morning waking, loss of appetite, and feelings of emptiness or despair.

Conventional treatment

Antidepressants are often prescribed, as well as counseling or one of many types of psychotherapy.

NATURAL TREATMENTS

- Homeopathic treatment should be constitutional, and based on a wide variety of factors
  - Aurum, for feelings of worthlessness or self-disgust. Your child may be intensely driven and competitive, but suddenly give up
  - Pulsatilla, for bursting into tears at the smallest slight
  - Arsenicum, if your child feels chilly, tired, restless and obsessively tidy
  - Ignatia, if depression has a specific external cause, such as bereavement, breaking up with a friend or exams
- Flower essences (see page 254) can be amazingly effective. Try the following:
  - Agrimony is for deeply held emotional tensions that are hidden from others
  - Gorse helps with feelings of great hopelessness
  - Gentian will help with a mild depression and despondency
  - Mustard is for blacker and deeper feelings when the joy is missing
  - Sweet chestnut should be taken if there is anguish and your child feels stretched beyond endurance
- There are a number of antidepressant oils that can be used in the bath, in a vaporizer, on a light bulb and in massage. Try geranium, melissa, lavender, rose, ylang ylang and chamomile.
- The best antidepressant and nervine (which have specific action for nerves) herbs include balm, borage, lime flower, oats, rosemary and vervain. These can be taken as herbal teas, added to the bath, or taken as pills or in tincture form. St. John's wort can be enormously useful, but see a

registered herbalist for appropriate applications. Ginkgo biloba has also been used in the treatment of depression. Offer it on a daily basis for as long as necessary.

DIABETES

Type 1 diabetes is the most common form of the disease in children. It is caused by the inability of the pancreas to produce insulin. The cause of diabetes is not yet known, but it is believed that both environmental and hereditary factors, as well as infections, play a part. It affects boys and girls equally. Type 1 diabetes is classified as an autoimmune disease. This process will have been developing for a long period before the symptoms of diabetes present themselves.

The onset of children's diabetes usually occurs in late childhood but can present itself from early infancy through to late adulthood. The symptoms develop in a matter of days or weeks, and include tiredness, excessive thirst, frequent urination, bedwetting, loss of appetite and weight loss, infections on the skin or around the mouth, or in extreme cases, nausea, vomiting and abdominal pain.

Conventional treatment

Children with diabetes are always treated through insulin and diet management. However, up to a year after the diagnosis is made, the child may need only a small dose of insulin. Insulin is injected into the skin either in the abdomen or the thighs, but can be injected anywhere there is sufficient skin.

NATURAL TREATMENTS

- Constitutional homeopathic treatment will be balancing and can be taken alongside conventional medication. In some cases the condition has been completely cured through homeopathy, but it must be undertaken by a registered practitioner.
- Brewer's yeast contains chromium, which helps to normalize blood sugar levels and metabolism. Add a tablespoon to your child's food every day.
- Onions and garlic lower blood sugar levels—

ensure that your child eats plenty in her diet, or offer a garlic supplement daily.

- An Ayurvedic practitioner would recommend oral preparations from herbs that act upon the levels of glucose in the blood. There have been good results from treatment.
- Chromium picolinate has been enormously successful in the treatment of diabetes (several clinical trials have shown very promising results). It does, however, have a dramatic effect on blood sugar levels and should never be offered unless under the supervision of a registered nutritional therapist.
- Research indicates that supplementation with the hormone dehydroepiandrosterone (DHEA) may help to prevent diabetes.[2] See a registered nutritional therapist for details of DHEA therapy.

Useful therapies

Acupuncture, nutritional therapy, traditional Chinese medicine, herbalism, homeopathy, Ayurveda.

SELF-HELP

- Measure blood glucose levels and teach the child how to do this as soon as she is old enough.
- Teach your child how to give herself insulin injections as soon as she is old enough (about nine).
- Make sure sugar is always nearby for the treatment of low blood sugar.
- Make sure your child's teacher can recognize signs of hypo and hyperglycemia, and knows what to do.
- It's important to give your child a healthy and balanced diet that is high in fiber and carbohydrates. Before any type of exercise, it is important that she has some extra bread or juice and other carbohydrates. Three main meals and two to three snacks, where the whole family eats the same, are recommended.

DIAPER RASH

Diaper rash is caused by contact with urine or feces, causing the skin to produce less protective oil and therefore a less effective barrier to further irritation.

Friction may also exacerbate the condition. Diaper rash may extend up over the abdomen, and down across the legs. White patches may indicate thrush (see page 389).

Conventional treatment

Your doctor will recommend changing your baby more frequently, and allowing periods of time without a diaper. In severe cases, an ointment containing a mild corticosteroid drug may be prescribed to suppress the inflammation. This may be prescribed in combination with an antifungal drug, to kill any candida present.

NATURAL TREATMENTS

- Rub a little calendula (marigold) ointment onto the cleaned diaper area to soothe and reduce inflammation.
- Bach Rescue Remedy (see page 260) cream may be gently massaged into the affected area to reduce inflammation and ease any pain or itching. A few drops of Rescue Remedy on pulse points will calm a baby who is distressed.
- Egg white can be painted on the sore bottom and allowed to dry before putting on a diaper. This will encourage the skin to heal and prevent further irritation.
- Powdered goldenseal can be applied to a clean diaper area before putting on the diaper.
- Add a few drops of tea tree to the rinse cycle of your machine when using cloth diapers to disinfect. Cloth diapers are much kinder to your baby's skin.
- A drop of lavender or rose oil in a peach kernel carrier oil can be gently rubbed into the diaper area. Use this to protect against diaper rash as well.
- A drop of oregano or thyme oil in a light carrier oil can be used to discourage thrush.
- Homeopathic remedies can help, but see a homeopath if your child suffers from regular rashes in the diaper area, or if you suspect thrush.
  - Use Rhus Tox., for an itchy, blistered rash
  - Sulfur may be appropriate if the skin is dry and scaled
  - Merc. Sol. can help to reduce the acidity of the urine

- Try Cantharis, when the urine is scalding and the skin is raw.
- Live yogurt can be spread on the diaper area to soothe, and to prevent thrush from occurring in the skin folds.

Useful therapies

Homeopathy, herbalism, traditional Chinese medicine, aromatherapy, nutritional therapies.

SELF-HELP

- Avoid using soap or other detergents on the diaper area. Rinse carefully with clean water at each diaper change. Frequent diaper changes are suggested, and using a disposable diaper liner may help to reduce irritation. Allow your baby to go for as long as possible with a bare bottom, to allow it to dry and heal.
- Give your baby lots of soothing drinks, such as diluted chamomile tea, to reduce the acidity of the urine. There are many herbal formulas available for newborn babies—make sure they haven't included any sugar in the preparation.

> **CAUTION**
> Any diaper rash that does not heal within a week or so should be seen by a doctor.

DIARRHEA

Diarrhea is common in children, especially in warm weather. It may be accompanied by vomiting and abdominal pain, and is usually due to an infection or toxin in the bowel, when it is known as gastroenteritis. Avoiding solid foods and taking plenty of fluids for 24 to 48 hours will usually settle it, but close attention should be paid to hand-washing, food hygiene and refrigeration, so the problem does not spread to other members of the household.

Toddler diarrhea is a profuse diarrhea in an otherwise well toddler who continues to have a good appetite and gain weight. It often contains undigested food particles. No treatment is needed and the problem resolves when the child is toilet-trained.

Conventional treatment

In cases of prolonged diarrhea or diarrhea following foreign travel, medical advice should be sought so that a sample can be sent for analysis. Very occasionally the analysis will indicate that an antibiotic is needed.

If your child is becoming dehydrated because of the diarrhea, you may be advised to give him an electrolyte mixture to replace body salts and water being lost.

> **CAUTION**
> Call your doctor immediately if your baby or child shows symptoms of dehydration, including a sunken fontanel, unresponsiveness, drowsiness, prolonged crying, glazed eyes or a very dry mouth.

NATURAL TREATMENTS

- It is a good idea to avoid milk initially, and if you are bottle-feeding it may be recommended that you use a formula that is low in lactose.
- Children (not babies) may take a little herbal tea, such as peppermint or blackberry, which acts as an astringents to the gut and may help to ease the condition.
- Offer your child plenty of fresh, bottled water to drink, to help cleanse the system, and avoid fruit juices if possible.
- If the diarrhea is linked to gastroenteritis, the homeopathic remedy Arsenicum may be useful. Or you might try Colocynth, for diarrhea accompanied by gripping spasmodic pains, with copious, thin, yellowish stools. Chronic diarrhea should be treated constitutionally, but acute attacks may be treated with one of the following remedies:
  - Aconite for diarrhea that comes on suddenly, with a distended abdomen
  - Pulsatilla for diarrhea that is worse at night, and made worse by rich foods

- Argent. Nit. for diarrhea caused by anxiety, characterized by belching and cravings for sweet and salty food
- Carrot juice or soup is very helpful, especially for infants.
- Give plenty of fresh acidophilus for at least a month after an attack, to ensure the health of the bowels.

Useful therapies

Homeopathy, herbalism, Ayurveda, nutritional therapies, traditional Chinese medicine.

SELF-HELP

Make sure your child drinks plenty of fresh water, boiled if necessary, and does not eat or drink anything that might irritate the digestive tract (fruit juices and processed foods should be off the menu; although mashed overripe bananas should help).

DYSLEXIA

"Dyslexia" comes from the Greek and means "difficulty with words." Dyslexia affects reading, spelling, writing, memory and concentration, and sometimes math, music, foreign languages and self-organization. Some people call dyslexia "a specific learning difficulty." Dyslexia tends to run in families, and can continue throughout life. If your child is dyslexic, you are not alone. At least 10 percent of the population is dyslexic, 4 percent being severely dyslexic. Dyslexics may have many creative, artistic, practical skills, and can be extremely bright, which makes the condition all the more frustrating for your child.

According to the British Dyslexia Association, there are many ways to diagnose dyslexia at different ages.

What's the cause?

There are various theories about dyslexia, including the idea that there is some type of neurological damage. Dr. John Stein, from Oxford University, has found damage in the optic nerves of dyslexic children, and believes other areas of the brain's nervous system may also be affected. His controversial idea also appears to account for other trouble experienced by some dyslexic children, such as subtle hearing problems. According to New Scientist magazine, Dr. Stein also believes that the damage occurs in the brain of the developing fetus and may be caused by the mother's immune system. Dr. Stein believes that dyslexics suffer from a defect in a set of very large nerve cells known as magno-cells. These cells rapidly transmit electrical impulses from the retina in the eye to the brain, so that it can recognize rapid changes or movement. Other researchers have shown that the magno-cells in dyslexics operate more slowly than usual, and postmortem examinations have revealed abnormalities in the shape and position of the cells.

Other scientists claim to have found a gene for dyslexia, although having the gene does not guarantee that your child will suffer. Environmental factors are believed to play a part as well. It may, however, help diagnose dyslexia earlier than it is possible to now. According to recent U.S. research, dyslexia is primarily due to linguistic deficits—a difficulty processing language.

Conventional treatment

Cooperation with a specialist teacher or educational psychologist can be most helpful. Some educational authorities have been willing to allow dyslexic children extra time during exam, and others offer computers for learning, which seems to help in many cases.

NATURAL TREATMENTS

There is still little understanding of how and why dyslexia occurs, but various treatments do seem to have an effect, even if we are not sure why.

- Homeopathic treatment of dyslexia has been successful in many cases, but it will need to be tailored to your child's specific needs. While you are waiting for treatment, try Lycopodium, taken three times daily for up to three weeks.
- Nutritional medicine has a lot to offer, and some cases of dyslexia have been eased substantially by treatment. One 1998 study showed that dyslexic

children have lower amounts of zinc than children without the condition, indicating that zinc supplementation may help to reverse some symptoms.

- In some cases cranial osteopathy may help, particularly if your child was born during a long labor or suffered distress throughout. Some scientists and doctors believe that dyslexia may have something to do with an inner ear imbalance. Chiropractic or osteopathic treatment to make adjustments to the small bones of the inner ear appears to have some effect. It's interesting to note that most dyslexic children suffer from motion sickness, which is also linked to inner ear imbalance.
- The herb ginkgo biloba has been used in the treatment of dyslexia. It improves brain functioning by increasing cerebral and peripheral blood flow, circulation and oxygenation.
- Make sure your child has a good, nutritious diet, which can encourage brain health.

Preschool signs

- Family history of dyslexia problems
- Later than expected learning to speak clearly
- Jumbles phrases, e.g., "cobbler's club" for "toddler's club," "teddy-dare" for "teddy-bear"
- Quick "thinker" and "do-er"
- Use of substitute words or "near misses"
- Mislabeling, e.g., lampshade for lamp post
- A lisp—"duckth" for "ducks"
- Inability to remember the label for known objects, e.g., colors
- Confused directional words, e.g., "up/down" or "in/out"
- Excessive tripping, bumping and falling over nothing
- Enhanced creativity—often good at drawing—good sense of color
- Obvious "good" and "bad" days for no apparent reason
- Aptitude for constructional or technical toys, e.g., bricks, puzzles, Lego blocks, control box for TV and video, computer keyboards

continues

- Flower essences can do a lot to redress poor self-image, which may be making the problem worse (see page 254).

Useful therapies

Many therapies have claimed to help dyslexics, including cranial osteopathy, homeopathy, acupuncture, traditional Chinese medicine, reflexology and nutritional therapies, among others. The creative therapies, such as art and music have, also been successful. If you do decide to go natural on this one, talk at length to your practitioner and ask how it is treated and what can be realistically expected.

SELF-HELP

- One of the most important things to remember is that a dyslexic child is not stupid. Because your child might struggle with tasks that come easily to others, he may be negatively labeled and even teased. In some cases a diagnosis is not made until children are well into their school careers, which means that they probably believe they are academically substandard. For this reason, it is crucial that you build your child's self-esteem (see page 174), and offer plenty of praise for even small tasks completed—or attempted.
- Make home a safe place, with as little expectation or potential for failure as possible. His entire school career can be hard work, and he'll need to know that he can relax and be accepted at home. Never try to load up on extra work at home, or think that you can cure the condition by sheer perseverance. This is a big mistake. You'll need to be patient and loving, and to celebrate every small victory along the way. Keep your anxieties about his long-term education to yourself. Your child will have the best chance of doing well if he is calm, loved and happy.
- Allow breaks from homework, and give your child a night off every now and then. It can be exhausting struggling through school days, and he will be genuinely tired and in need of a break. Extra handwriting or reading practice at the end of the day will not make things easier, and it may put him off altogether.

- Enjoys being read to but shows no interest in letters or words
- Difficulty learning nursery rhymes
- Finds difficulty with rhyming words, e.g., "cat mat fat"
- Finds difficulty with odd-one-out, e.g., "cat mat pig fat"
- Did not crawl—was a "bottom shuffler"
- Difficulty with "sequence," e.g., colored bead sequence
- Appears "bright"—seems an enigma

Children of 9 or under

- Particular difficulty learning to read and write
- Persistent and continued reversing of numbers and letters (e.g., "15" for "51"; "b" for "d")
- Difficulty telling left from right
- Difficulty learning the alphabet and multiplication tables, and remembering sequences such as the days of the week and months of the year
- Continued difficulty with shoelaces, and ball-catching, skipping, etc. as above
- Inattention and poor concentration
- Frustration, possibly leading to behavioral problems

Children of 9–12

- Continued mistakes in reading, or a lack of reading comprehension
- Strange spelling, perhaps with letters missed out or in the wrong order
- Taking an above average time over written work
- Disorganization at home and at school
- Difficulty copying accurately from blackboard or textbook
- Difficulty taking down oral instructions
- Growing lack of self-confidence and increasing frustration

Children of 12 and over

- Tendency to read inaccurately, or without comprehension
- Inconsistent spelling
- Difficulty with planning and written essays
- Tendency to confuse verbal instructions and telephone numbers
- Severe difficulty with learning a foreign language
- Low self-esteem
- Difficulty with perception of language, e.g., following instructions, listening comprehension

- Encourage hobbies such as collecting stamps or fossils or anything else. Teach him in a casual way, so that he will have a wealth of fascinating facts at his fingertips. Remember that he is not in any way mentally deficient, and will probably relish other ways of learning—through travel, hobbies or even television and theater. Make information fun! Read aloud interesting articles from the newspaper. Create your own story tapes, reading books or plays out loud. Make things visual—draw out a story you are reading, or re-enact a part of history that he is studying. Buy tapes with mathematical concepts set to music. He can remember a song, even if the numbers are difficult on a page.
- One study showed that some dyslexic children find it easier to read when wearing tinted glasses or when tinted plastic is placed across the page (see Resources section).[4] It seems that some dyslexic children are light-sensitive, and the contrast of black words on a white page can be difficult to manage. One child who took part in the study claimed that when the pages were tinted, "the words stopped jumping around." Obviously, because no one can know what anyone else sees, it can be difficult to understand the problems that plague dyslexics, and this provided researchers with a glimpse of what it can be like.
- Make things easy for your child. If he finds it difficult to remember left or right, put a blue band on the right hand and a red one on the left. Offer easy ways to remember things: little rhymes for remembering sequences of things, for example.

Buy books and stories on tape or take your child to the movies or theater to see plays studied at school.

- Read to your child as often as possible. Even teenagers faced with exams or plenty of homework will welcome the break from a printed page. Remember, though, that it can be exhausting trying to remember facts without a visual memory, so study sessions together should be short, with lots of breaks. Never stop reading to a dyslexic child. You can encourage a love of books and learning that might otherwise be threatened.

- It's important to remember that dyslexia is not a disease to be cured, and children do not grow out of it. Early recognition and appropriate intervention can, however, make a big difference to the extent to which it affects your child. Dyslexic children learn to accommodate to a greater or lesser degree, depending on their own personality and the type of support they have received from both home and school. Many individuals will experience difficulties throughout their lives, and the majority learn to develop strategies to enable them to cope most of the time, although in stress situations all the original problems can recur. It's important, therefore, to teach your child ways to relax and to avoid stress (see page 386), which can make it much worse.

DYSPRAXIA

Dyspraxia is completely different from dyslexia, but your child will benefit from much the same approach at home. Dyspraxic children will not appear obviously different from other children, and this condition can be notoriously difficult to diagnose. Dyspraxia is an immaturity of the brain resulting in messages not being properly or fully transmitted. In the U.S., it is known as developmental coordination disorder, and has, in the past, been called "clumsy child syndrome." Estimates put the number of children to be at least 10 percent of the population (it could be more), and 70 percent of those affected are male. According to the Dyspraxia

Foundation, all dyspraxic children will be affected by some of these problems:

- Clumsiness.
- Poor posture, poor body awareness, awkward movement.
- Confusion over handedness.
- Sensitive to touch and find some clothes uncomfortable.
- Poor short-term memory, can forget tasks learned that day.
- Writing/reading difficulties, holding of pens can be awkward.
- Poor sense of direction.
- Physical activities are problematic, cannot catch, run, skip, ride a bike or use equipment easily.
- Phobias, obsessive or immature behavior.
- Organizational skills are poorly developed.
- Activities requiring a sequence are very difficult, e.g., math or any subject requiring a series of tasks.
- Problems with awareness of time.
- Energy drain, dyspraxic children appear to tire easily and need longer periods of rest and sleep.
- Lack of awareness of potential danger, especially important in practical and science subjects.

Children with dyspraxia have difficulty learning new and unfamiliar tasks. Since many tasks can be learned, albeit with great effort, the phrase "He could do it if he tried" is often applied to these children. These children are described as clumsy or awkward in their movements and usually find that they have to be constantly planning their movements. Dyspraxia can also be described as difficulty in planning and carrying out skilled, nonhabitual motor acts in the correct sequence. Motor skill deficits may be seen in the gross or fine motor areas, and sloppy handwriting is common. Some investigators have found articulation deficits in these children. This type of dyspraxia is known as developmental articulator dyspraxia. This is characterized by marked difficulties in producing speech sounds and in sequencing them together in words.

Madeleine Portwood, author of *Developmental Dyspraxia: A Manual for Parents and Professionals* (David Fulton 1999), suggests that the condition is caused by the failure of the neurones in the brain to develop correctly. This failure of the neurones to form adequate connections means that the brain takes longer to process information, and there is a greater likelihood of the brain losing the suggestion and the child therefore failing to respond to requests given to him.

She says that as the brain develops, children become more capable. Some of the milestones are well known, such as crawling, walking, first words, etc., but there are many more. Many dyspraxic youngsters fail to achieve these expected levels of development.

Useful therapies

Osteopathy, cranial osteopathy, acupuncture, homeopathy, herbalism. Many of these therapies are unproved, but there have been some spectacular results.

SELF-HELP

- Madeleine Portwood suggests taking children through developmental milestones that they have missed in a series of exercises (starting when your child is about three), which take about 20 minutes a day. She claims that not only the motor skills but also the perceptual and handwriting skills develop. "The child may never be an Olympic athlete," she says, "but at least he can join in with the sports and games of his peers and reach an average standard."
- Physiotherapy can improve the coordination of children with dyspraxia by up to 97 percent, according to new research. In London, England, a Chartered Society of Physiotherapy study of 60 children with dyspraxia showed that, after five months of physiotherapy, their coordination and muscle strength improved by between 47 and 97 percent. Children had weekly physiotherapy sessions over eight weeks, involving exercises to strengthen their muscles and games to increase their coordination skills. The children were also given intensive daily programs to follow at home. In addition to improvements in coordination, the children also appeared to be more self-confident and better able to tackle school work.

- Michèle Lee, a U.K.-based physiotherapist has a great deal of success treating children with the condition. She offers the following advice to parents: ensure there is positive feedback/encouragement; set up strategies for revising and carrying out instructions and tasks; encourage extra sports to maintain muscle strength; use games to help overcome difficulties, improving hand-eye coordination, short-term memory and planning; be consistent about where things are kept, and keep to routines; and help with dressing, layer by layer. Advice and support by Lee and other experts is available on the Dyspraxia Foundation website, www.dyspraxiafoundation.org.uk.
- If handwriting is a real problem, consider purchasing a laptop computer for your child. Many dyspraxic children find it much easier to work a keyboard than they do a pencil! They are much more likely to be able to keep up with notes in class and produce readable work, and this helps to encourage the creative process.
- Take steps to build your child's self-esteem. Boys in particular find it difficult if they do not succeed at sports or games and they may feel "useless" and may become the subject of taunts from class or team-mates. Do your best to make sure your child feels good about himself, and understands that he has a condition that makes some things more difficult. Work with your child to increase coordination and skill as much as possible; he'll feel encouraged by your support and less likely to give up.
- Consider flower essence therapy for any negative emotional states that develop (see page 254).
- Make sure your child gets plenty of sleep (see page 116), and get him into bed before he becomes overtired and finds it difficult to settle. Dyspraxic children appear to need more sleep than many of their peers.
- Join a support group. You'll keep up to date on the newest treatments and theories, and you'll have the opportunity to share your experiences.
- Some children with dyspraxia also suffer from dyslexia. Have your child assessed if you are concerned.

EARACHES AND EAR INFECTIONS

Earache may be caused by inflammation of the lymph nodes in the neck, or by another illness such as mumps. There may be an ear infection in the inner, middle or outer parts of the ear. Occasionally a boil can crop up in the outer ear, which can be very painful. The most common causes of earache in children are middle ear infections (see below). These are usually caused by the transmission of infection from the nose or throat by the Eustachian tube. Because this tube is short and small in babies and young children, it is easily blocked, and infection does not have far to travel to the middle ear itself. Ear infections can cause a great deal of pain, and the pressure may burst the eardrum, causing a discharge. There may be fever and a sore throat. Children may complain of or appear to have earache when they are teething, or if they suffer from sinusitis.

Conventional treatment

Treatment with antibiotics and acetaminophen is usually effective, but some deafness may persist for a week or two until all the pus has drained away via the narrow tube to the throat.

NATURAL TREATMENTS

First and foremost, don't panic if your child's eardrum splits and discharges. Repeated perforation may be alarming and your child may run the very slight risk of developing further infection or scarring that may cause some hearing difficulties, but most children heal quickly and efficiently, and the release of built-up pus can be an enormous relief. Many natural practitioners see this discharging as an enormously healthy sign. Remember that inserting ear tubes (see page 353) involves perforating the eardrum, and in the vast majority of cases these perforations heal without trouble. Secondly, and most importantly, don't be tempted to go for antibiotics unless you are strongly advised to do so.

- One of the best treatments appears to be cranial osteopathy, which uses tiny, gentle manipulations to adjust the bones of the skull. Studies show that it can cure chronic ear infections, and glue ear, successfully with only a few treatments.
- If your child suffers from chronic ear infections, take a look at her diet. During cold and flu season

---

The facts about middle ear infection

- Over the past 15 years there has been a notable increase in the number of children diagnosed with otitis media (middle ear infection). Otitis media is the most common reason for visits to the doctor by children under age 15. Children under two have the highest rate of visits to doctors for otitis media and the greatest increase in visits. Otitis media is increasingly prevalent in Western society. So common is it that an increasing number of people accept it as a normal part of growing up. It is clear that current conventional treatment is not addressing the problem.

- The standard medical treatment of otitis media involves a two-tiered approach of drugs and surgery (grommets for chronic conditions). Antibiotic treatment is the standard conventional treatment for acute otitis media and otitis media with effusion (glue ear). Other common drugs used are antihistamines and decongestants.

- Dr. Cantekin, a researcher at the University of Pittsburgh, maintains that watchful waiting in acute otitis media is the best approach, with more than 90 percent of infections resolving within a few days. Cantekin also contends that the antibiotic amoxicillin for otitis media with effusion is no more effective than placebo and increases the risk of recurrences up to sixfold.

- The medical literature also supports watchful waiting. A 1981 Dutch study found no difference in outcome between antibiotics, myringotomy (inserting grommets), antibiotics combined with myringotomy and placebo. That study had a major effect in the Netherlands where a 1990 survey found only 31 percent of general practitioners treated acute otitis media with antibiotics. Nearly 98 percent of U.S. doctors in the survey prescribed antibiotics.

it is suggested that you take your child off milk as much as possible (see page 29), which can cause mucus to build up. Make sure your child's diet is rich in foods containing vitamin C and zinc, to boost the immune system and help treat infection.

- Offer echinacea, goldenseal and astragalus two to three times a week during cold and flu season. These herbs offer a more aggressive way of preventing illness than just a healthy diet. Echinacea and goldenseal stimulate the immune system and help keep the body clear of infections, and astragalus, with its rich concentration of trace minerals and micronutrients, also helps strengthen immunity.

- Wrap some ice cubes in a damp facecloth and apply to the ear and the surrounding area, to encourage decongestion of the ear, which will cause it to clear. Although heat can be comforting for a child, it tends to increase the congestion and in the end makes the infection worse.

- Chamomile tea can be drunk to soothe any pain and distress.

- Soak a cotton ball with a few drops of warmed garlic oil and press gently into the ear canal to draw out infection.

- Homeopathic treatment for chronic ear infections should be constitutional, but there are a variety of remedies that work for acute attacks. For example:
  - Hepar sulf. is useful for acute attacks, with an earache accompanying a sore throat; the child will feel chilly
  - Pulsatilla, if the pain feels like the eardrum is being pushed out and your child is weepy
  - Aconite, for an earache that comes on suddenly
  - Belladonna, when the affected ear is red and hot and the child is feverish and perhaps delirious
  - Chamomilla, when the child is inconsolable, and the pain is worse with a draft. This is a good first remedy for most earaches.

- Rub a little Bach Rescue Remedy Rescue cream (see page 260) into the painful parts just below the ears to stop panic and reduce inflammation. Rescue Remedy or Rock Rose will ease panic. Olive can be used while recuperating.

- A few drops of neat lavender oil can be placed in the ear on a cotton ball, or gently eased in with a cotton bud. If there is an external ear infection,

---

The facts about outer ear infection

An inflammation or infection of the outer ear can cause severe pain, possibly including a discharge and impaired hearing. Such infections may be due to a number of factors; boils or abscesses; bacteria entering the ear from polluted water (this is known as swimmer's ear and may become a chronic condition); fungal infection; damage from constant prodding and probing of the ear or an allergic reaction to a foreign body.

Try the following treatments:

- Homeopathic remedies are appropriate:
  - Belladonna for pain and redness
  - Mercurius, when there is a smelly discharge
  - Aconite for an acute infection with sharp shooting pains

- Give Bach Rescue Remedy (see page 260) or to ease symptoms and calm.

- Mullein oil will reduce external pain and encourage healing. St. John's wort oil will have the same effect.

- Wash the ear canal with a warm infusion of antiseptic herbs, such as chamomile, elderflower or goldenseal.

- Apply a little tea tree oil to the end of a cotton bud and gently swab the outer ear canal, and the ear itself. This is good for fungal or bacterially caused infections.

- Warm a little marjoram oil in grapeseed oil, and massage around the ear and dab a few drops into the ear canal. Apply a little more to a cotton ball, insert into the ear and leave overnight. This will reduce pain and encourage healing.

- Boost your child's immune system if she has recurrent boils or abscesses in the ear canal or outer ear (see page 207).

this will help to encourage healing. Gently massage the neck and head on the affected side with a few drops of mullein or lavender oil in a light carrier oil.

- Witch hazel can be added to a teaspoon of oil of St. John's wort, and dropped into the ear until relief is obtained. This will take away the pain and inflammation.

Useful therapies

Homeopathy, herbalism, cranial osteopathy (for chronic ear infections), reflexology, aromatherapy, Ayurveda, nutritional therapies.

EATING DISORDERS

Eating disorders are responsible for the highest number of deaths from psychiatric illness. According to Eating Disorders Awareness and Prevention in the U.S., 5 to 10 million adolescent girls and women struggle with eating disorders and borderline conditions, and a million boys also suffer. It claims that eating disorders affect at least three times as many people as schizophrenia (2.2 million people are living with schizophrenia). At one time, eating disorders were thought to affect primarily preteen and teenage girls in upper socioeconomic groups. But according to the latest statistics, eating disorders are increasingly appearing in younger children and boys, and have infiltrated all socioeconomic groups. The most common eating disorders are anorexia, bulimia and compulsive overeating. But other disorders exist. For example, some people severely restrict the range of food they eat, and some children have a psychological fear of food. Anorexia, which involves depriving the body of food, is more common in young people. Children as young as three have been treated for it. Bulimia, characterized by a cycle of starving and bingeing, is more likely in teens and adults.

ANOREXIA NERVOSA

Around 5 percent of young girls in the U.K. are estimated to have anorexia nervosa, and although this figure is slightly lower in the U.S. (about 1 percent), it still represents a huge proportion of the population. Boys are much less likely to be affected, although that situation is changing. The condition results in death in 20 percent of cases after 20 years of onset of the illness. Only around 60 percent of anorexics recover. The illness is also one of the most controversial areas in mental health, but what is clear is the fact that a poor self-image is almost always at the root of an eating disorder, and it is this that needs to be addressed before there can be any hope of a cure. The media and its emphasis on super-thin models is also blamed by some for influencing the way people, particularly girls, see themselves and making them believe looks are all-important.

Anorexia nervosa is a form of intentional self-starvation. What may begin as a normal diet is carried to extremes, with many reducing their intake to an absolute minimum. It is also characterized by obsessive behavior. The majority of anorexics deny they have a problem (see Warning signs, below). Lack of food deprives the body of protein and prevents the normal metabolism of fat. The effects of this can include

- An irregular heart beat caused by a change in the heart muscle. This can lead to heart failure and death.
- Cessation of or failure to begin menstruation.
- Dehydration, kidney stones and kidney failure.
- The growth of fine downy body hair, called lanugo, on the face and arms.
- Wasting away of muscles, leading to weakness.
- Constipation or bowel irritation.
- Osteoporosis due to lack of calcium.

Symptoms of anorexia

Symptoms of anorexia range from extreme weight loss for no discernible medical reason; ritualistic food habits, such as excessive chewing; denying hunger and exercising excessively, to choosing low-calorie food and hiding feelings. A person with anorexia may be excessively thin but still see herself as overweight.

The average age for onset of the illness is thought to be 16, although the age range of anorexia is between 10 and 40. Around 90 percent of cases are female. Most have no history of being overweight.

Warning signs

- Does your child seem obsessed by the fat or calorie content of food? Has she put herself on a "diet" for any reason, from which she cannot be swayed?
- Does your child exercise obsessively, carefully calculating the number of calories burned during physical activity?
- Is your child frequently "not hungry" or "too busy" at mealtimes?
- Does your child disappear into the washroom after meals?
- Have you noticed any mood changes, including angry outbursts, isolation from friends, withdrawn behavior, chemical abuse or depression? Studies indicate that starvation tends to increase feelings of depression, anxiety, irritability and anger. Of course, many teens are subject to mood swings, so if this is the only symptom, look elsewhere for a cause.
- Has your daughter failed to start her period at a normal time, or has it stopped?

- Apart from weight loss, does your child suffer dry skin, hair loss, rashes and itching?

Preventing eating disorders

- Anorexic children are much more likely to be a product of a family that is overconcerned about weight and diet. Avoid talking about weight or diets, even if your child does have a weight problem. Parents send strong messages to their children when they constantly complain about their bodies, discuss diets and obsess over the fat, calorie and sugar content of food.
- Make family meals a daily occurrence. Many parents are surprised to find a child is anorexic because they have not eaten with them, or seen them eating, for many weeks or even months. Studies in the U.K. show that in the majority of families, children no longer eat with their parents on a regular basis. Children should not be made responsible for their own food choices. Apart from the fact that they can make unacceptable choices that can damage their health, parents need to model positive eating habits, which will go a long way toward instilling healthy attitudes to food.

Bulimia nervosa

Bulimia is thought to be two to three times more common than anorexia, but is not generally as physically dangerous. However, excessive use of laxatives and self-induced vomiting can cause rupture of the esophagus, mineral deficiency and dehydration, which can have serious effects on health.

Bulimia was officially recognized only in the 1970s and is characterized by a cycle of bingeing and starving. Many bulimics seem fine, but experts say that, under the surface, they often suffer from poor self-esteem and self-image. Bulimics may have irregular periods or stop having periods at all because of excessive use of laxatives and vomiting. Using laxatives can also cause kidney and bowel problems and stomach disorders. It can be more

difficult to recognize this condition, because your child may stay around the same weight, or lose weight more slowly. She may, however, have a puffy face, swollen fingers, muscle weakness and stomach pains, which can be an indication that there are problems when associated with an obsession with weight and obvious signs of bingeing and purging.

Excessive vomiting can cause tooth decay, bad breath, mouth ulcers, sore throats and stomach disorders and may have serious long-term health implications. Some experts believe bulimia is the result of an imbalance of chemicals to the brain, but others think the illness is more likely to be linked to a lack of self-worth. It is thought that up to half of anorexics also suffer from bulimia and some 40 percent of bulimics are reported to have a history of anorexia.

- Always provide a variety of fresh foods from all food groups at meals. Don't force a child to eat, and give small helpings. They can always ask for more.
- Parents have a powerful influence on their children's self-esteem and body image. In one study, measured self-esteem scores of kids aged 9–11 were lowered when they thought their parents were dissatisfied with their bodies. Encourage your child to feel good about herself, no matter what her weight. Even if she is fat, she needs high self-esteem (see page 173). Make sure your child feels loved and accepted for what she is, not what she looks like. Children with high self-esteem naturally gravitate toward habits that are good for them—exercising, good hygiene habits, dressing well, and taking pride in their appearance (flaws and all!).

Conventional treatment

Over 25 percent of anorexics are so weak that they require hospitalization. This may involve force feeding, as well as advice on healthy eating and counseling. Many doctors believe that once a person's body weight has fallen below a certain level, she is no longer capable of making rational decisions. Other forms of treatment range from group therapy, family counseling and psychotherapy to antidepressants. Around one-third of patients recover fully; another third improve significantly; and the last third do not recover. Bulimics have the same range of therapies, including behavior modification in some cases.

NATURAL TREATMENTS

- Most of the complementary therapies will help address this condition, mainly because they take into consideration emotional factors that play a very real part. It can be difficult to encourage an anorexic to be honest with a therapist, and most anorexics will deny that they are in any way ill, or in need of treatment. You will have to provide as wide-ranging a picture as possible in order to give the therapist all the necessary information.
- Zinc, whether part of the diet or in supplemental

form, has been successful in helping many individuals with anorexia to regain normal appetite and weight. There are numerous studies showing a link between zinc deficiency and anorexia.[5] The first case of anorexia treated with zinc occurred in 1984, and a cure was produced within two months of zinc supplementation. Scientists worldwide are now testing the effects on anorexia.
- All anorexics should be given a good multivitamin and mineral complex. All nutrients are needed and must be taken in extremely high doses because they are passed through the gastrointestinal tract rapidly and are poorly assimilated.
- Acidophilus is also important, in that the friendly bacteria will have been lost through vomiting and/or laxatives, or from the absence of food. It will also help nutrients be assimilated better, even if they are in supplemental form.
- Talk to a nutritional therapist about vitamin B12 injections, which increase appetite, prevent loss of hair and damage to many bodily functions. If injections are not available, use a lozenge form.
- Extra vitamin C is required for the impaired immune system, and to alleviate stress on the adrenal glands.
- Some studies indicate that essential fatty acids might be at the root of some cases; offer evening primrose oil at 500 mg per day.
- Flower essences are an important addition to any anorexic treatment, given the nature of the negative emotional state that accompanies the condition. For example, Crab Apple is for those who feel infected or unclean, who are revolted by eating, or have a hygiene fixation. The remedy helps to put everything in perspective. Rock Water is for those who are strict with themselves and demand perfection. Or try White Chestnut, if you think your child might be tormented by persistent worries and unwanted thoughts. A good flower therapist will create a blend that will help your child.
- Homeopathic treatment would definitely need to be constitutional, but it can make a big difference. While you wait for treatment, try Aurum at 200C strength, in two doses, to help alleviate some of the emotional causes.

- Herbal treatment should also be supervised by a registered practitioner, but the following herbs are appetite stimulants: ginger, ginseng, gotu kola and peppermint. St. John's wort may help with the emotional problems underlying the condition.

SELF-HELP

- If your child does suffer from an eating disorder, you will need to address emotional issues to uncover problems affecting self-image and self-esteem (see page 173). The most important thing you can do is to support and love your child. Showing disgust when she is overly thin or fat will reinforce a poor self-image. Let your child know that you love and care about her. You can certainly show concern about her health, but make sure your child is aware that your love and concern are not judgmental.

- Encourage hobbies and activities that will help your child to feel good about herself—choose something at which she is bound to succeed. Draw attention to successes, and overlook failures of any kind.

- Get some help for yourself. Join a support group with other parents in the same situation. Try not to blame yourself. There is a great deal of finger-pointing going on about eating disorders, and parents often take full brunt. Even secure children can suffer from self-esteem and emotional problems after an upset, or there may be problems at school you know nothing about. The best advice is to get to the root of the problem, and to find ways of addressing it.

ECZEMA

This subject deserves a book to itself, given the increasing incidence of the condition and the huge number of cases that are misdiagnosed. Also called "atopic dermatitis," eczema is a skin disorder characterized by an allergic rash. Interestingly, the allergy may have nothing whatsoever to do with the skin. For example, many children with food allergies also suffer from eczema, or in a person with dust allergy, inhaled dust can cause the skin to erupt in an eczema rash. Frequently, the true cause of your child's eczema may remain unknown, which can make it frustrating to treat.

In typical childhood cases, eczema produces a rough, red area in the creases of the arms, behind the knees and on the cheeks. In some cases it can cover the whole or most of the body. The rash can be itchy, and it can crack and weep, in some cases leading to a bacterial or fungal infection; it can be very itchy. Most cases are made worse by frequent bathing, and the itching will increase in hot conditions. Sweating and contact with wool also aggravate eczema. Children commonly outgrow eczema, but some children develop asthma as the eczema fades away. Why? Natural therapists believe that the traditional treatment of eczema, including steroid preparations, drives the condition deeper into the body, where different types of allergic reactions result. Many children with asthma also suffer from eczema, partly because they are both allergic conditions with the same root, and partly because the condition of the skin often mirrors the health of organs such as the lungs. The key to treatment is dealing with the underlying allergies (there may be many) and balancing your child's system so that he can deal more effectively with allergens.

- Atopic eczema (linked with the family of allergies that includes hay fever and asthma) is the most commonly diagnosed form of the condition.

- Contact dermatitis is present on or near the skin exposed to the allergen; for example, nickel dermatitis is found where cheap jewelry is in contact with the skin under necklaces, bracelets or earrings. Biological soap powders produce dermatitis under clothes, sparing the hands and face.

- Eczema, often severe and widespread, can be due to a protein in cow's milk. The common infant formula milks are based on cow's milk so it is worth trying a soy-based or goat's milk infant formula to see if the eczema settles. In older children, switching to a different milk or dropping it altogether may ease the problem.

Conventional treatment

Your doctor will probably prescribe antihistamines, which help with the itchiness or scratching, or antibiotics, if the skin becomes infected. As a rule, steroid ointments are prescribed only when the itching is so severe that it prevents the child from sleeping, or if the skin is severely infected, although there is no doubt that they are overprescribed.

NATURAL TREATMENTS

- In traditional Chinese medicine, the cause of childhood eczema is seen as due to a malfunctioning digestive system. Emotionally, eczema is believed to arise from hidden feelings, and the inability to communicate feelings and be understood. When a child is in a stressful situation and cannot express herself, it can affect digestion and give rise to eczema. It's important to note that in almost every case of natural treatment, your child's eczema will get worse before it gets better. It "comes out" of the skin, if you like. So a mild case of eczema may temporarily become bright red, itchy and may even weep. Don't be alarmed. These symptoms are always short term and mark the end of what could be a lifelong condition. Try to remember that conventional medicine offers no treatment for eczema, although it can reduce the symptoms. Natural treatment can offer a cure.

- Since eczema is believed to be related to digestion, pay particular attention to your child's diet, and look into the possibility of a food allergy or intolerance (see page 344). Offer plenty of foods that help the body to detoxify (see page 145), and avoid artificial colorings, flavorings or preservatives. For older children it may help to mix flaxseed (linseed) oil into food each day (see page 13).

- For dry skin that feels hot, use calendula cream or Bach Rescue Remedy cream (see page 260). To relieve itching, urtica urens lotion or ointment will help.

- The most nourishing gentle moisturizer is olive oil, which can be rubbed into the skin following a bath. Never put moisturizing oils in the bath until after your child has soaked for some time. Otherwise, the oil forms a barrier between the water and the skin, preventing rehydration. Drop olive oil into the bath after about five to ten minutes of soaking, or apply it afterward. Add a drop of lavender oil to soothe.

- Add a cup of chamomile tea to your child's bath water to soothe inflammation and itching, or try a few drops of Bach Rescue Remedy (see page 260).

- Offer a good multivitamin and mineral pill to prevent any minor deficiencies that may be exacerbating the problem.

- Evening primrose oil has been used successfully in the treatment of eczema, reducing itching and encouraging healing. A study carried out by the Department of Dermatology at Bristol's Royal Infirmary showed a significant improvement in patients with atopic eczema. These improvements were recorded after just three weeks of taking 4,000 mg of evening primrose oil a day (2,000 mg for children). The evening primrose oil was shown to lessen itching by 36 percent, scaling by 33 percent and redness by 29 percent.

- Eczema requires constitutional homeopathic treatment, but the following remedies may be useful in the meantime:
  - Sulfur, when the skin is burning, red, hot and itching
  - Graphites, when the skin appears infected
  - Petroleum, when there are deep cracks with a watery discharge
  - Urtica urens, for a hive rash-type itchiness
  - Rhus Tox., for blisters that are worse at night and improve with warmth

- Aloe vera gel, from the leaf of the plant, will encourage healing.

- Flower essences can be very useful, and will help babies and children, particularly because eczema is so strongly linked to emotions. Consider Impatiens, which is useful for itching, and can be taken internally or mixed into a neutral cream. Bach Rescue Remedy (see page 260), taken internally, or used externally in a cream or wash is useful in most skin problems.

- A gentle massage with a blend of chamomile,

lavender and/or melissa in a little carrier oil can be used to treat eczema.

Useful therapies

Acupuncture, homeopathy, herbalism, traditional Chinese medicine, Ayurveda, nutritional therapies and any of the stress-relieving therapies (see page 386).

SELF-HELP

- Try to keep your child's room as dust free as possible (see page 150), and remove toxins from the environment.
- Dress your child in clothes that "breathe"—cotton, for example, or hemp—which will reduce symptoms.
- Make a careful note of situations, foods or chemicals that seem to make it worse and try to avoid them, or offer treatments to balance the effects (during exams, for example). All children will benefit from having their immunity boosted (see page 207), to help reduce the allergic response. Similarly, dealing with stress (see page 386) can prevent attacks and exacerbation of symptoms.

ENCEPHALITIS

Encephalitis is an inflammation of the brain tissue. Primary encephalitis is caused by direct infection of viruses including herpes simplex, herpes zoster or mosquito- and tick-borne viruses. Secondary encephalitis usually occurs as a complication of a viral infection such as mumps, measles, rubella or chicken pox. Encephalitis can be fatal within hours of onset, although many children make full recoveries, even from serious attacks.

In mild cases the symptoms are similar to those of other viral infections:

- fever
- headache
- loss of appetite
- lethargy and drowsiness

In more severe cases your child may experience:

- double vision
- mental confusion and impaired speech
- nausea and vomiting
- loss of balance
- stiff neck and back
- epileptic fits

Conventional treatment

This condition is very serious and must be dealt with by a conventional doctor and treated as a medical emergency. Depending on the cause, strong anti-viral drugs such as acyclovir will be offered, usually by intravenous drip (IV).

NATURAL THERAPIES

While natural therapies and treatments may not be appropriate during the infection itself, there are many ways to help your child on the way to recovery.

- Homeopathic remedies can be safely taken alongside conventional medication, and you can place a pill between your child's lip and her gum, even if she is groggy or asleep:
  - Belladonna, if she has a flushed face, with delirium and staring eyes
  - Nux Mosch., for drowsiness, particularly in an infant
  - Gelsemium, for dizziness, a tight band around the forehead and weakness with trembling
- Get the advice of a good homeopath, who understands the need for conventional intervention.
- Offer your child plenty of vitamin C and zinc, to help the immune system. Again, this will not interfere with treatment, but you must tell your doctor what you are doing.
- Echinacea is antiviral, and can be taken alongside orthodox treatment to boost the immune system and treat the infection.
- Offer plenty of fresh garlic following the illness to speed recovery and treat the immune system.
- Chamomile tea can be sipped when your child feels restless and uncomfortable.
- Essential oils of chamomile, lavender, peppermint or tea tree oils can be dropped on a cold compress

and used to bathe the forehead to soothe and encourage healing.

Epilepsy

Childhood seizures can be caused by a variety of common childhood illnesses that result in abnormal electrical activity in the brain. Recurrent seizures (i.e., those that occur more than once) are known as epilepsy. Epilepsy can be diagnosed only if more than one seizure has occurred. A child who has only ever had one seizure cannot be said to be epileptic because he may never have another. Epilepsy affects approximately 8 out of 1,000 children of school age.

In the majority of children no cause for the seizure is found. Occasionally, epilepsy may have a genetic basis and run in families. More rarely, brain injury at or around the time of birth may result in epilepsy.

- Primary generalized epilepsy is also called "grand-mal" or "tonic-clonic" epilepsy, and is by far the most common type of childhood epilepsy. The child loses consciousness, falls to the ground, and the body, arms and legs become stiff. This phase usually lasts for only a few seconds, and, as breathing stops, the child often turns blue in the face. A rhythmic jerking of the arms, legs and often the entire body follows, which may be violent and alarming to parents. These are involuntary movements. During this stage, breathing resumes and a normal color returns to the child's face. This stage normally lasts less than five minutes and may be associated with tongue biting and incontinence of urine. On coming around, the child is confused, drowsy and often tearful, but does not remember what happened.
- Absence seizures, also known as "petit mal" attacks, are episodes of loss of consciousness without falling or involuntary movements. The child stops whatever he is doing, looks vacant for 5 to 20 seconds and then continues what he was doing as if nothing had happened. These attacks occur after the age of two and are most common between five and nine years of age. Most children grow out of them by their teenage years.

- Juvenile myoclonic epilepsy is a condition that runs in families. There are episodes of jerking of the hands, arms or entire body without alteration of consciousness. The jerks occur most frequently in the early morning. It usually begins in late childhood, and the affected child may also suffer from separation anxieties or generalized seizures. It is important that this condition is correctly diagnosed as some anti-epileptic medications may make it worse.
- Temporal lobe epilepsy may be difficult to recognize and diagnose in children, as they find it difficult to describe the sensations experienced. Outward signs of a child experiencing this type of epilepsy include making strange faces, swallowing, lip-smacking, chewing and muttering while being apparently awake but not in touch with what is going on.

Conventional treatment

Epilepsy is normally controlled by one anti-epileptic medication (e.g., carbamazepine, ethosuximide) usually taken two or three times each day. Common side effects include drowsiness and rashes. More than 60 percent of children grow out of their epilepsy, and medication can be stopped if the child has not had a fit for at least two years.

Natural treatments

- Vitamin B complex, taken three times daily, is extremely important for the functioning of the central nervous system. Injections, under a doctor's supervision, may be necessary.
- Extra magnesium is indicated, as it is required to calm the nervous system and muscle spasm.
- Homeopathy can be offered alongside conventional treatment, although some of the drugs used may antidote remedies. See a registered, experienced homeopath for constitutional treatment. There are remedies that can be offered following a fit, when twitching and jerking stops. Offer every minute for up to ten doses. These remedies will quickly work to reduce the effects of the seizure on the body and brain. Try:

- Chamomilla, when a seizure is brought on by teething or after an outburst of anger. It's particularly indicated if your child has one red cheek and one white cheek, with thumbs clenched into palms.
- Ignatia, for a fit brought on by emotional upset. The twitching may start in the face and your child may be very pale.
- Aconite, for a seizure brought on by fright or fever, or when one occurs very suddenly without any obvious stimulus
- Belladonna, when your child is red-faced and feverish, with wide, staring eyes
- Cuprum, if your child's seizure is very violent and he has blue lips and face, and thumbs clenched inside fists
- Glonoinum, for fits brought on by exposure to sun or intense heat. Fingers and toes might be spread wide.
- Zinc, for fits brought on through illness, with fidgety, restless movements of the limbs and a bad temper
- Aconite, for fits brought on by fright or fever

- The source of the problem is believed to be excess heart mucus, internal damp and stagnant chi or blood. Sweet flag root and the juice of the young bamboo can prevent attacks in some cases. See a Chinese herbalist for details.
- Studies show that extremely small doses of rosemary might be helpful in treating epilepsy, but this must be done only under the supervision of an aromatherapist with a medical qualification. There are a number of oils to avoid if your child has epilepsy, and these include sage, fennel, hyssop and wormwood.
- Flower essences can be very useful, and if you can catch "states" before they begin to affect physical health, you may be able to prevent most attacks. See a good therapist who will put together the most appropriate blend. Try to encourage your child to recognize the warning signs, and to keep a bottle of Rescue Remedy (see page 260) handy to take as soon as that feeling appears. This will calm, and hopefully abort, an attack.
- Herbs to relax the central nervous system, including vervain and valerian, may be useful by reducing the frequency and severity of attacks.

Useful therapies

Reflexology, acupuncture, homeopathy, herbalism, traditional Chinese medicine, cranial osteopathy. Some of these may simply reduce stress levels, which can prevent attacks; others have a good record of cure. Talk to your therapist about what can reasonably be expected, and choose a treatment that is both safe and effective.

SELF-HELP

- If seizures are frequent or difficult to control, which is unusual, your child should not ride a bicycle in traffic, should not swim unaccompanied, and should take showers instead of baths to prevent the risk of drowning should a seizure occur while bathing. To help prevent seizures it is important to ensure that your child does not become overtired.
- You should make sure that those who look after your child, including you, teachers and older brothers and sisters, know what to do if your child has a seizure. This includes laying the child on her side to prevent the tongue from obstructing breathing. No objects must be placed in the mouth. Any tight clothing around the neck should be loosened. The child should be left undisturbed until the seizure has calmed down. Young children may be very frightened on coming around and require comforting.
- If a seizure does not stop after five minutes, an ambulance must be called.

FEBRILE CONVULSIONS (see Fevers)

FEVERS

Fevers are a fact of life for most children. In most cases they are nothing to worry about, but it is important to monitor the symptoms closely and to seek medical advice if they persist. Fever has been defined as a body temperature elevated to at least 1°F above the "normal" of 98.6°F (37°C). A baby's temperature normally varies by as much as 2°F, depending on the temperature of her surroundings, clothing worn, degree of stress, level of activity or time of day.

In most cases a fever is the body's reaction to an acute viral or bacterial infection. Raising the temperature helps create an inhospitable environment for viral or bacterial invaders, and stimulates the production of disease-fighting white blood cells.

The child with a raised temperature will feel hot or cold, may perspire or shiver, will feel hot to touch and usually look flushed. She will lack energy, wanting to flop around or sleep rather than run everywhere as usual, and be miserable and off her food. Babies may cry despite being cuddled, and be difficult to settle. If untreated, a high temperature will commonly cause a child to vomit, and rarely the child may have a seizure (febrile convulsion).

The fever can be confirmed by measuring the temperature with a thermometer. A mercury thermometer should first be shaken down so that all the mercury is below the beginning of the scale. With a baby or young child, the bulb should be put in the armpit and the arm held to the child's side to keep it in place for at least a minute, preferably two, before it is read. With an older child, the bulb should be placed under the tongue with instructions to close the mouth without biting. After removing it, rotate the thermometer between your fingers until the mercury can be seen clearly against the scale. The temperature is raised if it is greater than 98.4°F (37°C).

The body's temperature control system is not well developed in babies, which is why fevers are so common at this age. Infant and childhood fevers can be caused by a number of different factors including:

- overexertion
- dehydration
- mosquito bites
- bee stings
- allergic reactions
- viral or bacterial infections

Conventional treatment

Most doctors recommend acetaminophen to bring down fever. A child with a temperature of less than 102°F (38.8°C) does not normally require immediate medical attention, unless there are other symptoms, such as a stiff neck (see Meningitis), sensitivity to light or a rash.

NATURAL TREATMENTS

- A number of homeopathic remedies are useful, according to the symptoms. The most useful one is usually Belladonna, for fever, a bright red rash and hot face; Phytolacca helps when there are painful ears and swollen glands, which feel better after drinking cool liquids; Aconite should be tried if there is a high fever and not too much mucus; Merc. Sol. is suggested where there is yellow discharge from the ears, nose, throat or lungs with a fever.
- Bach Rescue Remedy (see page 260) can be taken to ease any distress and calm the child. Chicory, Hornbeam and Cherry Plum are useful for all childhood illnesses that may cause fever. In children and babies, the relationship between mind, emotions and body is very direct, so anything that they find disturbing can cause a fever, as unbelievable as that may sound. For example, after a temper tantrum, many children develop a fever. Therefore, flower essences can be appropriate in many cases.
- The best herbal remedy for reducing fever in children is catmint, which can be sipped regularly to cool the children as well as address the root of the problem. Lime flowers are calming, and elderflower is also useful. Both are normally available in syrup form, or they can also be sipped throughout the day. When the fever has abated, offer gentian or tincture of oats before meals, to encourage the recovery process. Goldenseal or elecampane will help to address any mucus that has built up.

Useful therapies

Aromatherapy, homeopathy, herbalism, traditional Chinese medicine, acupuncture.

SELF-HELP

- Dehydration is a risk for infants, and a feverish baby should always be given lots of fluids.
- Your child should be cooled down by removing clothes and excess blankets, and if necessary sponging with tepid (not cold) water, which is then allowed to evaporate.
- Keep food to a minimum, so that your child's energy is not used for digestion, but is free to fight infection. There is some evidence that fevers can be prolonged by giving too much food, particularly food that is hard to digest (spicy foods, for example).

> ### CAUTION
> Children should not be given aspirin. Several studies link aspirin use in children with Reye's Syndrome, a severe illness that is often fatal.

FLU

Influenza is a viral disease of the upper respiratory tract, spread by the contaminated droplets (via coughing and sneezing) of other sufferers. There are a number of types of flu, some of which confer immunity once your child overcomes them, and others that mutate constantly so that your child's body cannot build up a resistance. The conventional response is to push for antiflu vaccines (see Immunization, page 213) and drugs. What many natural practitioners believe is that our collective immunity is becoming increasingly lower due to overuse of drugs, a poor diet and a generally unhealthy lifestyle. The bottom line is that flu viruses will always exist, and if you want your child successfully to fight the infection, his immunity must be high (see page 207). Incubation of the virus (new ones appear all the time, so don't be fooled into thinking a vaccine will take care of them all) is generally one to two days, during which time it is infectious, and therefore notoriously impossible to contain.

Symptoms include a high fever, possibly accompanied by shivering, a sore throat, possibly a cough, a running nose and sneezing, breathlessness, weakness, headache, aching joints and muscular pains, nausea and loss of appetite, and sometimes accompanying sleep problems and even depression.

Conventional treatment

Symptom-reducing drugs, such as acetaminophen, cough suppressants and occasionally antihistamines. Antibiotics should never be offered for flu, as they have no effect on viruses.

NATURAL TREATMENTS

- Homeopathic remedies can be dramatically effective. My youngest son had the flu during the "epidemic" and was transformed from screaming with abdominal pain, a high fever and some delirium, to playing football in the front room some 15 minutes later. He had one relapse, which was as quickly taken care of, and although he was tired and quieter than usual for a few days, the flu had gone! Try:
  - Gelsemium, when muscular weakness, aching and heaviness are the most predominant symptoms. There may be shivering.
  - Rhus Tox., for flu that comes on after getting wet. There is a lot of aching in the joints rather than the muscles; the child is restless and can't find a comfortable position.
  - Bryonia, for a bad headache, and dry cough. Your child will want to lie quite still and may be intensely irritable.
  - Eupatorium Perfoliatum for very intense aching in the back and limbs with shivering chills
  - Belladonna for a high fever, with red cheeks and staring eyes
  - Chamomilla, when your child cannot be comforted and seems to be in intense pain
  - Arsenicum, when your child feels debilitated, often with loss of fluids; watery diarrhea and sometimes vomiting
- Barley water is a traditional remedy for high fever—particularly when the cause of the fever is infection and inflammation.
- Use a eucalyptus or peppermint essential oil inhalation to unblock sinuses and chest.

- Massage tea tree and geranium oil into the chest and head to reduce symptoms and fight infection. Oils that act to bring down fever include chamomile, melissa and tea tree.
- Fenugreek, with lemon and honey, will help to bring down fever and soothe aching limbs.
- See also remedies for fever, headache and sore throat (pages 341, 356 and 384).

Useful therapies

Aromatherapy, acupuncture, herbalism, traditional Chinese medicine, homeopathy, flower essences, nutritional therapy and more. Anything that works to boost immunity or balance the body will be useful in the long term for prevention, and most therapies will help to encourage recovery time.

SELF-HELP

- Follow the instructions for nursing a sick child (see page 225) and for boosting immunity (page 207).

FOOD ALLERGIES AND INTOLERANCE

Food allergies are on the increase, and intolerance to one or more foods may be the cause of many common health disorders.[6] So many of us suffer from allergies of one sort or another that it's difficult to imagine how serious a food allergy can be. Take a look at the Food Allergy Facts box on page 346. Allergies can kill adults and children alike, and the U.K. and U.S. governments are so concerned that both have initiated campaigns to make the food industry more aware of the dangers involved.

Not only are food allergies at the root of a number of health conditions in children, there is also mounting evidence that children who suffer food allergies or sensitivities in their early years are more likely to develop health problems in their adult lives.

According to recent research, babies can be sensitized to foods before they are born, because some food molecules from the food eaten by their mothers can reach the womb. The foods most likely to cause problems are often those craved by women while they were pregnant, or foods that were eaten in large quantities. Don't assume that milk is the problem. It can be a sensitivity factor for many babies, but it is not the only one by far. Food molecules are also transmitted via breastmilk, which makes the mother's diet critical in the fight against allergies. Formulas, based on cow's milk, goat's milk or soy, can also cause problems.

Be very careful of elimination diets in very young children. Many experts recommend undertaking dietary programs only under the supervision of a doctor, and this is probably a fairly good rule of thumb. If you are careful to include the right balance of proteins, carbohydrates, fats, vitamins and minerals in your child's diet throughout an elimination period, it is certainly possible to undertake a program at home. If you are not sure what this involves, take expert advice.

FOOD ALLERGIES

Food allergies should be distinguished from intolerance, and involve different parts of the body. According to the Food Allergy Network in Fairfax, Virginia, a food allergy occurs when the immune system mistakenly treats a harmless substance, in this case a particular food, as harmful. In its attempt to protect the body, it creates specific antibodies to that food. The next time the individual eats that food, the immune system releases massive amounts of chemicals and histamines in order to protect the body. These chemicals trigger a cascade of allergic symptoms that can affect the respiratory system, gastrointestinal tract, skin, or cardiovascular system.

Symptoms range from a tingling sensation in the mouth, swelling of the tongue and the throat, difficulty breathing, hives, vomiting, abdominal cramps, diarrhea, drop in blood pressure, loss of consciousness to death. Symptoms typically appear within minutes to two hours after the problem food has been eaten. Their onset is dramatic, and will effect either respiration, the skin (hives, for example) or the digestive tract (full-blown diarrhea or pain, for example).

Is there a cure?

Strict avoidance of the allergy-causing food is the only way to avoid a reaction. Reading ingredient labels for all foods is the key to maintaining control over the allergy. If in any doubt, allergic individuals should not eat that food. Fortunately, labeling has improved over the past few years, and manufacturers must state whether products contain nuts, for example. Other foods are less carefully labeled, which means that for some severe sufferers, all processed foods are out.

Most children outgrow their food allergies, although allergies to peanuts, nuts, shellfish and fish are often considered lifelong. This belief is, however, being challenged. New research from the Kaiser Permanente Medical Center in San Diego indicates that the most common food allergies—to milk and eggs—tend to disappear by ages three to five. This research also suggests that allergies to peanuts and fish may be present up to at least age seven.

What should I do?

Experts suggest that randomly withdrawing foods from a child's diet can be dangerous, leaving it unbalanced at a time when nutrients are required most. If you suspect a food allergy, keep a food diary for a week or two, and if your child shows a reaction to a food, drop it completely. But take care to replace it in the diet with a food or group of foods with similar nutrient content. For example, if you drop wheat or other gluten-containing foods, you must ensure that your child has another source of good-quality unrefined carbohydrates, as well as B vitamins, among other things.

- Any significant symptoms should be reported to your doctor. There are natural ways to deal with food allergies (see page 348), but you will need to learn emergency treatment, and perhaps have some medication on hand, should your child suffer a serious reaction.
- Your child will probably need to have an allergy test to confirm the allergy, and to test for other foods that may cause similar problems. Many children suffer from more than one allergy, and pinpointing it early is important.

- Practically speaking, there are many things that parents can do:
  - Be aware of common allergens and take care when introducing these foods (see page 344), particularly if there are allergies in your family
  - Send a supply of "safe" snacks with your child to school, and teach her not to swap
  - Talk to your child's school about what foods are suitable and ensure that there is plenty of "safe" food on the menu. If you are concerned, send a packed lunch. Above all, and once again, teach your child what she can and can't eat and explain what can happen if she is tempted to eat the wrong foods.
  - Make your child's school aware of any allergies. Write a letter and highlight problem foods in bold, or in a different-color ink.
  - Ask your child's teacher what projects (in art, or the science lab, for example) might contain foods that could cause a reaction. Find an alternative well in advance.

Allergy tests

There has been controversy about the efficacy of allergy tests. Which?, a consumer association in the U.K., found them unreliable and, they decided, a waste of money. Other experts don't agree. All severe allergies will be picked up by one of two tests (see below). What can be difficult to assess are food intolerances, the symptoms of which often show up much later.

There are two main types of tests:

- The skin prick test is normally done in a doctor's or consultant's office, and involves placing a drop of the substance being tested on the patients' forearm or back and pricking the skin with a needle, allowing a tiny amount to enter the skin. If the patient is allergic to the substance, a weal will form at the site within about 15 minutes.
- A RAST (radioallergosorbent test) requires a blood sample. The sample is sent to a medical laboratory where tests are done with specific foods to determine whether the patient has antibodies to that food. This test is often used on young children who might become distressed by frequent

"pricks" and for those with eczema or another skin condition that might make the results difficult to assess.

Ban the peanuts?

Some parents of allergic children have suggested banning products, such as peanuts, from schools. This idea has been greeted with some favor, but many of the experts believe that this is unrealistic and, in the long term, unhelpful. According to the Food Allergy Network, education is the key to avoiding an allergic reaction and successfully living with an allergy. Banning one or more products from a school creates a false sense of security. Peanut butter sandwiches and peanuts may be successfully withdrawn from children's lunchboxes and the school menu, but nuts may still appear in baked goods and processed foods, and they are equally dangerous in this form.

The Network also believes that children need to learn how to live in the real world. They must learn to make choices, know what they are eating, know how to take precautions and how to treat themselves should a reaction occur. Children don't want to be labeled "different" at any age, and being the cause of a ban could put them at a disadvantage socially. Obviously the possibility of saving their lives carries more weight than the possible social ramifications, but there is some evidence that a ban will do more damage than good, given that children will think it's safe to eat anything when it may not be. Furthermore, children do need to learn how to live with an allergy.

Can my child eat that food again?

When you have removed the danger food from your child's diet for a year or so, your doctor may agree to a food challenge test.

- For children between the ages of 2 and 4, with allergies to foods such as eggs, wheat or milk, a skin prick test will tell immediately if the offending food still causes a reaction. Allergies to shellfish and peanuts, which tend to be longer lasting, should not be attempted until your child is at least seven.
- Some parents notice that a child has eaten the "danger" food by accident, and has shown no sign

Food allergy facts

According to reports in the *Journal of Allergy and Clinical Immunology*:

- Up to 3 million Americans suffer from peanut or tree nut (walnuts, pecans, etc.) allergy. It is estimated that as many as 125 people die in the U.S. each year from food allergy-related reactions.

- In the U.K., as many as 1 in 200 people has a severe allergy to peanuts, and at least 6 people die from it every year. Thousands more suffer from reactions to other foods, including milk, fish and eggs.

- Eight foods account for 90 percent of allergic reactions. They include peanuts, tree nuts, fish, shellfish, eggs, milk, soy and wheat.

- Peanuts are the leading cause of severe allergic reactions, followed by shellfish, fish, tree nuts, and eggs.

- Individuals with food allergies and asthma appear to be at an increased risk of severe allergic reaction.

- Most individuals who have had a reaction ate a food that they thought was safe.

- One study showed that high-risk infants who did not consume cow's milk, eggs and peanuts during infancy, and whose mothers also avoided those foods during the perinatal period, had a reduced incidence of food allergy and eczema in the first two years of life.

- One report showed that of 76 hyperactive children treated with a low-allergen diet, 62 improved and a normal range of behavior was achieved in 21 of these. Other symptoms such as headaches and fits were often improved. Forty-eight foods were incriminated, and artificial colorings and preservatives were the most common provoking substances. The study reported that benzoic acid (preservative E210) and tartrazine (Yellow Food Coloring E102) had a bad effect on nearly 8 out of 10 children involved.

of reacting. In these circumstances, you can try a small amount of the food a week or so later, or, better still, ask for another skin prick test in your doctor's office.

- Don't be tempted to reintroduce foods without checking that the allergy has disappeared. Even well-prepared parents can be caught out by a severe reaction and that's not a risk any of us would want to take.

Will my child be allergic?

Research by Dr. Robert S. Zeiger of the Kaiser Permanente Medical Center in San Diego indicates the following:

- Children have a 40 to 70 percent chance of developing allergies if both parents have allergies, depending on whether the parents share the same allergy. The risk drops to about 20 to 30 percent with one allergic parent and to 10 percent if the parents have no allergies.
- Avoiding the early introduction of potentially allergenic foods is the basic step in the primary prevention of food allergies in children who are at high risk, but some infants may still become sensitized or allergic to a food. Signs of food allergy in infants include eczema, hives, wheezing or vomiting from formula. Fortunately, early detection of a food allergy can help reduce its severity.
- Children with food allergies are several times more likely to develop a respiratory allergy as they get older. The earlier we can identify food and other allergic conditions, the earlier we can step in to prevent allergic disorders like asthma and allergic rhinitis.

Intolerance

By contrast with allergies, an intolerance does not involve the immune system. It is an adverse reaction caused by specific foods. For example, lactose intolerance occurs when the sufferer lacks an enzyme that is needed to digest milk sugar. When that child (or adult) eats milk products, she will experience symptoms such as gas, bloating, diarrhea and/or abdominal pain.

Interestingly, research shows that it is almost al-ways the most commonly eaten foods that are the source of the problem. In Britain and in other Western countries, wheat and milk are key culprits, largely because they are consumed several times every day. In the U.S., wheat and milk are equally suspect, but sensitivity to corn is also very common, partly because it is present in so many prepared foods in the form of cornstarch and corn syrup. Peanuts are a very common allergen in the U.S.—possibly because peanut butter is so popular, but also because peanuts are a very common snack food. There is less sensitivity in the U.K., but, as the peanut butter and snack food revolution begins to take hold, cases are on the increase. Soy beans and soy flour are now more widely used in processed foods, and, not surprisingly, sensitivities have increased.

Dr. Jonathan Brostoff and Linda Gamlin, authors of *Food Allergy and Intolerance*, reported a remarkable link between the overconsumption of particular foods, and subsequent sensitivities in patients. They claim that a large intake of any food, regardless of what it is, can trigger intolerance of that food. When a mother is breastfeeding, large amounts of any food can have a sensitizing effect on her baby.

How will I know if my child is intolerant?

Symptoms are often difficult to pinpoint, largely because they can seem innocuous in the early stages. The time it takes for symptoms to appear can also make it harder to link a reaction with a specific food. Some children become intolerant after a course of antibiotics, or being exposed to pesticides or other toxins. Symptoms may become worse in periods of stress, or after illness, which also clouds the issue.

Some of the most common symptoms are listed in the box opposite.

The best way to test for intolerance is to look for any changes in your child's health, even if it has been a slow, progressive change.

Eliminating foods

Elimination diets are a good idea for older children, and for younger children under the supervision of a doctor or good nutritionist. Food intolerances can be vast or they can be limited to just one or two key foods. Try the obvious ones first—for example, milk or wheat. If there is no obvious change in symptoms, put them back into the diet one at a time and try another suspect food, such as eggs, corn or oranges.

Children need a varied diet and it's important not to cut out more than one or two foods at a time. If you cut out milk and milk products, for example, make sure your child is getting enough protein and calcium from other sources (plenty of green vegetables and legumes, for example). An elimination diet should have a fairly immediate effect, and you should notice that the symptoms are alleviated within a few days. Take out one food at a time for a week or so. Reintroduce that food on its own so that any reaction can be assessed. The reaction time after a period of elimination is normally much faster than it would have been when the food was a regular part of the diet. In some children, there is an almost immediate reaction—sneezing, vomiting or flushing, for example.

Children can go on to eat foods that cause sensitivities in many cases. You may find that they become sensitive again after an illness or course of antibiotics, or when they are simply run down and tired. In these situations, withdraw the offending food or foods for a week or so and then try them again later. Take steps to ensure that problem foods never form a big part of your child's diet, which can set off the problem again.

Top tips for avoiding common allergens

- First foods should be introduced one at a time, and any reactions noted (see page 83).
- Do not give children eggs, fish, chocolate, wheat, orange, peanuts or other nuts for at least the first six months, or preferably for the first year of life. These are the most common allergens. Tomatoes, eggplant, potatoes and peppers should also not form a part of a baby's diet until his first birthday. These vegetables are members of the "deadly nightshade" family, which contain toxins that are now being linked to a variety of health conditions, including headaches and depression. Your child may not be

---

Craving the worst foods

This is an unusual feature of food intolerance, and it may be something that you have noticed in your own diet. There is plenty of evidence to suggest that we crave the foods to which we are intolerant. Some studies show that at least 50 percent of us suffer food cravings for problem foods. We may even be unaware of it. Look at the foods your child chooses, particularly if she is a picky eater. Children who refuse to eat anything other than peanut butter sandwiches, or pasta and cereal, show clear-cut tendencies for suspect foods.

This interesting perspective provides us with an even stronger reason to vary our children's diets. First of all, a varied diet is less likely to cause allergies caused by overeating certain foods. Secondly, a varied diet provides the vitamins, minerals and other nutrients that can help to ensure your child's body is working at optimum level. Thirdly, it helps to balance out food cravings that might be exacerbating a problem.

Common symptoms of food intolerance

- anxiety
- asthma
- bedwetting in children over the age of three or four (although this may have other causes, including emotional factors)
- behavioral problems
- bloating
- chronic sniffling
- constipation
- coughing
- Crohn's disease
- diarrhea
- eczema
- excess mucus
- facial puffiness
- fatigue
- flatulence
- headaches
- hives
- irritable bowel syndrome
- indigestion
- insomnia
- itchy eyes
- itchy skin
- mood swings
- mouth ulcers
- muscular aches
- nausea
- skin rashes (around the mouth, particularly, although the whole body may be affected)
- sore throats
- water retention
- wheezing

Food intolerance facts

- Food intolerance is believed to cause or exacerbate such conditions as asthma, migraine, nasal congestion, eczema, hyperactivity, irritable bowel syndrome and Crohn's disease.
- Between 6 and 10 percent of children under the age of three will have symptoms associated with food—probably milk. But most of those will disappear as they become older.
- The Allergy Research Foundation (ARF), based in Western Australia, believes a change in diet can help alleviate the problems in 50 percent of cases of children with irritable bowel syndrome.
- Evidence shows that 50 percent of those suffering from Crohn's disease feel better when a particular

food is eliminated from the diet.

- Most children who are food intolerant are sensitive to between 1 and 5 foods, although older children who have had their intolerances undiagnosed for many years, may be intolerant to many more (up to 20 or 30, in some cases).
- The Children's Centre in Surrey, England, has used diet management to tackle a range of problems in children, including attention deficit disorder, irritable bowel syndrome and migraine.
- Professor Joseph Egger, professor of neurology at the Children's Hospital, Munich, Germany, has used brain mapping to show changes that take place in children suffering from attention deficit disorder after they have eaten certain foods, such as milk, chocolate and cereals.

---

one of those who is susceptible to the toxins contained in these vegetables, but it is wise to play safe.

- Test out beef and eggs cautiously, as these can cross-react with milk. If they seem to cause no problems, include them in your child's diet.
- Infant formulas commonly contain corn and tapioca, as well as cow's milk, so there is a possibility that your child has become sensitive to these foods. Avoid including them in your child's diet until she is at least nine months of age (and watch out for hidden ingredients—corn, for example, is found in cornstarch, corn oil, corn syrup, corn, popcorn and cornflakes).
- Gluten grains, such as oats, rye and barley, can be introduced at about a year, but hold off wheat

until your child is between a year and two years of age (in other words, as long as possible).

- Soy products and ground nuts and seeds can be introduced, one by one, at about a year, but make sure you try them out, one at a time, and watch carefully for any reaction.
- Dairy products can be introduced singly after a year, but, again, leave them out as long as possible.
- Shellfish and strawberries can be introduced after your child's second birthday.
- Whole nuts should not form part of your child's diet until he is at least five. Quite apart from the possibility of allergies, nuts are responsible for an alarming number of deaths caused by choking.
- No food should be eaten in large quantities and it is a good idea to avoid giving any one food on a daily basis. This does mean being imaginative with your child's diet, but if you try to eat a varied diet as a family, it should be easier to achieve. Try out fruits, vegetables and grains that you may not normally consider buying: sweet potatoes, kale, legumes (such as lentils, black beans), dried unsulfured fruits soaked and puréed, millet, rice, parsnips, kiwi fruit, mango, quinoa, chickpeas (even very young children like humus, for example), buckwheat, split peas, barley and tofu.

Childhood problems caused or exacerbated by food sensitivities include colic, eczema, asthma, chronic runny nose, glue ear (see page 353), headaches, migraine, behavioral problems, chronic diarrhea, rheumatoid arthritis, some kidney problems, urticaria (nettle rash), skin problems, sleep disorders, persistent stomachaches.

GASTROENTERITIS (*see also* Nausea and vomiting)

Gastroenteritis is an acute inflammation of the stomach and intestine causing violent upset. It may be due to bowel organisms such as salmonella or other bacterial toxins or viruses that may contaminate food or water. Food intolerance or allergies may also cause the condition, and it can be a side effect of certain drugs. Gastroenteritis is most serious in babies because of the danger of dehydration through vomiting and diarrhea. Symptoms may include fever, abdominal pain, nausea and vomiting and diarrhea.

Conventional treatment

If dehydration is a concern, your doctor may offer electrolyte compounds (rehydration therapy). If bacteria is present, antibiotics may be indicated.

NATURAL TREATMENTS

- Homeopathic remedies can be taken hourly, as required:
  - Arsenicum, for burning pains in the abdomen and great thirst
  - Pulsatilla, for symptoms worse at night, and tearfulness
  - Baptisia, if a salmonella infection is

Is soy milk the answer?

Soy milk and other soy products have been put forward as the answer to food allergies and sensitivities, and as the ideal protein supplement for a vegetarian or vegan diet. There are, however, many differing views on this approach, and it's worth taking them into consideration when adding soy to your child's diet:

- Overeating or drinking any one food can lead to sensitivities and intolerance (see page 344). In fact, infants allergic to cow's milk are, in 40 to 50 percent of cases, also at risk of developing allergy to soy.

- Soy can be healthy as part of a varied diet, but it is not a complete food and should not be relied upon too heavily.

- There is growing evidence that soy protein might help lower blood cholesterol levels in some individuals, including children.

- Before replacing cow's milk with soy milk in your child's diet, read the labels carefully. Soy milk is not naturally high in calcium, which children need to build strong bones. Look for a soy milk fortified with at least 30 percent of the daily value of calcium, which is the same amount of calcium in cow's milk.

- Soy milks also vary in protein and fat content. A good choice contains at least 6 to 8 g of protein per cup and less than 3 percent fat. Many soy milks are also fortified with vitamins D and A, which are important for healthy growth and development.

- Soy is a food product that has been heavily involved in genetic modification. Ensure that any soya product you purchase is GM-free, and preferably organic.

- Soy is not naturally sweet, and many formulas and milks have added sweeteners to make them more palatable. Watch out for artificial sweeteners, which have been linked to health problems (see page 154), and high levels of sugar or corn syrups, which can damage teeth.

- Soy is a prime source of "phytoestrogens," which are natural compounds that act as weak estrogens. While phytoestrogens have been shown to have a dramatic effect on health in adults (they may offer some protection against conditions such as breast, bowel, prostate and other cancers, cardiovascular disease and menopausal symptoms), there are concerns over the long-term effects of phytoestrogens given to infants and young children, largely on the grounds that they can play havoc with hormonal activity. Currently, breastmilk or cow's milk formula are recommended for infant feeding, unless there is a clear indication that soy milk formula is required on medical grounds.

suspected—stools dark, bloody and smelly, nearly liquid

- Phosphorus, for a burning sensation when stools are passed, with vomiting and cravings for cold water, which is then vomited
- Sulfur, for burning diarrhea that is worse around 5 A.M., with a red and itchy anus
- Arrowroot or slippery elm tea can be sipped during the worst symptoms to soothe the digestive tract, and afterward to help restore bowel health.
- Offer acidophilus to restore the healthy flora in the intestines, which will help to fight infection.
- Very ripe bananas will ease nausea, act as a gentle constipant, and help to restore the healthy bacterial growth in the intestines.
- Live yogurt, taken by the teaspoon throughout the day, can help to restore bacteria to the stomach and digestive tracts. This is not appropriate for babies who have not been weaned.
- Honey is a natural antibiotic and anti-inflammatory. Mix a few teaspoonfuls in a cup of warm water and encourage your child to sip. Freeze into ice cubes if your child finds hot drinks difficult to manage.
- Massage chamomile and geranium oils into the abdomen to bring relief from pain and discomfort.

Useful therapies

Homeopathy, herbalism, acupuncture, traditional Chinese medicine.

> **CAUTION**
> If symptoms persist for more than 12 hours, or are accompanied by severe pain, call for emergency help.

GERMAN MEASLES (RUBELLA)

Rubella is a viral infection characterized by symptoms that mimic a cold, and go on to include loss of appetite, sore throat, mild fever and swelling of the lymph nodes in the neck. There is an accompanying rash, made up of pale pink spots that usually cause only mild discomfort. The incubation period is 14 to 21 days. The condition itself lasts only three to five days.

Conventional treatment

Your doctor will suggest acetaminophen to bring down any fever and reduce discomfort. Creams and ointments can be prescribed if the rash is very itchy; these include calamine and mild steroid preparations.

> **CAUTION**
> The symptoms in small children may be mild but if a pregnant woman who does not have immunity to German measles (either by having had the disease or by being immunized against it) comes in contact with the condition, there is a serious risk of miscarriage and birth defects.

NATURAL TREATMENTS

- Hot yarrow tea, cooled and drunk several times daily, will relieve symptoms.
- An infusion of elderflower, combined with peppermint, will help cool a fever and calm your child.
- Very high fever can be treated with an infusion of catmint, taken as required.
- Homeopathic remedies are appropriate. Consider:
  - Pulsatilla, when there is thick yellow discharge and hot, red eyes
  - Belladonna, for fever, a bright red rash and hot face
  - Phytolacca, for painful ears and swollen glands, which improve on taking cool drinks
  - Aconite, if there is a high fever and not too much mucus
  - Merc. Sol., where there is yellow discharge and a fever
- Bach Rescue Remedy (see page 260) will ease any distress, and calm the child. Chicory, Hornbeam and Cherry Plum are useful for all childhood illnesses.
- Acidophilus should be taken after any illness, to encourage the healthy bacteria in the gut.

- A few drops of lavender oil on the bedclothes, or on a tissue near the bed, will help ease symptoms and calm your child.
- If there is a buildup of phlegm, use a few drops of tea tree or eucalyptus oil in a vaporizer to encourage easier breathing.

Useful therapies

Herbalism, homeopathy, aromatherapy, flower essences, acupuncture, traditional Chinese medicine, nutritional therapies.

SELF-HELP

- Frequent, tepid baths will relieve any itchiness and bring down a fever.
- Eat plenty of raw fruits and vegetables to cleanse the system.
- Increase the intake of foods containing vitamin C and zinc to aid the action of the immune system.

GLANDULAR FEVER

Glandular fever, or infectious mononucleosis, as it is also known, is caused by the Epstein-Barr virus (EBV—a herpes virus). The virus multiplies in the white blood cells, eventually harming the immune system's efficiency. Glandular fever is usually transmitted via saliva, hence its nickname, the "kissing disease." While symptoms may last for only six weeks, recovery is slow, and fatigue and low energy levels may linger for months. The virus spreads more rapidly among children in closed or overcrowded conditions. Most adults have been exposed to EBV by the age of 18 years and are immune.

Most young children infected with EBV show no symptoms, unlike older children and adults, who may have fever, fatigue, enlarged neck lymph nodes, and inflamed throat and tonsils. In many cases, it is diagnosed in children who appear incredibly lethargic, with little energy to undertake even their favorite activities. There may be some indication of swollen glands or a mild rash of small slightly red raised spots. A blood test may be necessary to diagnose the condition if it is suspected.

Conventional treatment

Almost all cases resolve within about four to six weeks without any drug treatment. Rest is suggested. If antibiotics are wrongly given (the condition may be misdiagnosed), symptoms can worsen and a rash may appear. In rare cases corticosteroid drugs are required to reduce severe inflammation, particularly if tonsils are swollen.

NATURAL TREATMENTS

- Constitutional homeopathic treatment is recommended, but the following remedies may be useful, taken up to six times daily, for two days:
  - Belladonna, for sudden high fever, with red face and agitation
  - Merc. Sol., for tender glands and smelly sweat
  - Calcarea, for chilliness, sweating, a sour taste and fatigue
  - Cistus, for chilly feeling, with painful neck and glands, exacerbated by cold air and mental exertion
  - Baryta Carb., for swollen glands—this remedy is particularly useful for children
- Evening primrose oil has a beneficial effect on the immune system and can encourage healing.
- Royal jelly will help fight feelings of fatigue and depression, and stimulate the immune system. Look for a preparation designed for children, but don't offer this treatment if your child is allergic to bee stings.
- Essential oils can be used in the bath, or in massage, which also has therapeutic benefits. Oils to consider are eucalyptus, lavender, rosemary and tea tree, to encourage the immune activity and fight the virus.
- Herbs to promote healing include cleavers, echinacea and nettles, all of which stimulate immune activity, as well as fighting infection.
- Balm, oats and skullcap are suitable if your child seems to be depressed (depression is a common symptom during the healing process; see also page 323).
- Infusions of yarrow and elderflower will help to control fever, and induce sweating.

- Tonic herbs, such as astragalus and ginseng, will help your child's recovery.
- Bach flower essences are often used by practitioners to help cope with the physical and emotional effects of glandular fever. For example, Olive will help if you feel exhausted on all levels; Mustard will help with any accompanying depression; Gorse will help with feelings of hopelessness.

Useful therapies

Homeopathy, herbalism, aromatherapy, traditional Chinese medicine, acupuncture, Ayurveda, nutritional therapy.

SELF-HELP

- Make sure all children and adults in your household do not share eating or drinking utensils, or toothbrushes.
- Make sure all children and adults follow good handwashing practices.
- This condition represents a fairly profound attack on the immune system, and you will need to work on building it back up again, probably for several months.

GLUE EAR

Also called serous media with effusion, glue ear is a chronic condition affecting a large number of children. It is characterized by a thick, often smelly mucus that builds up in the middle ear, impairing hearing. The condition arises mainly because the middle ear is unable to drain its secretions into the nose by way of the Eustachian tube. Unlike the other common forms of earache, glue ear is not primarily caused by infection and will not respond to antibiotics.

It may be caused by chronic nose or throat infection, but can also be due to allergies or exposure to drafts. It may also be associated with chronically enlarged tonsils and adenoids causing Eustachian tube obstruction.

The condition is usually symptomless, apart from occasional "deafness," which may not be apparent. Most children are unaware that anything is wrong and may be accused of being inattentive.

Conventional treatment

Glue ear is often treated by a simple operation in which a tiny cut is made in the eardrum and a small plastic drainage tube is inserted. This allows immediate equalization of pressure on the two sides of the drum and free drainage of middle-ear secretions. Some studies show that this does nothing to affect the course of the condition (see page 332), and you may want to consider alternatives.

NATURAL TREATMENTS

- Cranial osteopathy has been enormously successful in treating this condition, probably because it can improve Eustachian tube drainage.
- Chronic infection can be caused by a buildup of catarrh (see page 312).
- Clean away discharge with a warm infusion of antiseptic herbs, such as chamomile or goldenseal.
- Herbs to help clear the catarrh include elderflowers, euphrasia, goldenrod and hyssop.
- Homeopathic remedies can be very effective. Constitutional treatment will be indicated as this is a chronic condition, but the following remedies might help in the interim. Try:
  - Kali. Mur. when there are cracking sounds in the affected ear, accompanied by swollen glands in the neck
  - Lycopodium when there is deafness and a roaring sound in the affected ear
  - Pulsatilla for a full feeling in the ear, and weepiness
  - Mercurius when there is thick, smelly discharge
- The remedies for ear infections may also be appropriate (see page 332).
- For feelings of congestion, massage the area around the ear and the neck with lavender and eucalyptus oils (one drop of each) diluted in two tablespoons of olive oil. Swab out the ear canal with tea tree oil when there is effusion.

Useful therapies

Cranial osteopathy, homeopathy, acupuncture, herbalism, traditional Chinese medicine, nutritional therapies.

SELF-HELP

- Diet may be a big cause of persistent glue ear. Look out for food allergies and intolerance (see page 338), and consider reducing consumption of dairy produce and any other possible allergens, including wheats.
- Remember that your child may be frustrated by having hearing difficulties. Try to be patient.
- Building up your child's immune system can have a good long-term effect, and can help to prevent the condition from recurring (see page 207).

GRINDING TEETH

Habitual grinding or clenching of the teeth is known as bruxism. It is usually performed unconsciously, but is audible to others. It is common among children, particularly during sleep. It's not dangerous, but in severe cases it can wear away the enamel of the teeth. Many children who grind their teeth do so because they are anxious or under stress.

Conventional treatment

If emotional problems cannot be resolved, or the habit broken, a biteplate worn at night may minimize the damage.

NATURAL TREATMENTS

- Constitutional homeopathic treatment will be appropriate, particularly since this condition seems to have an emotional basis. But try Arsenicum, for grinding of teeth during sleep, especially between midnight and 2 or 3 A.M.
- Herbal remedies would be used to calm the nervous system and to relax your child. Valerian is a gentle herb, which encourages the health of the nervous system and helps to keep him calm.

Encourage your child to sip this several times daily during periods of stress. Lime blossom may also work to ease anxiety and tension that may be exacerbating the condition.

- Bach flower essences (see page 258) are particularly useful, but treatment should be aimed at your individual child. You might want to consider Elm for anxiety accompanying a feeling of being unable to cope, or Red Chestnut for anxiety over the welfare of others. Anxiety for no apparent reason might be treated with Aspen.
- A relaxing blend of essential oils of lavender, geranium and bergamot in sweet almond oil or peach kernel oil may be used in the bath to calm and prevent attacks.

Useful therapies

Cranial osteopathy, homeopathy, herbalism; indeed, any of the therapies that help to address emotional issues.

SELF-HELP

If your child grinds his teeth during sleep, try to keep the bedtime routine as calm and reassuring as possible. Try to work out what might be making your child anxious—something at school, for example, or perhaps trouble with a sibling or his peers. Younger children who grind their teeth may do so for a short period during stages of developmental change. Try not to be anxious. Most of the time, it passes quickly, and if you show concern, your child will pick it up, which may make things worse.

GROWING PAINS

There is considerable debate about whether growing pains actually exist as a condition in its own right, or if it is simply a symptom of another underlying disorder. What we do know is that growing pains are often the diagnosis for leg aches in children. These pains typically occur at night (after your child has gone to bed), affecting both legs with no clear localization. They come and go without any other symptoms.

The most common explanation for this complaint is that a child who is very physically active has a buildup of lactic acid in the leg muscles. This build-up causes no discomfort during the day, but when your child takes a hot bath before bedtime, the heat seems to activate this acid, irritating the muscles. There may even be some accompanying spasm. Other potential causes may be subclinical (slight) mineral deficiencies.

Conventional treatment
None.

NATURAL TREATMENTS

- Homeopathic constitutional treatment may alleviate the problem in many children, particularly if it is common. For rare occurrences, try one of the following remedies:
  - Calcarea, for dragging pains in the ankles and knees that are worse for walking
  - Phosphoric acid, when your child feels weak and the pains come on after prolonged stress. It might be worse after exertion.
  - Guajacum, for pains that are worse in cold, wet weather, and made worse by heat, but normally better when pressure is applied to the area
- During an attack, warm a little olive oil and add one drop of lavender oil. Massage into the legs, working from top to bottom and then bottom to top, to improve circulation, release tension and encourage flow of any lactic acid buildup.
- Offer your child Bach Rescue Remedy (see page 260) during an attack.
- Ensure that your child has plenty of calcium, vitamin D and magnesium in the diet, which may be lacking.
- The tissue salts Calc. Fluor. and Calc. Phos., taken three times a day, are often helpful.
- If your child seems agitated or overexcited at bedtime, offer a little valerian tea to calm and relax.

Useful therapies
Massage, homeopathy, herbalism, aromatherapy, yoga.

SELF-HELP

Hot baths at night can make the condition worse, as the heat seems to activate the acid, irritating the muscles. If your child is prone to growing pains, try switching bathtime to the morning and offer a shower or a sponge bath in the evenings instead.

HAY FEVER

Hay fever (also known as allergic rhinitis) is an allergic reaction to airborne irritants such as grass, tree or flower pollens. These allergens (and others including dust, animal fur, feathers, spores, plants and chemicals) trigger a reaction that causes swelling of the nasal membrane and the production of the antibodies that release histamine. It is this chemical substance that is responsible for the characteristic allergic symptoms, including a runny nose, congestion, sneezing, red, itchy eyes, a sore throat, wheezing and a general feeling of malaise.

Conventional treatment
Antihistamines would be the first course of action, and nose or eye drops might also be offered, as well as a decongestant if there is difficulty breathing. There are a number of over-the-counter medications available, but you should be aware that these simply suppress symptoms and do not do anything to cure the condition itself.

NATURAL TREATMENTS

- Hay fever can be deep-seated and take some time to cure, and treatment should be undertaken on the basis of your child's individual symptoms. Homeopathic remedies have been particularly effective in curing hay fever, and in reducing symptoms, but you should see an experienced practitioner for constitutional treatment. In the meantime, there are remedies that will help. Try:
  - Allium for hay fever with a burning nasal discharge
  - Sabadilla for hay fever with a sore throat

- Arsenicum when there is a constant need to sneeze
- Euphrasia when the eyes are itching and red
■ Blend a drop of lavender, eucalyptus and chamomile essential oils with five tablespoons of carrier oil and add to your child's bath, or use in massage. This will help sneezing, congestion and a runny nose, and help your child feel better. The essential oil melissa, used in a vaporizer, may soothe and calm the allergic reaction.
■ Strengthen resistance with elderflower tea for some weeks before the pollen season starts.
■ Soothe itchy eyes with a chamomile compress.
■ Eat plenty of fresh garlic to boost the immune system; it also acts as an anticatarrhal agent.
■ Vitamin C, combined with bioflavonoids, will act as a natural antihistamine to control symptoms. Diet is important in all allergic conditions (see page 344).
■ Bach Rescue Remedy (see page 260) will help to ease symptoms during an attack, and help to produce a more positive frame of mind.

Useful therapies

Nutritional therapy, Ayurveda, homeopathy, traditional Chinese medicine, herbalism, acupuncture, reflexology.

SELF-HELP

All allergic conditions represent a breakdown of immunity, and it is important that you take steps to keep your child's immune system as strong as possible (see page 207). All of the treatments suggested for allergies (page 301) are also effective, and you may also want to consider some of those suggested for stress (see page 386).

HEADACHES

Most headaches in children are due to infections such as a cold, ear infection, gastroenteritis or tonsillitis. Some children also suffer headaches when they are stressed or upset, or when teething. However,

headache and fever can also be the signs and symptoms of the much rarer meningitis, which can cause brain damage, fits or even death, if untreated.

> **CAUTION**
> In meningitis typically there is headache, fever, vomiting, neck stiffness and photophobia (dislike of bright light). In the dangerous form, meningococcal meningitis, there may also be a faint rash but this is an unreliable sign. Not all the signs and symptoms are present in every case. If meningitis is suspected, medical help must be sought at once because a child with meningitis can worsen rapidly.

Headache without fever may be due to:
■ stress (tension headache) caused by problems at home or at school (see page 386)
■ squinting or straining to see properly
■ food allergies or intolerance (see page 344)
■ hormonal changes—in puberty, for example
■ lack of sleep
■ overconsumption of caffeine (in cola drinks, for example) or processed foods
■ problems with the teeth or jaw
■ allergies (see page 301)
■ toxic overload (see page 141)
■ sinusitis
■ low blood sugar

Conventional treatment

Analgesics may be suggested for chronic headaches, but your doctor will investigate to uncover the cause before prescribing anything. If your child is troubled and is getting tension headaches as a result, some family counseling may help. Meningitis should be treated as a case of extreme medical emergency, and will be addressed in the hospital.

NATURAL TREATMENTS

■ In all cases of headaches, the cause should be investigated and treated. Headaches are just a symptom of an underlying disorder—usually not sinister! If your child suffers from chronic headaches, it is important to see a natural therapist to establish what the cause might be. If you are fairly certain of the cause, by all means go ahead and offer treatment based on that knowledge—by treating a food allergy, stress and tension or allergies, for example. For acute headaches, many of the following remedies will be appropriate.

- Frequent headaches could be a signal that your child is low on some important vitamins and minerals. Low levels of niacin and vitamin B6 can cause headaches, for example, and all the B vitamins are needed to help combat stress and avoid tension headaches.

- A relaxing cup of mild herbal tea is often good for a tension headache. Good choices are peppermint, spearmint, chamomile, rosehip, meadowsweet or lemon balm.

- Valerian root tea can also be helpful, but it may make your child sleepy, so use it at night, or when she has time to take a nap.

- Researchers are studying the benefits of the herb feverfew for treating chronic headaches and migraines. The leaves of this plant contain a substance that relaxes the blood vessels in your brain. Studies suggest that children who eat a few fresh feverfew leaves or take an extract of the leaves every day have fewer and less severe migraines;[7] the herb has no unpleasant side effects.

- Homeopathic remedies can be very effective, particularly for chronic headaches. In the short term, try some of the following remedies:
  - Ignatia, for headaches caused by emotional stress
  - Nux vom., for headaches caused by overindulgence or stress (after a birthday party, for example!)
  - Nux vom. or Pulsatilla, for migraine
  - Aconite, for a sudden headache that feels worse when exposed to cold, and is characterized by a tight band around the head
  - Apis, for stinging, stabbing or burning headaches, where the body feels tender and sore
  - Belladonna, for throbbing, drumming headaches with a flushed face

  - Bryonia, for sharp, stabbing pain when the eyes are moved
  - Hypericum, for a bursting, aching headache with a sensitive scalp
  - Ruta, for a pressing headache caused by fatigue, and made worse by reading

- The relaxing qualities of lavender oil make it a good treatment for a tension headache. This essential oil is very gentle, so you can massage a drop into your child's temples and at the base of the neck (dilute it in a carrier oil first), or add to her bath.

- Chamomile tea is soothing and will ease the symptoms.

Useful therapies

Dependent upon the cause, but most therapies will help with both chronic and acute headaches.

HEAD BANGING

Head banging and body rocking are normal in children under the age of three, who seem to find the rhythmic back-and-forth movements a soothing way to fall asleep. Head banging can start as early as four months or as late as the second year and can last for several months. Some therapists suggest that head banging has an emotional basis, but chances are that your child is simply "rocking" himself to sleep. Remember that for many months your baby is gently rocked in the womb, in a small space. He may enjoy the feeling of being rocked against a hard surface.

While it may look painful, your child will rarely hurt himself. Some parents find that their child will stop if they put a ticking metronome in their child's bedroom; the rhythmic sound seems to soothe and distract them from their head-banging behavior. If your child's head banging starts after 18 months or continues into the third or fourth year, see a practitioner for some help. Although most cases are not due to emotional problems, strong head banging that lasts for longer than 10 or 15 minutes, and recurs throughout the night, may be a sign that all is not right.

Very occasionally head banging in young babies can be a sign of earache, so get that checked out if you are concerned.

Conventional treatment

In severe cases, protective headgear and behavioral therapy might be offered.

NATURAL TREATMENTS

- Ensure that your child has a good sleep routine and that he feels confident and relaxed at bedtime. Gentle music, a drop of lavender oil on a tissue, tied to the bedpost, and a prebed massage can all help.
- If you feel that this behavior has become a problem, contact a homeopath, who can provide constitutional remedies. In the mean time, offer one of the following remedies last thing at night, for up to a week:
  - Millefolium (usual dosage is 30C)
  - Chamomilla, for when your child is angry and impossible to please. He will prefer to be carried and may be furious when you put him down to sleep.
  - Silicea when head banging has become an obsession
- Flower essences may be appropriate for children whose head banging has an emotional root. Consider Red Chestnut for children who are anxious, White Chestnut for persistent worries, Walnut in periods of change and Mimulus for fear of known things (the dark, school or the dog next door, for example).
- If your child cannot relax at bedtime, offer a warm cup of chamomile or valerian tea with a little organic honey.

Useful therapies

Depending on the cause, any of the stress-relieving therapies, or those appropriate for sleep problems (see page 380) may be useful. The important thing is to discover the cause, if there is reason for concern.

SELF-HELP

Try to keep bedtime as stress-free as possible, and encourage relaxation long before it's time to sleep. If you are stressed or anxious about anything, try not to let it show. Your child will pick up on your feelings and it will make him feel more insecure or stressed. Take steps to build up your child's self-esteem (see page 174), which can help to deal with any emotional problems that might be developing or troubling him.

HEAD LICE (see Lice)

HICCUPS

A hiccup is an irritation of the diaphragmatic nerves, which causes involuntary inhalation of air. A lowering of the diaphragm and the sudden closure of the vocal cords results in the characteristic hiccup sound. There is rarely anything sinister about hiccups, although they can become painful if they carry on. Some children get them frequently, perhaps after eating or drinking. If you are concerned, see your doctor who can assess whether there is anything causing the problem.

NATURAL TREATMENTS

- There are homeopathic remedies for everything! Here are some of the best ones to try during an attack:
  - Nux vom., for hiccups after eating, accompanied by belching
  - Ignatia, when hiccups come on after emotional upset
  - Cicuta, for violent, noisy hiccups
- Squirt some lemon juice to the back of your child's throat, or ask him to suck a piece of fresh lemon. If nothing else, the shock will stop the hiccups! For babies, offer a sip of warm, previously boiled water laced with a drop of lemon juice.
- If hiccups are persistent and causing pain, give your child a gentle massage with a drop of lavender oil. It will help to relax her.

- One trick that always works: look intently at your child and ask her to produce another hiccup. Suggest firmly that you have cured them, and that they are gone. Your child will concentrate hard on repeating the hiccup, and will find they have disappeared. Who knows why this works, but it always does!

HIVES (URTICARIA)

Urticaria is an itchy, blotchy rash commonly called hives. It is a harmless form of allergic reaction that will not make your child feel unwell, but can be very irritating. The causes of urticaria are many and vary from person to person. In some, a particular food or drink may provoke it, in others simply getting hot or too cold may bring it on. In these cases the rash recurs whenever the stimulus recurs, but sometimes the rash is manifested only once. Your child may brush against a plant in the backyard, for example, and get the characteristic rash, or he may get it after eating a specific food. If he's rundown, he may be allergic to a food, but chances are that the allergy will cease when he's feeling stronger. If your child suffers repeated urticaria after eating a food, leave it out of the diet for a while. It may be an indication that he is severely allergic (see page 301). Sometimes children suffer from urticaria when they are stressed, and when there seems to be no apparent external cause. Under these circumstances, you will want to boost your child's immune system, and ensure his diet is good, and that he is getting plenty of sleep.

Conventional treatment

Your doctor may prescribe antihistamines to ease the itching, or a topical cream.

NATURAL TREATMENTS

- The best homeopathic remedies to try are:
  - Apis, for burning or swelling, particularly of the lips and eyelids
  - Urtica, for a rash that results from a sting made worse by touching or scratching

  - Rhus Tox., for burning, itching and blisters. These remedies should be taken every three hours.
- The Bach flower remedy impatiens is very useful for itching. Take internally or mix into a neutral cream and apply to the affected area.
- Urtica urens cream, which is available from health food stores and some good pharmacists, will soothe and promote healing.
- Aloe vera can be used topically to soothe the rash.
- A warm bath with essential oil of chamomile or melissa will soothe the skin and help to prevent stress-related attacks.
- Add a few tablespoons of baking soda to the bath to relieve itching.
- For urticaria brought on by anxiety and stress, offer an infusion of valerian at bedtime.

Useful therapies

Homeopathy, aromatherapy, Ayurveda, traditional Chinese medicine, acupuncture, flower essences, nutritional therapy and any of the therapies suggested for allergies or stress (see page 301 and 387).

SELF-HELP

Chronic urticaria can be sign of a food allergy, or another allergy that might be caused by a diet that is deficient in certain vitamins or minerals. Ensure that your child gets a good multivitamin and mineral pill daily, and add acidophilus to the diet to ensure that he is absorbing what he needs from his food. Build up his immune system, to ensure that his body is balanced and working at optimum level (see page 207).

HYPERACTIVITY (*see* Attention Deficit Disorder)

IMPETIGO

Impetigo is a highly contagious skin infection caused by bacteria such as streptococci and staphylococci. It usually first appears around the mouth and nose, but can spread rapidly if other parts of the body are touched after touching a blister. It can be passed on to others by direct contact or by sharing towels. In the past, many people considered impetigo a sign of poor hygiene, but many healthy, clean children suffer from the condition, so don't be alarmed or embarrassed. Scratching a cut on a face can do it!

The condition makes itself apparent with areas of red, inflamed-looking skin that soon become small fluid-filled blisters that burst and weep. They dry to form a yellow crust.

Conventional treatment

This usually involves antibiotics, orally and topically. Some doctors also prescribe a type of liquid soap to sterilize the rest of the skin and scalp, too, where the bacteria may be lurking with no outward sign.

NATURAL TREATMENTS

- Suitable homeopathic remedies include:
  - Antimonium tart., for blisters around nostrils and mouth
  - Arsenicum, for blisters, with exhaustion and restlessness
  - Depending on the type of infection, streptococci or staphylococci can be taken in potency. See a homeopath for details.
- A few drops of tea tree oil, applied neat to the affected area, will encourage healing and prevent the infection from spreading; it also has immunostimulant properties to help your child's body fight infection.
- Heartsease can be used internally or as a wash to treat impetigo; it is both softening and drying, and can soothe the skin.
- I have a regular concoction that I make when my children or their friends are hit by this condition. I wash the area first with cider vinegar, and then blend together 2 drops of tea tree oil, 2 drops of lavender oil, 5 drops of propolis, the contents of 5 vitamin E capsules and 3 tablespoons of Bach Rescue Remedy cream (see page 260). Apply with a

cotton ball to the affected areas two or three times a day. It may sting a little, but it works every time.

Useful therapies

Homeopathy, aromatherapy, nutritional therapy, herbalism, Ayurveda.

INSECURITY

Insecurity is an emotional symptom that affects most children from time to time. It can be caused by problems at school, a stressful situation, hormonal changes that cause confusion and mood swings, parental divorce and, in the long term, by poor self-esteem. The main way to deal with insecurity is to raise your child's self-esteem, whatever the situation (see page 174), and ensure that he feels good about himself and confident enough to cope with situations as they arise. Encourage hobbies with like-minded friends, and sports at which he can take part with some pride. Spend time with your child and try to get to the bottom of any negative feelings or experiences. Regular chats can do a great deal to ease insecurity.

Insecurity is, of course, a symptom rather than a health condition, so it's important to get to the root of whatever is making your child feel insecure. Young children may experience insecurity at key developmental stages (when starting school, when learning to walk and during separation anxiety), and they will need constant reassurance, no matter how irritating you may find their behavior. While young children cling and demand attention, adolescents and older children may withdraw and you may find it more difficult to draw them out. Work on their self-esteem, ensure that they know that you love them (no matter what!) and that you will always be there for them. Adolescents may shrug off your attentions, but they will be reassured.

NATURAL TREATMENTS

- There are natural treatments for insecurity, but they will be most effective when the whole picture is taken into consideration. For example, homeopathic treatment should be constitutional, although some of the following remedies may help:

- Aconite, for insecurity brought on by a traumatic experience
- Ignatia, for insecurity stemming from a particular incident or cause, such as a bereavement
- Pulsatilla, if your child feels tearful and longs for company

■ Marjoram essential oil is cheering and can boost self-image. It can also put your child to sleep, so use it at night in a vaporizer for best effect.

■ Flower essences can work wonders for insecurity. One of the best options is mimulus, for insecurity caused by fears of any sort. Larch is great for children who have little confidence and may feel inferior. Elm can help if your child feels overwhelmed or inadequate. Use Walnut in times of change (house moves, new school, adolescence, for example).

Useful therapies

All therapies can help with emotional problems.

INSOMNIA (*see* Sleep and wakefulness)

JUVENILE ARTHRITIS

Arthritis means joint inflammation, and refers to a group of diseases that cause pain, swelling, stiffness and loss of motion in the joints. The term "arthritis" is often used as a more general term to refer to the more than 100 rheumatic diseases that may affect the joints, but can also cause pain, swelling, and stiffness in other supporting structures of the body such as muscles, tendons, ligaments and bones. Some rheumatic diseases can affect other parts of the body, including various internal organs. Children can develop almost all the types of arthritis that affect adults, but the most common type of arthritis affecting children is juvenile rheumatoid arthritis.

According to the National Institutes of Health, juvenile rheumatoid arthritis (JRA) is arthritis that causes joint inflammation and stiffness for more than 6 weeks in a child of 16 years of age or less. Inflammation causes redness, swelling, warmth and soreness in the joints, although many children with JRA do not complain of joint pain. Any joint can be affected and inflammation may limit the mobility of affected joints. Doctors classify three kinds of JRA by the number of joints involved, the symptoms and the presence or absence of certain antibodies in the blood. Pauciarticular is the most common form of JRA; about half of all children with JRA have this type. Pauciarticular disease typically affects large joints, such as the knees. Girls under age eight are most likely to develop this type of JRA. Many children with pauciarticular disease outgrow arthritis by adulthood, but it can cause eye problems that continue into adulthood, and joint symptoms may recur in some people.

About 30 percent of all children with JRA have polyarticular disease. In polyarticular disease, five or more joints are affected. The small joints, such as those in the hands and feet, are most commonly involved, but the disease may also affect large joints. Polyarticular JRA often affects the same joint on both sides of the body.

Besides joint swelling, the systemic form of JRA is characterized by fever and a light pink rash, and may also affect internal organs such as the heart, liver, spleen and lymph nodes. Doctors sometimes call it Still's disease. The systemic form affects 20 percent of all children with JRA. A small percentage of these children develop arthritis in many joints and can have severe arthritis that continues into adulthood.

The main difference between juvenile and adult rheumatoid arthritis is that many people with JRA outgrow the illness, while adults usually have life-long symptoms. Studies estimate that, by adulthood, JRA symptoms disappear in more than half of all affected children. Additionally, unlike rheumatoid arthritis in an adult, JRA may affect bone development as well as the child's growth.

JRA is an autoimmune disorder, which means that the body mistakenly identifies some of its own cells and tissues as foreign. The result is inflammation marked by redness, heat, pain and swelling. Doctors do not know why the immune system reacts the way it does, but there is some evidence that it can have a genetic basis. If your child has a predisposition to JRA, an environmental factor, such as a virus, can trigger the condition.

The most common symptom of all types of JRA is persistent joint swelling, pain and stiffness that typically is worse in the morning or after a nap. The pain may limit movement of the affected joint, although many children, especially younger ones, will not complain of pain. JRA commonly affects the knees and joints in the hands and feet. One of the earliest signs of JRA may be limping in the morning because of an affected knee. Besides joint symptoms, children with systemic JRA have a high fever and a light pink rash. The rash and fever may appear and disappear very quickly. Systemic JRA also may cause rashes. Eye inflammation is a potentially severe complication that sometimes occurs in children with pauciarticular JRA. In most cases there are periods where the symptoms improve or disappear (remission) and flare-ups. The pattern is different in every child. Some children's growth may be slowed.

Conventional treatment

Doctors recommend treatments to reduce swelling, maintain full movement in the affected joints, relieve pain, and identify, treat and prevent complications. Drugs commonly prescribed include nonsteroidal anti-inflammatory drugs (NSAIDs, which can include ibuprofen, naproxen, or even aspirin). If these drugs don't relieve the symptoms, disease-modifying antirheumatic drugs (DMARDs) may be suggested. These can include hydroxychloroquine, oral and injectable gold, sulfasalazine, and d-penicillamine and methotrexate (the most popular for children). In children with chronic JRA, cortico-steroids like prednisone may be added to the treatment plan to control severe symptoms. Physical therapy is also an important part of a child's treatment plan.

Useful therapies

Homeopathy, herbalism, traditional Chinese medicine, acupuncture, nutritional therapies, reflexology, hypnotherapy. Also any of the therapies that help to boost immunity and reduce the effects of stress that can bring on an attack.

NATURAL TREATMENTS

- Homeopathic treatment can be very effective for arthritis. Treatment will need to be undertaken on a constitutional basis. In the meantime, some of the following remedies may help:
  - Bryonia, for arthritis where stitching pains occur in swollen pale or red joints
  - Colchicum, when it is worse in warm weather, with inflamed joints that are sensitive to touch. Your child may feel irritable.
  - Rhododendron, when symptoms are worse in stormy weather
  - Rhus Tox. when symptoms include pain and stiffness, made worse after rest and in cold damp weather; symptoms improve with movement
  - Pulsatilla, when pain moves from one joint to another. Your child may be tearful.
  - Apis, for hot, stinging pain
- If your child was immunized, see a registered homeopath for postvaccination cleansing, which can reverse damage that may have been caused.
- Traditional Chinese medicine, which uses herbs and acupuncture to balance the body, has a good record of treating arthritis. In Chinese medicine the problem is considered to be caused by wind damp, with painful joints caused by wind cold. This basically means that parts of the body have become invaded by these elements, which can then be addressed.
- Herbs that work to heal arthritis include feverfew, meadowsweet, celery seed and white willow. They can be taken internally, or used externally, as required. It is a good idea to see a registered herbalist for specialist advice and blends that will address the cause in your individual child.
- Siberian ginseng is beneficial for rheumatoid arthritis.
- Lemon and cypress oils are detoxifying and can be used in the bath and in massage to help the body eliminate poisons. These are powerful oils

and not normally suitable for children, but if you use a tiny drop of each, they will help relieve symptoms in children over the age of six.

- Chamomile and lavender oils are anti-inflammatory and pain-relieving and can be used in local massage or compresses.
- Eucalyptus will improve the circulation in the area and reduce stiffness.
- There is some evidence to show that the antioxidants—Vitamins A, C and E, plus selenium—may have beneficial effects on arthritis. Vitamin C in particular is a powerful free radical destroyer that also aids in pain relief because of its anti-inflammatory effect. Ensure that your child has plenty in her diet, or consider a good supplement if not.
- Any immune condition can be exacerbated by a food allergy, so it's important that you take a good look at your child's diet as a first course of action (see page 344).
- Furthermore, any condition that is caused by the immune response can be improved and even cured by ensuring that your child's immune system is working at optimum level (see page 207).
- Consider whether your child could be suffering from leaky gut syndrome (see page 364), which is at the root of many autoimmune conditions.
- Research into the claim that evening primrose oil (see page 283) combats arthritis has been under way for some time. GLA is known to increase production of prostaglandins, which work to reduce inflammation. In one study,[8] 60 percent of patients given evening primrose oil were able to stop taking drugs completely, and a further 25 percent were able to halve their doses without any harmful effects.
- Fish oils may also be beneficial. Numerous studies have established the value of these supplements in reducing tender joints and morning stiffness in patients with rheumatoid arthritis.
- Bromelain is a digestive enzyme that helps to stimulate the production of prostaglandins, and it helps the body to digest proteins. It is available in supplement form (or in fresh pineapples), and is safe for children.
- Glucosamine is classified as an "amino sugar,"

involved in the formation of nails, tendons, skin, eyes, bones, ligaments and heart valves. It has been shown to be extremely helpful in the treatment of arthritis and many allergies, and is available in supplement form. It is safe for children, but should be taken only under the guidance of a registered practitioner.

- Avoid the nightshade vegetables (peppers, eggplant, tomatoes and white potatoes). These contain solanine, to which some people suffering from arthritis are highly sensitive. This chemical interferes with the enzymes in the muscles and may cause pain and discomfort.
- It is suggested that children with JRA take a free-form amino acid complex regularly to help repair tissue. Amino acids should, however, be taken only under the supervision of a registered practitioner.

SELF-HELP

- Exercise is essential for reducing pain and retarding joint deterioration. Choose activities that do not put stress on the affected joints, but that strengthen the surrounding bones, muscles and ligaments. Bicycle riding, walking, swimming and even soccer or dancing are good forms of exercise for children with JRA.
- Try to treat your child as normally as possible. It is tremendously difficult for children to accept that they are unable to do what other children are capable of doing, and it can be very depressing to suffer from a chronic health condition. Consider using some of the flower essences to encourage a positive approach to life.
- Consider joining a support group to give your child the opportunity to interact with other sufferers, and allow you to discuss problems and solutions with other parents.
- Talk to your child's teacher and make arrangements for your child to be helped from classes, or be allowed to leave a few minutes earlier than the others to ensure that she makes it to her next class on time.

LEAKY GUT SYNDROME

According to Dr. Zoltan P. Rona M.D., M.Sc., a Canadian doctor and expert on immunity, leaky gut syndrome is the suspected cause of many of the most common untreatable chronic conditions, and it can dramatically affect immunity. Leaky gut syndrome is a very common health disorder in which the intestinal lining is more permeable (porous) than normal. The abnormally large spaces present between the cells of the gut wall allow the entry of toxic material, such as bacteria, fungi, parasites and their toxins, undigested protein, fat and other waste, into the bloodstream that would, in healthier circumstances, be repelled and eliminated. Leaky gut syndrome is almost always associated with autoimmune disease, and reversing autoimmune disease depends on healing the lining of the gastrointestinal tract.

Autoimmune diseases occur when the immune system makes antibodies against its own tissues. Some of the diseases in this category include lupus, alopecia, rheumatoid arthritis, olymyalgia rheumatica, multiple sclerosis, fibromyalgia, chronic fatigue syndrome, Sjogren's syndrome, vitiligo, thyroditis, vasculitis, Crohn's disease, ulcerative colitis, urticaria (hives), diabetes and Raynaud's disease. Doctors are increasingly recognizing the importance of the gastrointestinal tract in the development of allergic or autoimmune disease.

Because of the spaces between the cells of the gut wall, larger than usual protein molecules are absorbed before they have a chance to be completely broken down as occurs when the intestinal lining is intact. The immune system starts making antibodies against these larger molecules because it recognizes them as foreign, invading substances. The immune system starts treating them as if they have to be destroyed. Antibodies are made against these proteins derived from previously harmless foods. It is believed that the antibodies created by the leaky gut phenomenon against these antigens can get into various tissues and trigger an inflammatory reaction when the corresponding food is consumed or the microbe is encountered. According to Dr. Rona, an expert on the syndrome, auto-antibodies are thus created and inflammation becomes chronic. If this inflammation occurs at a joint, autoimmune arthritis (rheumatoid arthritis) develops. If it occurs in the brain, myalgic encephalomyelitis (chronic fatigue syndrome) may be the result. If it occurs in the blood vessels, vasculitis (inflammation of the blood vessels) is the resulting autoimmune problem. If the antibodies start attacking the lining of the gut itself, the result may be colitis or Crohn's disease. If it occurs in the lungs, asthma is triggered on a delayed basis every time the individual consumes the food that triggered the production of the antibodies in the first place.

The inflammation that causes the leaky gut syndrome also damages the protective coating of the IgA family normally present in a healthy gut. Since IgA helps us ward off infections, with leaky gut problems we become less resistant to viruses, bacteria, parasites and candida.

In addition to the creation of food allergies by the leaky gut, the bloodstream is invaded by bacteria that can overwhelm the liver's ability to detoxify, and create a long list of mineral deficiencies because the various carrier proteins present in the gastrointestinal tract that are needed to transport minerals to the blood are damaged by the inflammation process.

Why is this important for children?

Autoimmune conditions are becoming increasingly common in children, and the number of cases of asthma, eczema, juvenile arthritis, allergies and bowel problems are on the rise.

What causes it?

The syndrome is caused by the inflammation of the gut lining, which can be brought about by the following:

- antibiotics, because they lead to the overgrowth of abnormal flora in the gastrointestinal tract (bacteria, parasites, candida, fungi)
- caffeine and many soft drinks, which are strong gut irritants and can be particularly dangerous for younger children

- chemicals in fermented and processed food (dyes, preservatives, peroxidized fats)
- enzyme deficiencies (e.g., celiac disease, lactase deficiency causing lactose intolerance)
- NSAIDS (nonsteroidal anti-inflammatory drugs, such as ibuprofen)
- prescription corticosteroids (e.g., prednisone)
- a highly refined carbohydrate diet (including chocolate bars, candy, cakes, biscuits, soft drinks and white bread)

Symptoms

- Many nutrients are poorly absorbed, leading to a host of mild deficiency symptoms (see page 286).
- The inflammation can cause swelling, and there may be bloating, gas and cramps.
- Constipation alternating with diarrhea is common (often diagnosed as IBS, or irritable bowel syndrome). It is interesting to note that in well over 80 percent of cases, IBS sufferers have an overgrowth of fungi, parasites or bacteria.
- Complaints like fatigue, headaches, memory problems, poor concentration or irritability often follow.
- Eventually symptoms of arthritis, migraines, eczema, asthma or other forms of immune dysfunction present themselves.

Conventional treatment

Leaky gut syndrome is not a widely recognized condition, and many doctors treat it symptomatically—in other words, they address the symptoms of the conditions as they occur. Common treatments include corticosteroids, prescription antibiotics and immunosuppressive drugs.

NATURAL TREATMENTS

- To reverse leaky gut syndrome it's crucial that you change your child's diet to one that is as hypoallergenic as possible. Sugar, white flour products, all gluten-containing grains (especially wheat, barley, oats and rye), milk and dairy products, high-fat foods, caffeine products and any other allergenic foods (determined by testing) must be eliminated for long periods of time (in children, it can take up to a year; in adults sometimes longer).
- According to Dr. Rona, natural antibiotics, such as echinacea and garlic, are extremely important; antiparasitics, such as cloves and black walnut, may be offered; and natural antifungal agents such as grapefruit seed extract might be appropriate, depending on the type of infection that shows up in tests.
- Experts suggest that your child should chew food more thoroughly, and eat small, frequent meals.
- Gastrointestinal function can be improved with supplements like lactobacillus acidophilus and bifidus.
- Natural digestive enzymes are indicated (bromelain or papain are safe for children), and aloe vera juice can also help a great deal.
- Some natural therapists may use amino acids, such as glutamine, but this should not be undertaken at home.
- Essential fatty acids, including flaxseed oil and evening primrose oil, as well as fish oil and blackcurrant seed oil, will help a great deal.
- All of the antioxidant nutrients (including Co-Q10, see page 285) will help to heal some of the damage done.
- Some experts recommend green foods, such as spirulina or blue-green algae (see page 285), for their concentrated nutrient content. These will help to ensure that basic nutrient needs are met to help the body function better.

If you suspect that your child may be suffering from leaky gut syndrome, the most important thing is to have him tested by a natural health practitioner, and by your doctor. If your doctor is reluctant to consider the possibility that your child may suffer from this condition, find one who will. There are many tests that can assess gut permeability, and most of them are not invasive. Put your child in the hands of an experienced natural practitioner, such as a naturopath, or a good nutritional therapist with a knowledge of herbs and other products.

LICE

Head lice is an infestation of tiny insects that bite the skin to feed from the blood. These parasites lay their eggs, which are visible as tiny gray dots, on the hair shafts. Head and body lice are itchy and are highly contagious. They are a common problem among schoolchildren and seem especially to like clean hair.

Conventional treatment

A shampoo, purchased from your pharmacist, will be suggested to deal with the problem, but wash all towels, clothing and bedding in boiling hot water, and disinfect combs and hair brushes after treatment. There is some evidence that treatments containing organophosphate (permethrin) can cause some neurological damage in a small percentage of children, so it is worth consulting your doctor before purchasing anything.

NATURAL TREATMENTS

- Blend some lavender, tea tree and eucalyptus oils in some warmed olive oil, and apply to your child's head. Leave overnight, and rinse off in the morning. Apply every 48 hours as required. This works as a strong insecticide, and also helps to prevent infestation.
- Alternatively, add a few drops of tea tree oil to your child's conditioner. Leave on for an hour or so, and then comb through the hair carefully with a fine-toothed comb. Add tea tree oil to your child's rinse water as a preventive method when nits are about.
- Children who are prone to nits may benefit from a single dose of the homeopathic remedy psorinum, at 30C dilution.

Useful therapies

Aromatherapy, herbalism, homeopathy.

MEASLES

Measles is a highly infectious disease caused by a virus that is normally inhaled. The incubation period is about 14 days, and just before the rash appears, spots can be seen in the mouth. It begins like a cold, with runny nose or cough, then a fever and occasionally conjunctivitis occurs. Fever tends to become high as the rash comes out. The rash is characterized by flat, brown-red spots, which begin usually behind the ears and on the face. The lymph nodes will become swollen and there will be little or no appetite, perhaps vomiting and diarrhea. Measles spots are not itchy, but your child will feel profoundly unwell. Complications of measles include pneumonia, middle ear infections and bronchitis, and in rare cases encephalitis.

Conventional treatment

Fever is generally controlled with acetaminophen, and plenty of liquids should be taken. Antibiotics are not prescribed for the measles itself, but may be necessary if any additional complications develop. In the unlikely event of encephalitis, a brain infection that may occur secondarily, strong antiviral drugs may be used in hospital. In the U.K. and the U.S., children are routinely offered the combined MMR (measles, mumps, rubella) vaccine between the ages of 12 and 24 months (see page 213).

NATURAL TREATMENTS

If you have decided not to immunize your child against measles, it is important that you take him to a good homeopath, who will offer Morbillinum, a nosode that works to reduce the harmful effects of the condition. This is particularly important if you believe that your child has been in contact with someone with measles.

It is also important to note that natural practitioners often see measles as an important illness, in that it is one of the best ways for your child's body to expel toxins. Indeed, the severity of the condition may reflect your child's toxicity. Chinese practitioners in particular see measles as a "transition" disease, in which children mature on an emotional and physical level. Many parents comment that their children seem to change after a bout of measles.

Some children will have mild cases, and others will become seriously ill. The best way to help your child is to offer consistent natural treatments, and it is advised that you stay in close contact with a registered practitioner throughout. Although complications are rare, they can occur, and you need to be in good hands.

- On a preventive basis, all children should be given the best chance of fighting any infection by having a strong immune system. From an early age, you should take steps to boost your child's immunity, particularly when she is under stress, a little run-down, following illnesses, including colds and coughs, and during the cold and flu season.
- During the condition itself, offer garlic and echinacea (see page 207) to improve the action of the immune system and to act as antiviral agents.
- Catmint and yarrow can be sipped as teas to bring down fever and ease discomfort. Elderflower is also useful.
- Add chamomile or marigold to the bath water to calm and soothe your child.
- A compress of crushed ginger (heat it a little to make it less powerful, and wrap it in several layers of gauze to protect skin) may be used to help encourage the toxins to be released from the body.
- Homeopathic remedies are appropriate for measles, but you may want to talk to a good homeopath about the best remedies for your child. In the mean time, consider:
  - Aconite and Belladonna for high fever
  - Pulsatilla when there is diarrhea, yellow discharge and a cough
  - Bryonia when there is a hard, painful cough and a high temperature accompanied by thirst
  - Stramonium when there is a high fever, a red face and convulsions
- Flower essences will also help. Bach Rescue Remedy (see page 260) can be used to ease distress and discomfort. Rub Rescue Remedy cream into sore skin. Cherry plum, hornbeam and chicory are suggested for all childhood illnesses.

- A few drops of Roman chamomile in the bath will ease symptoms and help encourage sleep.
- Lavender oil can be dropped on the bedclothes or on a tissue by the bed to calm. It can also be applied neat to spots, to encourage healing.
- When there is a buildup of phlegm, and other symptoms of a cold, a gentle chest massage with a few drops of tea tree oil in a light carrier oil base will help.
- Essential oil of eucalyptus, tea tree or chamomile can be used in a vaporizer.

Useful therapies

Nutritional therapies, homeopathy, herbalism, Ayurveda, traditional Chinese medicine, flower essences, aromatherapy, reflexology.

SELF-HELP

- Offer plenty of fresh water to encourage flushing of toxins, and to prevent dehydration, particularly in the case of fever.
- Acidophilus should be taken following the illness, to encourage the healthy bacteria in the gut.
- Keep your child in a darkened room. Many children are sensitive to bright light during measles, and there have been cases of eye damage caused by the condition. This measure helps to prevent eye damage.
- Spend plenty of time with your child, offering reassurance and comfort (see page 225).
- If your child is not hungry, don't force him to eat. Offer nutritious, highly diluted blends of fresh juices (fruit and vegetables) and simple foods like mashed ripe bananas, stewed unsweetened apples and oatmeal.
- Don't be tempted to send him back to school too early. Your child will be very run-down after this condition, and will need time to get his strength back. Offer plenty of healthy, restorative foods during this period to boost nutrient levels and help the healing process.

CAUTION
If fever recurs several days after the spots have begun to heal, see your doctor.

MENINGITIS

Meningitis is an infection of the lining of the brain (menges) and is a serious condition that must be identified and treated quickly. It affects people of all ages, but is most common in preschool children. Meningitis can be caused by several different viruses or bacteria. The outcome can vary from a mild infection, which clears up after a few days' illness, to a serious and frequently fatal condition. If meningitis is suspected, it is important to contact a doctor immediately.

Meningitis can occur in perfectly healthy people. However, if your child is run-down, has a condition that suppresses immune activity, has had a trauma to the head causing skull fracture, or suffers from any inflammation or infection of organs near brain (the ear, for example), she may be more susceptible. The viruses and bacteria that cause meningitis are commonly found in the throat and may cause infections there. If these organisms get into the blood, they can travel to the brain where they may cause meningitis. These organisms are common, and they rarely cause life-threatening infections. The bacteria and viruses that cause meningitis are spread through the air or by close contact, such as kissing. Other rarer types of meningitis can be caused by fungi and parasites; however, these usually occur only in people whose immune systems are suppressed. Viral meningitis, which accounts for about half of meningitis infections, often causes a mild illness and is not usually life threatening, although in a small proportion of people, the illness is severe. Bacterial meningitis is a severe and life-threatening illness. Your child will become extremely unwell and may die within a matter of hours if treatment is not immediate. However, if the infection is treated early, the chances of survival and recovery are good.

All parents should be aware of the symptoms of meningitis in children of all ages.

In older children, look for:
- Fever
- Neck stiffness (your child may find it hard or painful to bend her neck forward)
- Headache, which may be severe
- Photophobia (sensitivity to light)
- Vomiting
- Drowsiness
- A patchy rash that does not turn white when pressed (press down a clear glass over the rash; if it remains red, chances are your child has meningitis)
- These symptoms often develop rapidly over a period of hours

In babies and very young children the early symptoms of meningitis are not specific. They include:
- Fever
- Irritability, which may be made worse by holding or hugging
- Loss of appetite
- Vomiting
- Unusual lethargy or sleepiness
- Resisting bending her neck, even if you try to encourage her to look down or up

Later, babies and young children with meningitis may have seizures. In babies, the fontanels (the spaces between the bones of the baby's skull) may bulge or feel tense to the touch.

If you suspect meningitis, call an ambulance immediately and make it clear that you believe your child has the condition.

Conventional treatment

The treatment for bacterial meningitis is antibiotics given directly into the vein. A drip is usually employed to keep your child well hydrated. Viral meningitis does not usually require specific treatment, over and above bed rest, fluids and pain killers, although antiviral medication may be required. Children are now offered vaccines against two types of meningitis (see page 223).

NATURAL TREATMENTS

Don't consider meningitis to be anything other than a medical emergency. No matter how natural you have managed to make your family, this is one occasion where conventional help is not only required but also essential. You can, however, use many natural treatments alongside conventional drugs to help your child to heal.

- After you have called an ambulance, you can offer the following homeopathic remedies:
  - Arnica for symptoms arising after a head injury
  - Aconite for restlessness, fear and great thirst
  - Bryonia for a severe headache, made worse by eye movement
  - Belladonna for staring eyes, delirium and fever
- An experienced homeopath will also be able to supply other remedies to help your child through the illness. Don't consider using them as a substitute for conventional medicine.
- Offer Bach Rescue Remedy (see page 260) (apply to the temples or moisten the lips if your child is very young, delirious or unconscious) to help your child's body overcome the trauma it is undergoing.
- When your child is on the mend, use one or two of the herbs suggested on page 231. Remember that your child will be very fragile following this illness, and you should not bombard her system with too many remedies—natural or not. The best idea would probably be to stick with a good homeopath, who can offer different remedies as the condition changes.
- Use flower essences to boost her emotional health (see page 254), which will affect her recovery.
- Use some gentle essential oils, such as Roman chamomile or lavender in a vaporizer in your child's room to calm and encourage good, restful sleep.
- Above all, no matter how serious your child's con-

dition, try to remain as calm as possible while you are with her. She will need your reassuring presence, and it is important that she not pick up on any anxiety, which can make things much worse. Use any of the herbs suggested for stress yourself, including Bach Rescue Remedy (see page 260) for the shock and trauma.

Remember that a child who has a strong immune system, and a healthy, balanced lifestyle will be much less likely to succumb to meningitis. The best medicine is always prevention.

MIGRAINE

Migraine in children is much more common than you might think, and it can be as debilitating for them as it is for adults. In fact, it can be worse, in that they may feel very frightened and confused by the symptoms and the accompanying pain. The classic feature of a migraine headache is pain on one side of the head only. This is caused by the narrowing and dilating of the blood vessels to a part of one side of the brain. An attack may last for up to two days in adults, but they are usually shorter in children.

Migraine can be hereditary, but may also be triggered by many other factors including stress, menstruation (particularly in adolescent girls), food allergies and intolerance (see page 344), as well as foods that are not normally suspect. These are foods that contain tyramine, an amino acid that affects the blood vessels; foods rich in tyramine include bananas, cheese, chocolate, eggs, oranges, spinach and tomatoes. Other triggers include stress, hormonal changes (in adolescence, for example), and changes or extremes in temperature, lighting or noise level.

There are two main types of migraine, common and classical. A common migraine consists mainly of a headache and perhaps one or two other symptoms (see below), but not visual disturbance. A classical migraine is preceded by an aura, which is a warning of what is to come. An aura generally takes the form of a visual disturbance, or a strange feeling, almost a second sense. The visual disturbance, which may consist of focusing problems, blind spots or flashing lights, is often accompanied by speech problems and occasionally weakness or temporary paralysis of the limbs or extremities. Migraine occurs in about 10 percent of people, and is more common in women and girls, although it is increasing in young boys, particularly those who are competitive and push themselves hard.

Common symptoms include:

- severe headache, usually confined to one side of the head (but not always)
- nausea and vomiting
- blurred vision
- other visual disturbances
- intolerance to light
- numbness and tingling in the arms

Some children suffer from abdominal migraine, which is characterized by periodic attacks of abdominal pain. The child will become very pale and want to lie down. There may be nausea and vomiting, and even a high temperature. The condition is often caused by stress or periods of emotional upset.

Conventional treatment

During an attack, vasoconstrictors, antihistamines and antiemetics may be suggested to minimize the symptoms. Alternatively, combinations of other drugs can be offered long term to prevent attacks.

NATURAL TREATMENTS

- Homeopathic treatment can be dramatic in the long run, but in order to address the root cause it will need to be constitutional. The following remedies may help during an attack:
  - The best first remedy is Aconite, if symptoms come on suddenly, particularly if they are worse after exposure to cold
  - Then offer Belladonna, which is most useful if your child is red-faced and staring
  - Pulsatilla for migraines that seem to be worse in the evening, and aggravated by rich or fatty foods. Your child may be tearful, and not thirsty.

- Thuja for a left-sided headache, with the sensation of a nail being drilled into the skull
- Lycopodium for pain that is worse on the right side, and painful temples and dizziness. This is a good remedy for many children.
- Nat. Mur. when the headache is blinding, and throbs, is worse for warmth and movement, and the attack was preceded by numbness around the mouth and nose

- Consider cranial osteopathy, or osteopathy to adjust the temperomandibular joint in the jaw, which can help a large number of sufferers.
- Feverfew is an effective remedy for reducing the frequency of migraine. Give your child two or three small leaves, between slices of fresh bread daily. Pills are also available, but watch the dosage for children.
- Peppermint and lavender oils, applied to the forehead and the base of the neck as a cool compress, will help to relieve symptoms.
- A dab of lavender oil, at the base of the nostrils, can be used at the first signs of an attack. It will help to ease symptoms and allow the child to relax. Some children are extremely sensitive to smells during an attack, so if your child objects vehemently, give it a miss.

Useful therapies

Osteopathy, cranial osteopathy, Ayurveda, herbalism, homeopathy, reflexology, nutritional therapies, aromatherapy and any of the therapies suggested for stress (see page 386) might help.

MOLLUSCUM CONTAGIOSUM

These very small skin-covered warts are easily spread from one skin area to another through contact, hence the name "contagiosum". These smooth-topped warts are almost always grouped together, perhaps on the side of the chest with another grouping on the skin of the inner arm where it has had repeated contact with the warts on the chest. While they may spread quickly and become fairly widely distributed, the cure is often worse than the problem. Since recent studies show that molluscum contagiosum eventually disappears on its own, you may want to choose to wait it out. You may also be interested to know that molluscum has become more common in recent years, and has been linked with the MMR vaccine.

Conventional treatment

When there are relatively few warts a corrosive medication works well with a minimum of discomfort. Other treatments include cutting them away with a sharp curette or burning them off with an electric needle.

NATURAL TREATMENTS

- It's important to remember that molluscum is cosmetic, and there is no point in going for aggressive conventional treatment unless your child is in discomfort or embarrassed by the warts. Many natural therapies will work to address the root cause, balancing your child's system so that he fights off the virus himself. In all cases the treatment should be undertaken by an experienced practitioner, who can look at the whole picture. Constitutional homeopathy treatment, herbalism and traditional Chinese medicine are extremely effective.
- The homeopathic remedy Thuja is ideal for this type of wart. Offer it twice a day for several weeks.
- Paint the spots with tea tree and lavender oils (one drop of each, diluted in vitamin E oil) after bathing every day.
- Bach Rescue Remedy cream (see page 260) can help with any warts that become inflamed and painful.

Useful therapies

Homeopathy, herbalism, aromatherapy, traditional Chinese medicine, acupuncture and any of the therapies that boost immunity (see page 208).

SELF-HELP

- This condition is amazingly contagious, but it will affect only children with a predisposition to it. Some parents can bathe children together for the duration of the warts without it being passed on. In other families, all children come down with it, and it can be notoriously difficult to cure. To be on the safe side, bathe your children separately. Use different towels and face cloths, and put a drop of tea tree oil in each child's bath on a nightly basis.
- Take steps to boost your child's immune system to help reduce the duration of the condition.

MOUTH ULCERS

Mouth ulcers are white, gray or yellow open sores with an outer ring of red inflammation that can appear on the inside of the lips, cheeks or sometimes at the base of the gums. In children, they are often a sign of being run-down, accidentally biting the side of the mouth, eating hot food, or eating too many candies or sweet foods. In some cases children who have the virus that causes cold sores will get mouth ulcers instead, and when they are older, cold sores may appear in periods of stress or ill health (see page 315). In some cases mouth ulcers can be a feature of digestive conditions, such as Crohn's disease.

Conventional treatment

This will be based on rectifying the cause. Dietary changes may be suggested, as well as gargling with salt water.

NATURAL TREATMENTS

- To prevent attacks in susceptible children, keep your child's diet as pure and varied as possible, including plenty of fresh, whole foods. Avoid strong spices, which can irritate the delicate lining of the mouth, and processed or refined foods, carbonated soft drinks, caffeine and refined sugar. Acidic foods, such as oranges, and foods that contain arginine (chocolate, peanuts, coconut, oats, wheat and gelatin) should be avoided.
- Keep your child's immune system strong (see page 207). If an attack does occur, offer immune-boosting herbs, such as astragalus, echinacea and garlic. Other herbs, including nettles, yellow dock

and burdock, help with the elimination of toxins. The latter are available as teas.

- Tincture of myrrh can be added to a cup of cooled boiled water and used as a mouth rinse to destroy infection or infestation. Use the tincture neat and apply to sores in the mouth with a cotton swab.
- Rub a little aloe vera gel into the affected area.
- For recurrent ulcers, constitutional homeopathic treatment is indicated. For attacks, try:
  - Arsenicum when ulcers are on the edges of the tongue, with burning pains
  - Mercurius when ulcers are on the palate or tongue, and are yellow and spongy
  - Kali. Bich. when the ulcers feel thick and firm, and sting

Useful therapies

Any of the therapies that boost immunity and help your child to cope with stress (see page 386) are appropriate. If the cause is dietary, nutritional therapies will be the best course of action. Recurrent mouth ulcers will respond to homeopathy, herbalism, Ayurveda, reflexology, aromatherapy and traditional Chinese medicine.

MUMPS

Mumps are a viral infection, usually affecting children and causing fever and swelling of the main salivary glands, the parotids. This swelling produces the characteristic chipmunk appearance. The condition rarely occurs in children under two or three years of age, and takes about two to three weeks to incubate. It is infectious for a day before the glands begin to swell until about a week after they have gone down. Symptoms include a general malaise, and then a fever with headache and pains around the neck. Swallowing will be painful.

Conventional treatment

Fluids, acetaminophen for the pain and fever, and rest. Complete resolution is usual in a week or two. Children are now offered a vaccine to protect against measles, mumps and rubella (MMR vaccine) between the ages of 12 and 24 months (see page 213).

NATURAL TREATMENTS

- To help resolve the infection and any fever, offer garlic and echinacea, combined with yarrow and peppermint (which can be taken as a tea, sweetened with honey or blackcurrant juice).
- There are herbs that can help to reduce the congestion and swelling, including red clover and marigold. You can add tinctures of these to any drink, or offer as a tea. Poke root is also good.
- Very, very gently massage the neck and jaw with one drop each of chamomile, eucalyptus and lavender oils in about six tablespoons of olive oil. It might help to gently warm the oil first. Use these same oils in a vaporizer or steam inhalation.
- Offer plenty of fresh fruit and vegetable juices to cleanse. If your child finds it difficult to swallow, use a straw or freeze juices as popsicles that can be sucked.
- If the temperature is high, use tepid water to sponge the child down, adding an infusion of chamomile to calm.
- If your child has not had mumps, the homeopathic remedies Phytolacca or Parotidium can be taken during an epidemic to reduce severity of symptoms. If he does succumb, try:
  - Rhus Tox. when the left glands are more severely affected than the right
  - Belladonna when there is high fever, shooting pains, and a bright red face and throat
  - Merc. Sol. when there is heavy sweating and a coated tongue
  - Pulsatilla to help prevent orchitis, and is useful if fever continues
- Bach Rescue Remedy (see page 260) can be used to ease distress and discomfort. Rub a little into the pulse points, or drop some into a warm bath. Cherry Plum, Hornbeam and Chicory are suggested for all childhood illnesses.

Useful therapies

Homeopathy, herbalism, traditional Chinese medicine, Ayurveda, nutritional therapies, aromatherapy.

NAUSEA AND VOMITING

Nausea (a feeling of sickness) and vomiting are symptoms of various disorders including gastroenteritis, inner ear infection, migraine, overeating (especially the wrong kinds of foods), and many, many other causes. A constant feeling of nausea with no vomiting, but with a headache and abdominal pain, is most likely to be stress- or anxiety-related. A raised temperature can also cause vomiting in some children, and food poisoning may be at the root. Many children also vomit when they have colds or coughs (due to excess mucus). These conditions are not usually serious, unless they recur. Remember that babies and children can dehydrate quickly, and you must ensure that they drink plenty of liquids.

Whatever the cause, the treatment is initially the same—simple solids and fluid replacement. The best fluid replacement is fresh, clean water. If your child can't keep anything down, and seems to have diarrhea or to be suffering from dehydration, you can make your own fluid replacement. This is a mixture of clean water (2 cups/500 ml), sugar (one tablespoonful/15 ml) and salt (one or two pinches). Flavoring such as lemon-barley juice, or blackcurrant, may be added if your child refuses to drink without it. When the first batch has been drunk, another should be prepared. If this gets vomited, sips rather than a cupful should be offered . In this way the stomach can usually be persuaded to keep some down. Babies may be offered full-strength or half-strength milk.

If the vomiting has not stopped after 24 hours, the starvation needs to be continued for a further 24 hours. When feeding is restarted, it is wise to begin with a quarter of a slice of dry toast (no butter), then to wait for an hour. If it stays down, more can be offered. Then a small quantity of another food can be tried, followed by a further hour's wait. If a food causes vomiting, revert to the foods that were safe. If they cause vomiting as well, return to starvation and fluids.

Conventional treatment

Your doctor will probably suggest fluid replacement (see above), or if the condition is serious, your child may be admitted to hospital. In severe cases, antiemetic drugs will be prescribed.

If you are concerned about her vomiting, or it has no recognizable cause (an accompanying fever or excess mucus, for example), contact your doctor immediately.

NATURAL TREATMENTS

- The essential oils of peppermint or lavender can be used in a vaporizer and inhaled to alleviate nausea and vomiting.
- Make a cup of very weak blackcurrant or chamomile tea and offer to your child in small sips after it has cooled. This will help to soothe the digestive tract and boost the immune system.
- Chewing a little fresh ginger, or weak ginger tea, will help to settle the stomach, and is particularly useful for travel sickness.
- Homeopathic treatment can be very effective. If your child seems to suffer from nausea or vomiting on a regular basis, constitutional treatment is indicated. These remedies will help for acute attacks:
  - Arsenicum, for when nausea and vomiting are accompanied by diarrhea and symptoms seem to be worse between midnight and 2 A.M. Your child may be thirsty for small sips of water.

- Nux Vom., when nausea is made better by vomiting, and may be caused by overindulgence (after a party, for example)
- Tabacum, for nausea and vomiting relieved by uncovering the abdomen. This is a good one for travel sickness.
- Phosphorus, for cravings for cold water, which is then vomited, and burning pains in the stomach
- Pulsatilla, for vomiting after rich fatty food, with tearfulness
- Arnica, when vomiting follows a head injury
- Aconite, when vomiting and severe pain last for more than an hour, and pain is not relieved by vomiting

- Bach Rescue Remedy (see page 260) will be useful for prolonged or distressing vomiting; it will help to reduce panic and clam the mind and body. Holly or Beech may help if the vomiting is linked to emotional problems.
- Chamomile and vervain can be taken internally to soothe a child whose illness is exacerbated or caused by emotional upset, or who is distressed by the vomiting.
- Chamomile, echinacea, peppermint and thyme can be drunk as infusions, or added to a footbath when there is infection at the root of the illness.
- Massage the tummy and chest with a few drops of lavender or chamomile in a light carrier oil.
- Use essential oil of thyme or tea tree in a vaporizer for their antiseptic properties. A few drops of lavender in the bath or by the bedside will calm.
- Following an attack of vomiting or diarrhea, offer lots of live yogurt and very ripe bananas to restore the bacterial balance of the gut. An acidophilus pill, which comes in a vanilla flavor, can be taken for the same purpose.

Useful therapies

Homeopathy, herbalism, aromatherapy, traditional Chinese medicine, reflexology, Ayurveda, nutritional therapies.

NIGHT TERRORS (see Sleep and wakefulness)

NITS (see Lice)

OBESITY

We discussed obesity at length in chapter 3, and it should be clear that obesity in children is normally caused by a poor diet or overeating. There can be emotional problems at the root of this condition, and these need to be addressed if your child is to develop healthy eating habits in the long term. The causes of obesity in adults are not normally relevant to children, but in rare cases the following can affect weight: metabolic problems, digestive disorders, endocrine problems or side effects of certain drugs. Your doctor will advise you if there is a medical root to the problem.

Conventional treatment

Most doctors will suggest dietary changes, and will keep an eye on the problem. It is unusual for drugs to be prescribed for children.

NATURAL TREATMENTS

- Brewer's yeast will help to reduce cravings for food and drink, which may be helpful if your child is voraciously hungry all the time.
- Chromium supplements will help to ensure that your child's blood sugar levels are stable, and it also helps to regulate appetite. Do not offer these unless under the supervision of a registered nutritional therapist.
- Constitutional homeopathic treatment is most appropriate for all cases of excess weight, but some of the following remedies might be useful:
  - Graphites, if your child suffers from constipation and skin problems, and feels cold
  - Kali Carb., if your child has catarrh
  - Ferrum, if your child is oversensitive and flushes easily

- Capsicum, if your child tends to be lazy, has a red face and suffers from burning sensations in the digestive tract
- If your child's weight problem has an emotional basis, try flower essences. For example, Elm can be useful if your child feels inadequate or overwhelmed. Gentian may help if your child is pessimistic and easily discouraged. Larch is good for children who need to believe in themselves, and suffer from poor confidence and self-esteem.
- Uplifting aromatherapy oils, such as lavender or rosemary in a vaporizer, can help your child if she feels sluggish and even a bit depressed.

Useful therapies

Acupuncture, homeopathy, herbalism, aromatherapy, flower essences, reflexology, Ayurveda, massage, traditional Chinese medicine, nutritional therapies (the latter being probably the most effective).

PNEUMONIA

Pneumonia is an infection of the lung caused by bacteria or viruses, which enter the lungs via the upper respiratory tract, leading to inflammation of the lung tissue. There are two main types of the disease: bronchopneumonia, which is usually confined to areas of tissue surrounding the bronchi; and lobar pneumonia, which affects a whole lobe (or more) of the lung.

Inflammation and infection are normally caused by a virus or bacteria, although it can rarely involve a fungus, or be caused by inhaling irritating vapors or chemicals. In children pneumonia occurs following another respiratory infection, such as colds, flu, bronchitis or whooping cough, or after measles (bronchopneumonia). It is more likely to occur after illnesses when your child has not recovered completely, or rested sufficiently throughout the course of the illness, and it can also follow treatments that have suppressed the body's natural healing mechanism (cough suppressants or antihistamines, for example).

Lobar pneumonia can occur suddenly without warning, and in older children when there is no other infection. Normally one or more lobes of the lung are affected, usually by pneumococcus bacteria. When both lungs are affected, your child has "double pneumonia."

Some children are more prone to respiratory problems like pneumonia, and in others it can be the result of a consistently poor diet, lack of fresh air and exercise, pollution, passive smoking, or if your child is chronically ill and taking drugs regularly.

Symptoms can include rapid, shallow breathing; chest pain; sore throat and headache; cough with mucus (occasionally bloody); a dry cough, which becomes moister and more productive; high fever, sweating; shivering and a general feeling of malaise.

Conventional treatment

This is aimed at the cause. Bacterial pneumonia is treated with antibiotics, while antiviral drugs will be given for the viral form of the disease. Acetaminophen may be given to reduce fever, and, in severe cases, oxygen therapy or artificial ventilation may be required. Pneumonia is an emergency, and medical attention should be sought.

NATURAL TREATMENTS

- Constitutional homeopathic treatment is necessary after and during the illness, but the following remedies may help in a case of mild pneumonia:
  - Aconite, for sudden onset with anxiety and fever
  - Bryonia, for sharp chest pains worse for movement
  - Sanguinaria, for pneumonia after flu, with right lung affected and rust-colored phlegm
  - Phosphorus, for rust-colored phlegm, weakness, trembling and thirst for cold drinks
- Use a variety of herbs to boost your child's immune system (see page 207), to ensure that he fights the condition. This will also help prevent complications from developing.
- Try an infusion of coltsfoot, which soothes coughs and helps to fight infections—particularly respiratory infections. This may be quite strong-tasting for young children, but you can dilute it and add

it to a favorite juice. Blackcurrant is a good choice, as it has its own healing properties.

- Ginseng is a great all-around restorer and will help to bring down body temperature and fight infection.
- A steam inhalation of eucalyptus and tea tree oils will aid breathing, open lungs and help to fight infection.
- Massage (but not when there is fever) with niaouli and lavender can be used to fight infection and ease symptoms.
- Bach Rescue Remedy (see page 260) can be rubbed into your child's pulse points if he is distressed. Take some yourself if you are concerned.

Useful therapies

Homeopathy, herbalism, aromatherapy, reflexology, nutritional therapy, traditional Chinese medicine, acupuncture; all of these can be used alongside conventional medication, should that be required.

SELF-HELP

- When your child is on the road to recovery, offer plenty of fresh live yogurt to rebalance the flora in the gut (see page 284). An acidophilus pill should also be taken daily for some weeks.
- Offer a good multivitamin and mineral supplement throughout the course of the illness and afterward.
- Avoid mucus-producing foods (such as milk or wheat) during the infection, and for several weeks afterward. Give only light foods, with no milk or meat, except chicken. Give plenty of fresh vegetables and fruit, plus soups, juices and whole rice.

> ### CAUTION
> Seek urgent medical attention if pneumonia is suspected.

RASHES AND SPOTS

In a small baby, a rash on the body is often heat rash, as babies have ill-formed sweat glands. The rash disappears on cooling down. Rashes in children are very common, most of them being caused by acute viral illnesses or allergies (see page 301). Most of the viral rashes are accompanied by a fever, loss of appetite and malaise, although some (such as rubella) are not.

Many rashes have a typical appearance, such as sparse, itchy blisters in a spot of red skin (chicken pox). Others produce a generalized, nonspecific rash, frequently mimicking rubella (German measles). Eczema has its own characteristic rash as do dermatitis and urticaria, so these can be ruled out fairly easily. Some babies come out in a rash when they are upset, but these should subside as quickly as they arise.

Conventional treatment

Calamine lotion may soothe itchy rashes; acetaminophen is useful if they are accompanied by a fever. Your doctor may prescribe antibiotics if there is a risk of infection from scratching, or if there is a bacterial cause.

NATURAL TREATMENTS

Treatments are aimed at the cause, rather than being simply palliative. Consider the cause first: food allergies (see page 344); other allergies (see page 301); eczema (see page 337); one of the infectious diseases affecting children, such as measles or rubella (see page 366 and 351); heat; fever; emotional causes; diaper rash (see page 325) or a virus.

- Apply calendula cream to the affected area, to encourage healing and soothe inflamed or itchy skin.
- Bach Rescue Remedy cream (see page 260) soothes sore and itchy skin, and encourages the healing process.
- Add a handful of chamomile flower, or a drop or two of Roman chamomile oil, to your child's bath, to ease the symptoms.

- For viral infections causing rashes, use tea tree oil in a vaporizer in your child's room, or add a drop to her bath.
- For rashes brought on by emotion, any of the remedies suggested for stress will be appropriate. Or try one of the flower essences listed on page 254. Rock Rose, for example, might be good for terror or panic, and it will also help with accidents or sudden illness. Olive is good if your child is exhausted and run-down.
- There are a variety of good homeopathic remedies that can help. If your child suffers from rashes frequently, get some constitutional treatment from a good homeopath. Otherwise, try Belladonna for a rash that comes on with a fever, particularly if your child has flushed skin and staring eyes. Rhus Tox. is good when the skin is itchy with little blisters.
- In all cases, take steps to boost your child's immune system (see page 207).

Useful therapies

Homeopathy, herbalism, flower essences, aromatherapy, traditional Chinese medicine, reflexology, Ayurveda, nutritional therapies.

SCHOOL PHOBIAS AND TRAUMA

As dramatic as it may sound, school phobia is quite common in children and adolescents, and there can be a variety of reasons for this condition. First of all, young children may have a negative experience that they build up in their minds to be something traumatic. They associate school with trauma, even if it is on a subconscious basis, and no amount of rational discussion will sway them.

Consider whether there has been a traumatic event in your child's life—a parental divorce or the loss of a loved one can have a dramatic effect on your child's emotional health (see page 170).

Usually a school phobia masks something else, and the negative emotions surrounding whatever is causing the upset can translate themselves into headaches, abdominal pains, nausea and vomiting, and even fainting. Symptoms are normally worse on weekday mornings, better at weekends and during holidays. If there is any tension in the family, your child may feel that he needs to stay at home to prevent something terrible from happening (a fight, a divorce, violence or whatever he may have conjured up). For children who lack confidence, find schoolwork difficult, or have problems with their peers, home is the safest place to be, and they are right to head toward safety.

Never underestimate your child's concerns or fears. There may be a serious problem at school affecting his emotional health, or it may be something simple that has affected your child more dramatically than perhaps it should have done. Whether or not you consider a problem to be valid is irrelevant. If it is enough to cause your child to become upset, and to manifest physical symptoms, something has to be done about it.

What to do if your child has school phobia

- School phobia is not a medical condition, but it will affect your child's health. The most important thing you can do is to get to the bottom of it. Spend as much time as you can with your child talking things through. It may be that he is too traumatized or upset to talk about it, or he may be vaguely embarrassed or ashamed of his concerns. He may not even be able to pinpoint what the problem is—there may just be a general feeling of unhappiness and fear, or self-consciousness. Choose different times of the day for chats, and use personal examples to lead into discussions. For example, you can recount a childhood experience that upset you greatly. Children respond well to comparisons because it helps them believe that they are not weird or unusual.
- Talk to your child's teacher and, if necessary, other classmates, to find out what is wrong, and then work out a solution. If your child is being bullied, for example, the school will need to put a stop to it. Try inviting one of the bullies over, and see if the problem stops. Most bullies are insecure and feel emotionally threatened. If you change the nature of the relationship, chances are it will be resolved.

- Consider some of the flower essences (see page 254). For example, Mimulus is for the everyday fears of known things (school, other children, sports, teachers—anything). Aspen is for the vague and dark fears that play on the imagination. Rock Rose should be added when the fear is turning into terror and perhaps panic. Cherry Plum is for the fear that everything will fall apart (particularly useful if your child thinks he needs to be at home because he imagines that his presence is required) and Red Chestnut is for fear for others' safety. The most important Bach flower remedy for fear, anxiety and phobias is Rescue Remedy.
- Essential oils can be very useful in the treatment of school phobias. The effect of certain smells can help to release tension and induce a feeling of calm. Some of the best oils to try are chamomile, geranium, jasmine (for older children), lavender and ylang ylang, which are sedatives. They can be used in the bath, in massage with a light carrier oil (such as sweet almond), or in a vaporizer.
- A school phobia (or indeed any type of phobia) should be treated constitutionally by a good homeopath, but some of the best remedies are:
  - Arnica, when fears are brought on by an obvious trauma or accident
  - Argentum nit., when your child finds it difficult to concentrate, lacks self-confidence and cannot explain why school is so terrifying. He may suffer diarrhea.
  - Lycopodium helps children who are frightened or worried about new situations. They will feel insecure and may perhaps show off to compensate.
  - Gelsemium, for children who are tired and shaky, and who seem to dread things like speaking in front of a class of other children
  - Nat. mur., when your child is afraid to use the school toilets, and fears having an accident
- Watch your child's diet. If it is high in refined and processed foods, or if there is too much sugar, he may become more highly strung and sensitive to new situations.

- Also ensure that your child is getting enough restful sleep (see page 117), which can affect his emotions.
- Valerian tea, sipped at night before bed, can help to reduce tension.

SHINGLES

Shingles is an extremely painful disease caused by the herpes zoster virus (the same family as the chicken pox virus). Following an attack of chicken pox, the virus remains dormant in the body. Many years later a drop in the efficiency of the immune system may cause reactivation of the virus, this time in the form of shingles, causing acute inflammation in the ganglia near the spinal cord. Most children are not affected by shingles, although it can occur in some cases. The most likely candidates are adolescents, particularly during periods of great stress, such as during exams, or when their immune systems are impaired for any reason.

The first sign of shingles is sensitivity in the area to be affected, then pain. There may be fever and nausea, and a rash of small blisters develops on the fourth or fifth day. These turn yellow within a few days, form scabs, then drop off, sometimes leaving scars. In some cases there may be persistent pain for months or years (post-herpetic pain).

Conventional treatment

Antiviral drugs, such as acyclovir, are offered to reduce the severity of the active stage. Analgesic drugs may be offered.

NATURAL TREATMENTS

- The following remedies can be taken every two hours for up to ten doses:
  - Arsenicum, for burning pains worse between midnight and 2 A.M., with skin eruptions and a restless, chilly and anxious state
  - Lachesis, when the left-hand side of the body is affected with swelling
  - Rhus tox., for red, blistered and itching skin— better for movement and warmth

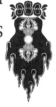

If you wish to receive a copy of the latest Shambhala Publications catalogue of books and to be placed on our mailing list, please send us this card, or e-mail us at:
info@shambhala.com

PLEASE PRINT

Book in which this card was found

NAME

ADDRESS

CITY & STATE

ZIP OR POSTAL CODE   COUNTRY

(*if outside U.S.A.*)

E-MAIL ADDRESS

- Fanunculus, for nerve pains and itching, worse for movement and eating
- Sponge blisters with a blend of hypericum and calendula tinctures in a little hot water.
- Make a combination of the following nervine herbs and offer as an infusion three times daily: oats, skullcap, St. John's wort and vervain.
- Offer plenty of foods rich in the B-complex vitamins to aid nervous health.
- Increase your child's intake of vitamin C, and give a supplement up to three or four times daily.
- Supplementation with vitamin E is now known to reduce the long-term symptoms associated with shingles. A usual dose for a child is about 600 mg a day, broken into three doses, with food. Vitamin E oil, applied directly to the sores, will encourage healing.
- An attack of shingles is a sign of general debility, and any of the treatments suggested for stress (see page 387) will help to tone the system. It's also important to boost your child's immune system (see page 207).
- Essential oils can combine analgesics with anti-viral properties, and can be applied as a compress, added to the bath or massaged into the skin. Try combining chamomile, eucalyptus, melissa, lavender and tea tree (a drop of each) in some olive oil, and use once or twice a day.
- Fresh lemon can be cut and applied to the affected areas to relieve the pain.

Useful therapies

Acupuncture is particularly effective, as well as reflexology, aromatherapy, flower essences, homeopathy, herbalism and any of the therapies that help to reduce stress (see page 387).

SHYNESS

Shyness is discussed in detail in chapter 8, but it is helpful to know what remedies are most appropriate for helping your child to feel more confident and secure, and for her to believe that her views, opinions and thoughts are valid.

NATURAL TREATMENTS

- Constitutional treatment with homeopathy is extremely helpful if your child is chronically shy, and it is affecting her interactions with others. There are also remedies that can help in different situations, according to your child's individual characteristics:
  - If your child is quiet and tends to cry a lot, Pulsatilla is most appropriate, particularly if she tends to blush
  - Lycopodium is good for children who are shy in new situations, although they tend to hide behind a false bravado (only you know how shy she is feeling, and prior to a situation she's made it clear)
  - Try Phosphorus if your child constantly seeks affection and reassurance, and is pale and highly strung
  - Silicea is useful if your child is bashful, with a tendency to burst into tears, although she can sometimes be obstinate. It's most appropriate if your child is one who feels the cold.
- Flower essences come into their own here. For some good examples, see page 254, or try Mimulus, which is suitable for children who are shy, nervous and blush easily. Your child probably feels uneasy with people she doesn't know, feels self-conscious and doesn't like parties. Larch is for children who suffer from poor confidence, which holds them back. They probably feel inferior and self-doubtful. Elm will help if your child feels overwhelmed and inadequate due to pressure from family, work, friends and other commitments. Cerato is good for children who constantly seek the reassurance of others because they do not trust their own judgment.
- Use therapies that boost a sense of well-being, including those suggested for stress on page 387.

SINUSITIS

Sinusitis is an inflammation of the sinuses—the air-filled cavities located in the bones around the nose. When this occurs the lining of the sinuses swells, causing blockage in the channel that drains them. A buildup of mucous discharge results and this becomes infected, creating intense pressure and pain. Sinusitis normally sets in after a sore throat, cold or flu, and it can become chronic, lasting for many months. Common symptoms include nasal congestion, nosebleeds and sneezing, loss of sense of smell, headaches with a sensation of pressure around the eyes, and even toothaches. There is often dripping catarrh into the throat, which can cause an irritating cough. Sinusitis is more common in older children, as the sinuses of babies are not fully developed.

Conventional treatment

Antibiotics are given immediately, and decongestant nosedrops or sprays may be offered. If sinusitis persists (rare in children), surgical drainage of the affected sinuses might be performed.

NATURAL TREATMENTS

- Most cases of sinusitis are due to excess mucus production, with or without a viral infection at the root of the condition. Many children suffer from excess catarrh (see page 312), which should be alleviated, particularly if your child suffers from chronic sinusitis.
- Elderflower is excellent for catarrh and sinusitis—offer as an infusion as required to reduce symptoms and encourage healing.
- During an acute attack, offer goldenseal.
- For particularly persistent infections, you will need to offer extra antibacterial herbs such as echinacea, garlic or myrrh. Most importantly, however, use every method possible to boost your child's immune system, to encourage healing, reduce mucus and prevent further attacks.
- Try steam inhalations of lavender, eucalyptus and tea tree, which are anticatarrhal and antibacterial. Lavender in particular will act as an anti-inflammatory and ease any painful symptoms.

- Homeopathic treatment should be constitutional, particularly if the condition persists or recurs, but the following remedies will help:
  - Kali bich. is the main remedy, particularly for thick, sticky mucus that accumulates in the throat and is difficult to clear
  - Hepar sulf., if Kali bich. doesn't help
  - Pulsatilla, for sinusitis accompanied by weepiness and pain above the eyes
- Many cases are exacerbated and even caused by food allergy or intolerance (see page 344).
- Place an ice pack across your child's face. At first it may be difficult to bear the cold, and you may be able to hold it there only for a few minutes, but within a short space of time, your child will begin to feel the congestion breaking up. This is one of the principles of osteopathy and it can make a dramatic difference.

Useful therapies

Cranial osteopathy, herbalism, homeopathy, Ayurveda, nutritional therapies, massage, aromatherapy, reflexology.

SLEEP AND WAKEFULNESS

In chapter 6, we discussed the importance of sleep, and various ways to help your child get what he needs. There are, however, many cases where children need a little help on the way—to break a bad cycle, for example, or to relax them enough to allow them to doze off into a good, restful sleep. There are also a number of common conditions affecting children's sleep patterns, and they may be preventing your child from getting the rest he needs. I'll focus here on common sleep disorders that affect children, providing details of what therapies work best for each condition. For general advice on sleep, see chapter 6. No matter what disorders affect your child, the basic advice remains the same: set up a good routine, be calm and firm, and create an environment in which your child will fall asleep comfortably and sleep until morning.

Breaking a bad cycle

Perhaps your child is jetlagged, or he's had a series of late nights. Perhaps he is under stress and can't get to sleep, pushing his bedtime later and later, and waking either too early or too late in the morning. In most cases a good routine will help to alleviate this problem, but sometimes it is necessary to offer your child a little help along the way.

NATURAL TREATMENTS

- Vervain is a gentle sedative, and can help children fall asleep—particularly if they are fighting it.
- Lime flowers will be useful for children who are nervous and sensitive.
- Motherwort can be useful for calming a frightened child or baby.
- A crying baby may be soothed with an infusion of chamomile, offered an hour or so before bedtime, or when he wakens.
- A strong infusion of chamomile, hops, lavender or lime flowers can be added to a warm bath to soothe and calm a baby or child.
- Tincture of catmint, added to a little honey, can be given to a distressed child as required.
- Homeopathic treatment should be constitutional, based on your child's exact requirements and symptoms. However, the following remedies may be appropriate for short-term problems, or while waiting for a consultation. Remedies can be taken an hour before going to bed, for up to 14 days. Repeat the dose if your child wakes in the night and cannot get back to sleep:
  - Calcarea and Antimonium tart for night terrors
  - Colocynthis or Bryonia may be effective for constant crying
  - Arsenicum, when your child wakes between midnight and 2 A.M., restless, worried and apprehensive
  - Rhus Tox., when your child cannot sleep, is irritable, restless and wants to walk around. He may complain that something "hurts."
  - Aurum, when your child has vivid dreams about dying, hunger or problems at school. He may wake depressed.

- Aconite, when sleep problems are worse after shock. There is restlessness, nightmares and perhaps even a fear of dying.
- Phosphorus is useful if there is thirst, and alternating anger and affection
- Pulsatilla, for a weepy, clingy child
- Chamomilla, if sleep is being disturbed by teething, or if your child cannot settle without being hugged, rocked or patted to sleep
- Nux vom., for irritability, and after a busy day, or too much food or fun
- Coffea, when your child's mind is overactive and he can't switch off
- Avoid cold energy foods such as bananas and cucumbers, which can cause colic and digestive problems.
- A warm glass of goat's milk will encourage sleep without causing digestive disturbance.
- Older children may suck a zinc lozenge before bedtime to help them sleep.
- Flower essences (see page 254) can be enormously useful. You may wish to create a blend of some of the most appropriate (see page 254), or see a flower therapist for advice:
  - White Chestnut will be helpful for children with overactive minds
  - a distressed child or baby can be given Bach's Rescue Remedy (see page 260) to calm him.
  - Offer Rock Rose for night terrors
  - Aspen is useful for fear of the dark
  - Walnut will be useful for change, such as a new baby, school or house
  - a few drops of Mimulus will soothe a distressed or fearful baby or child
- A few drops of chamomile, geranium, rose or lavender oil can be added to the bath water to calm and soothe.
- Lavender oil, on a hanky tied near the crib or bed, will help your baby or child to sleep.
- Lavender or chamomile can be used in a vaporizer in your child's room with the same effect.
- A gentle massage before bedtime, using a little lavender or chamomile blended with a light carrier oil, may ease any tension or distress.

Useful therapies

Cranial osteopathy (see page 251), flower essences (see page 254) (when there is something emotional keeping him awake), nutritional therapies, aromatherapy, homeopathy, herbalism, music therapy, Ayurveda, massage, reflexology—in fact, almost all of the therapies improve a sense of well-being and encourage relaxation. Just what your child needs.

Sleepwalking

Sleepwalking causes children to take nocturnal trips they don't remember, but navigate surprisingly well. It seems to be a temporary sleep mechanism malfunction that occurs during the deeper stages of sleep, and it tends to run in families. Sleepwalking usually begins between ages 6 and 12, and affects boys more often than girls. Most children outgrow the condition by puberty, although in some cases it can continue. There is no need for medical intervention, but it is important to protect habitual sleepwalkers from harm by keeping doors and windows closed. Sleepwalkers have an uncanny ability to maneuver in the dark, avoiding potential danger, but if you have a regular sleepwalker on your hands, it is a good idea to keep stairways gated, and traffic areas clear. If you find your child wandering at night, gently take him back to his bed, but don't try to wake him. He will remember little if nothing of the episode the following day.

If sleepwalking is becoming a regular occurrence, and is starting to affect your child's health or schoolwork, you may need to use some of the remedies suggested above, to ensure that your child is relaxed enough to fall into a deep sleep and stay there.

Sleeptalking

Sleeptalking can range from a word or two of nonsense speech, to whole conversations with someone else sleeping in the room (who may answer back, also in his sleep) or to an unknown party, as part of a dream. It can be distressing for parents to witness sleeptalking, as many children can become excited and agitated while speaking. They may also earnestly try to get across a point, and it can be upsetting not to be able to reassure them. This condition can be brought on by stress or illness, and can also be associated with sleep apnea or night terrors (see below). It is, however, harmless on its own and not cause for concern.

Again, if it is disrupting your child's sleep on a regular basis, you may want to ensure that your child's mind is calm before he goes to bed. Keep to a regular bedtime routine, and have a chat with your child before bedtime to ensure that there is nothing making him anxious. Try some of the natural remedies listed above, to soothe him off to sleep, or consider the remedies for stress (see page 387), if your child seems out of sorts and anxious. Flower essences can be particularly useful.

Night terrors

Night terrors are marked by a sudden awakening with physical behavior associated with intense fear. Your child may scream and try to escape, and appear extremely distressed—even hysterical. You may believe he is awake, but it is unlikely that he is. The fear and panic can continue for many minutes, and children will need a great deal of reassurance. Your child will have no recollection of what happened the following day. Like sleepwalking, night terrors are more common in children and typically do not continue into adulthood. Sleep terrors usually begin between ages 4 and 12, and they normally occur in the first third of the night—suddenly, from a deep sleep.

Many children suffer one or two a month and seem perfectly fine. Others have terrors more regularly, causing serious disturbance to sleep and occasionally injuring themselves or others, although they are unaware of what they are doing. Night terrors can be combined with sleepwalking, particularly in adolescence, and some children may run around the house, apparently terrified and inconsolable for many minutes. They may appear to awaken, confused and disoriented, and then fall asleep. Again, they will have little or no recollection of the event.

Night terrors are often considered to be an anxiety attack. Some children suffer night terrors after a frightening story or television program. Other children suffer from deeper-seated anxieties that will need to be brought to the surface and addressed.

The best advice is to remain calm during an attack, providing a reassuring and safe presence that your child can latch on to. Take steps to address any anxiety that your child might be experiencing (see page 303), and if the condition becomes more common, it might be a good idea to see a natural practitioner, who can treat the underlying cause on all levels—spiritual, emotional and physical. All of the remedies listed above will help to relax and soothe a child before bedtime and help ease any anxieties that are surfacing. It is a good idea to include a chat in your nighttime routine, when you can draw out any concerns. Many children can be encouraged to talk when they are relaxed and away from the distractions of toys, homework, television or siblings. Remember to never be judgmental. Just listen and offer solutions wherever possible. If your child wakes in the night with terrors, don't try to "talk things through." Just reassure your child and talk about it in the morning. If you are anxious, angry or frightened yourself, you will pass on your feelings to your child, which can make things worse. Last, avoid anything that can cause anxiety in your child before bedtime—arguments, scary stories or tapes, frightening television shows or games (such as murder in the dark, and even hide 'n' seek).

If night terrors occur night after night, some experts recommend waking your child about 15 minutes before they normally occur. Comfort your child, and stay with him for a few minutes while he goes back to sleep. This can normally break the cycle, and if the terrors do occur, they should be much less dramatic and distressing.

Nightmares

Nightmares are different from sleep terrors, and they normally take place during the latter part of the night, when we have our most vivid and memorable dreams. Many children will remember their nightmares, and they may even awaken during them. In night terrors, your child will remain asleep.

Nightmares often follow a traumatic event such as a bereavement, a disaster or a violent attack. They can also reflect anxieties that have not been resolved during the day, and that are preying on your child's mind.

Try to relax your child as much as possible before bed, and offer some of the remedies from page 381. Many of the listed remedies are suitable during attacks; check which one seems most appropriate in the circumstances. If your child wakes up, be rational and calm, reassuring him that everything is all right. If your child has recurrent nightmares, it is a good idea to talk about them the following morning, asking for a full description and encouraging your child to assess what it might mean. In the cold light of day, nightmares are rarely as frightening as they are at night, and you may be able to encourage your child to laugh about things that were terrifying only hours earlier. Be sensitive to her fears and concerns, and don't be tempted to make light of them, but point out the unrealistic parts of the nightmare (ghosts don't exist, for example, or burglars can't break into a house with an alarm), and try to reassure your child as much as possible. Avoid television prior to bedtime, which can disrupt sleep.

Sleep apnea

Sleep apnea is a condition in which people stop breathing while they sleep. Many studies have been conducted on this disorder, but the vast majority of them have focused on adults. Recently, it has been recognized that sleep apnea occurs in children, but the symptoms of sleep apnea are different from those of adults. For example, adults become drowsy and lapse into microsleeps during the day, whereas children seem to become hyperactive.

Obstructive apnea is the most common and severe type of sleep apnea. The muscles at the back of the throat relax to the point of obstructing the upper airway. Breathing can actually stop for ten seconds or more, causing mini-awakenings (usually not remembered) several hundred times a night as the sleeper gasps for air. Loud snoring is common in cases of sleep apnea, and your child may sleep with his mouth wide open, and seem to jerk awake frequently. Obstructive apnea is associated with heavy snoring and apart from enlarged tonsils, can be due to small oropharynx, obesity, chronic upper respiratory infections, rhinitis and hay fever. There are other forms of apnea (central and mixed), but these are less common in children.

In children, sleep apnea can cause irritability, poor grades, poor development and growth, aggression and daytime sleepiness or hyperactivity. In fact, researchers found one in five underachieving youngsters showed signs of sleep apnea.

Surgery to remove the tonsils and/or adenoids, which could be causing obstruction, is necessary for a large number of children, after which there can be a noticeable improvement in behavior and concentration. However, it may be worth investigating some alternatives before taking this route. Homeopathy, for example, can treat the underlying cause—allergies, hay fever, infections or chronically enlarged tonsils, for example—and there is some evidence that cranial osteopathy can help. The Buteyko method, which involves teaching children to learn to sleep with their mouths closed, can make a big difference to sleep apnea.

SORE THROATS

A sore throat (or pharyngitis) is an inflammation of the pharynx—the area of the throat between the back of the nose and the beginning of the trachea and vocal cords. It is usually caused by a bacterial or viral infection, but it can be caused by irritation (strong foods, second-hand smoke or cold weather, for example). A sore throat is a feature of illnesses such as tonsillitis and may also signal the onset of glandular fever, flu or scarlet fever. Many sore throats are caused by low humidity (common with central heating), and are worse in the morning, when the mucous membranes dry out and swell, causing irritation and inflammation.

Conventional treatment
If the condition is caused by bacteria, antibiotics will be prescribed. Otherwise, antibacterial and analgesic lozenges might be suggested.

NATURAL TREATMENTS
- Offer your child plenty of fresh garlic, which has antibacterial and antiviral properties.

- Tincture of calendula can be added to a cup of boiled water and used as a mouthwash to encourage healing and treat infection.
- Add echinacea tincture to some fresh water and spray the throat to fight infection and viruses. Offer echinacea and goldenseal (and any other remedies suggested on page 231) to boost your child's immune system.
- There are a number of useful homeopathic remedies, although chronic sore throats should be treated constitutionally. Try:
  - Belladonna, for sore throat accompanied by a red face and fever
  - Gelsemium, when swallowing is painful, and your child feels exhausted and weak with pain in the neck and ears
  - Apis, when the pain is worse on the right side, and it feels better for cold drinks
  - Lachesis, when pain is worse on the left side, there is a feeling of constriction, and pain is worse from swallowing saliva but better for swallowing food
  - Aconite, for a sore throat that comes on suddenly, with a burning throat and swollen tonsils
- Older children can gargle with salt water to ease the symptoms and reduce inflammation.
- A steam inhalation of benzoin, lavender or thyme will ease the discomfort and help to treat the infection.
- Massage a little lavender oil, blended in a light carrier oil, into the neck.
- Dab the throat internally with diluted tea tree oil on a cotton swab—it is analgesic and fights infection, which will help to ease symptoms and treat the cause.
- Osteopaths recommend using cold to cure a sore throat (with infection) within 24 hours. Offer plenty of ice-cold fruit juices (internal) and wrap the neck in a cold compress (with ice, if you can). Once again, while heat may make your child feel better, it increases congestion and slows down the circulation in the area. Ice is stimulating, and your child's body will fight off the infection more quickly.

Useful therapies

Aromatherapy, homeopathy, Ayurveda, reflexology, herbalism, nutritional therapies and traditional Chinese medicine.

SQUINT

A squint (or strabismus) is a condition in which only one eye focuses on an object of interest. In a divergent squint the other eye looks outward, while in a convergent squint it looks inward. A squint in children may be caused by congenital hypermetropia (long-sightedness), or physical defects in the cornea, lens, retina, nerves and muscles of the eye. It's important to note that many young babies have a squint because the normal mechanism for aligning the two eyes has not yet developed.

Conventional treatment

If the squint persists for more than two months, a complete ophthalmological assessment is recommanded. In children up to the age of about six, treatment may involve covering the normal eye with a patch to force the child to use the weak eye. If this does not work, surgery or glasses may be effective.

NATURAL TREATMENTS

- Constitutional homeopathic treatment would be accompanied by exercises for the eye. Specific remedies, to be taken 3 times daily for up to 14 days, include Gelsemium. If this does not work, try Alumina.

Useful therapies

Cranial osteopathy (this has proved enormously effective in children, see page 251), Ayurveda, acupuncture, homeopathy.

STAMMERING

Also called stuttering, stammering is a speech disorder in which there is repeated hesitation and delay in uttering words, unusual prolongation of sounds and repetition of different elements of words. It usually starts in childhood, beginning before the age of eight, in 90 percent of sufferers. Temporary stuttering is fairly common in children between ages two and four, but studies indicate that about half of all children whose stutters continue until the age of five will continue to stutter in adult life.[9] It's more common in boys, twins and left-handed children.

The cause of stuttering is uncertain, although the problem does tend to run in families. Some experts believe it is caused by minor brain damage, but most believe that it is related to stress and anxiety—made worse, of course, by trying not to stammer.

Conventional treatment

Speech therapy.

NATURAL TREATMENTS

- Constitutional homeopathic treatment can be important, as it will unroot the cause and treat the stammering as part of the overall picture. In the meantime, however, try:
  - Stramonium, when your child is excitable, given to muttering and to expansive movements of the limbs
  - Nux vom., for children who are irritable and overcritical
  - Hyoscyamus, for children who talk too quickly and trip over their words, making the condition much worse
  - Cuprum, when the condition is accompanied by nervous spasms of the face and limbs
  - Mercurius, when your child's tongue trembles, and he seems to have too much saliva in his mouth
- Flower essences (see page 254) can be very helpful. Consider one or more of the following: Mimulus when your child develops a real fear of speaking,

making the condition worse; Rock Rose for terror or panic that may set in; Impatiens for children who do everything in a hurry, and find their inability to speak as quickly as they think frustrating; or Aspen, for children who seem afraid for no obvious reason.

Useful therapies

Cranial osteopathy (this is a good one for children whose stuttering starts very young), homeopathy, music therapy and any of the therapies suggested for stress and insecurity.

SELF-HELP

It is extremely important that you never put pressure on a child to finish a sentence or to find the right word. Many children stumble over words and stammer as part of developing speech patterns, and you can draw attention to and create a problem that would otherwise be temporary. Be calm and patient, even if it seems an intolerable length of time before your child manages to spit out his words. If stammering does continue past age four or five, adopt the same methods, but don't pretend it isn't happening. Your child will feel self-conscious and insecure and he will need your reassurance. Let him know that stammering is normal and tell a funny story about yourself—stammering through your first public speaking engagement, for example. If you ignore it, your child will feel isolated and this can make the problem worse. Offer remedies and explain that they will help him when he needs it. Create relaxing situations where he can talk with no pressure. When he realizes that he can do it, and that it isn't a big issue, he will feel more confident in less relaxed circumstances. Don't hesitate to see a speech therapist, but if your child objects or feels uncomfortable, don't push it.

STICKY EYE

Sticky eye is a mild infection of the eyes causing a yellowish discharge and crusting. It is most common in the first week of life, and is usually the result of a blocked tearduct. This condition is not serious and usually rights itself without treatment. In an older child, sticky eyes are usually a sign of conjunctivitis, a condition in which the conjunctiva of the eye becomes infected (see page 318). There may be a blocked tear duct.

Conventional treatment

Most doctors simply advise bathing the eyes to clear away the discharge.

NATURAL TREATMENTS

- Homeopathic remedies can help, particularly if sticky eye continues past the first week of life. Try:
  - Pulsatilla, when there is mucus collecting in the corner of the eyes
  - Hepar sulf., to help to draw out any infection
- One or two drops of euphrasia tincture, diluted in cooled, previously boiled water, can also be used to bathe the eyes.
- A very mild infusion of chamomile can be used to clean the eye areas (from the inside corner to the outside of the eye, using a new cotton swab for each eye), and to reduce any inflammation.

Useful therapies

Homeopathy and herbalism.

STRESS

Not so long ago, it would have been thought absurd to consider treating a child for stress, but we now know that children are as susceptible to its effects as adults. In some cases, it can be worse, because they cannot always verbalize their emotions in the same way as adults.

It's important to remember that stress doesn't equate to overwork. Stress comes in many forms, and can be fairly safely described as anything that places undue pressure on the mind, body or spirit of a child. Stress can come from obvious sources—trouble at school, exams, peer pressure, too much homework, an overscheduled life, parental divorce, breaking up with a boyfriend or even insufficient relaxation time—but it can also stem from anything that causes the body to work harder, including a poor diet, inadequate sleep or exercise, constant noise, pollution, chemicals in food and the environment, and even injury.

Add them up, and you may find that your child is being faced with more than she can easily handle. To most parents the symptoms of stress are obvious:

- increased breathing and heart rate
- nausea
- tense muscles
- inability to relax
- irritability (including temper tantrums)
- insomnia
- allergies
- skin problems
- headaches
- fatigue

These are the same symptoms that can occur in children, but there are more. Watch out for hyperactivity, loss of appetite (or sudden cravings or bingeing on food), nightmares, night terrors, loss of interest in normal games, toys or activities, poor self-esteem and a loss of interest in appearance (in adolescents). Your child may also suffer from abdominal pains, inexplicable nervousness, tearfulness, sleep problems and irrational fears.

Stress is a major factor in diseases whose physical symptoms are induced or aggravated by mental or emotional problems. Stress-related disorders compose 50 to 80 percent of all illnesses, though stress may not be the only cause.

NATURAL TREATMENTS

- Essential oils are excellent for stress reduction because many of them work on the nervous system and the brain to relax and soothe. Other oils are uplifting, which can be invaluable in times of serious stress. Massage with aromatherapy oils is very comforting—particularly the physical element of touch—and a few drops of essential oil in the bath can offer an opportunity to "wash away" the problems of the day, while experiencing the benefits of the oil. Suitable oils include chamomile, geranium, lavender, neroli and rose. Oils that strengthen the adrenal system, which is weakened by stress, include rosemary and lemongrass. Don't apply these to your child's skin—use a vaporizer instead.

- Massage can be enormously stress-relieving (see page 274). If your child seems under pressure or reacting unusually, offer a massage. Babies and children will love it. You might have to convince a teenager that it's a good idea, but most will respond to a relaxing shoulder massage while they listen to music. Or rub their feet while they are watching television.

- Eating a good, balanced diet will make your child's body stronger and able to cope more efficiently with stress. B vitamins are often depleted by stress, so ensure that he is getting enough in his diet, or take a good supplement (see page 435).

- Vitamin C is a great stress reliever, and boosts immunity, making your child fitter and more healthy.

- Herbs that encourage relaxation and act as a tonic to the nervous system include balm, lavender, chamomile, verbena, passiflora and oats. Any of these can be drunk as an infusion—as often as necessary in stressful situations. Some of them have a fairly strong sedative effect, so save them for bedtime if you can.

- Ginseng is an excellent "adaptogenic" herb, which means that it lifts when your child is tired and relaxes when he is stressed. It also works on the immune system and energizes. Some therapists recommend that you take it daily in stressful times.

Useful therapies

Ayurveda, aromatherapy, massage, reflexology, cranial osteopathy, osteopathy, music therapy, meditation, hypnotherapy, homeopathy, herbalism, traditional Chinese medicine, acupuncture, art therapy, nutritional therapies, yoga.

SELF-HELP

- Some stress is healthy and invigorating, but in excess it can cause health to decline on all levels—affecting the function of all systems in the body, including immunity. Relaxation is essential. Ensure that your child has time for hobbies that interest him and give him satisfaction and pride. The feel-good factor will go a long way toward reducing the effects of stress in other parts of his life.
- Take care that your child isn't overstretched. He might be a determined child who likes to be busy, but all children need time to rest and recharge. If he suffers from any stress symptoms, it might be time to cut back on what he's doing.
- Make sure that you have family time together, and that there is time for play and friends.
- Watch your child's diet (see chapters 1 and 2), which can dramatically affect his ability to deal with external stress.
- Be physically affectionate with your child. The power of touch is well documented, and if your child feels loved and lovable, he'll feel good about himself and better able to withstand the effects of stress.
- Make sure your child isn't getting too much caffeine in his diet. Caffeine is found in chocolate and cola drinks, among other things, and it can increase adrenaline levels, enhancing the effects of stress.
- Encourage your child to think positively. Children are in training for facing the stresses of the adult world. Although all parents should make it their responsibility to keep their children's lives as stress-free as possible, it is important to teach life skills along the way. When things pile up, teach your child to plan ahead and to be optimistic, even when things go wrong.
- Have a watch-free day every week (or if you can't manage that, when on holiday). Let your child do whatever he wants (within reason!) whenever he wants, and don't push a schedule on him. Let him play, nap, do his homework, ride his bike, play the piano, hit a ball about, exercise or whatever he wants without demanding that he meet commitments.

- Ensure that your child gets plenty of exercise—and it should be fun!
- Encourage communication. The better your child is able to express his feelings and emotions, the more ably he will handle stress. If your child finds it hard to confide in you, see if you can find another family member or a teacher who can make some headway. Reassure him that it is OK to show how he feels—to cry or get angry. These are good ways of relieving tension and can make him feel better.
- Encourage your child to do things he enjoys, such as drawing, painting or writing, relaxing to music, or going to the movies. Seeing friends, taking part in a sport or activity, and having his "own space" to be alone are also important means of coping with stress.

See also chapter 8 for more on coping with stress.

STYES

A stye is a boil occurring around the root of an eyelash, usually caused by staphylococcal bacteria. A collection of pus at the base of the eyelash produces the characteristic small, yellow head. Styes usually last for around seven days, but the infection may spread to adjacent follicles. They tend to occur when general resistance is low.

Conventional treatment

A warm compress may be suggested to help the pus to discharge. Use of an eye ointment containing antibiotics may be suggested to prevent recurrence.

NATURAL TREATMENTS

- Recurrent styes should be treated constitutionally by a homeopath, but you can try the following:
  - Pulsatilla, in the first instance
  - If this doesn't work, try Staphisagria every hour, for up to ten doses
- Echinacea and poke root will boost the immune system, which is particularly useful if your child suffers from recurrent styes. Infusions of chamomile or eyebright can help to reduce swelling.

- A drop of lavender or tea tree oil, on a cotton swab, can be diluted and dabbed at the base of the stye. Hold a cotton ball beneath (or above) the lashes to ensure that no trace of the oils enters the eyes.

Useful therapies

Homeopathy, Ayurveda, herbalism, traditional Chinese medicine, reflexology.

> **CAUTION**
> Recurrent episodes of styes may be an indication of diabetes and should therefore be investigated.

TEETHING

Most babies get their first teeth between about four and six months of age, but there may be problems with teeth coming through until the age of two or three. The majority of children experience some discomfort, which can range from simply being clingy and fractious, to dribbling, loosened stools and problems sleeping. Many experts insist that there is no evidence to confirm that babies may become unwell with teething, but mothers have quite different experiences, and your happy baby may experience a variety of complaints.

Conventional treatment

Teething gels or teething rings may be suggested.

NATURAL TREATMENTS

- Offer your baby a cool teething ring (not PVC!) to gnaw on, and rub her gums with a clean finger. If she has trouble sleeping, gentle rocking may help.
- The homeopathic remedy Chamomilla is standard for teething, and can be taken as required for up to six times a day to ease symptoms and relieve the distress.
- Rub a little Bach Rescue Remedy (see page 260) directly into the gums, or apply to pulse points if your baby is crying inconsolably. A few drops at nighttime will help your baby to sleep, as will a few drops of lavender on the bedclothes.
- A little of the essential oils of chamomile and lavender can be added to the bathwater to calm a distressed baby.
- Rub the gums with a tiny drop of chamomile oil mixed with a teaspoon of organic, cold-pressed honey. Clove oil also acts as a local anesthetic and a minute amount (one drop) can be diluted in olive oil and rubbed into the gums.
- Syrup made from the marshmallow root will soothe inflamed gums, and a few teaspoons can be added to your baby's normal meals.
- Offer infusions of chamomile or fennel to calm and soothe.

Useful therapies

Herbalism, homeopathy, traditional Chinese medicine, cranial osteopathy, massage, reflexology.

> **CAUTION**
> Fever and vomiting are not symptoms of teething. See your doctor if your baby seems unwell.

THRUSH

Thrush, or candida albicans, is a fungal or yeast infection, which is very common in those with immature immune systems, or those with immune systems that are compromised or very stressed. Thrush takes many forms, the most common of which are oral and a form that develops in the diaper area. The immune system can be impaired by poor diet, pollution, injury or surgery, the overuse of drugs that suppress it and upset the balance of the intestinal flora, causing candida or thrush to flourish, among other things. In babies, it usually occurs in conjunction with diaper rash. Oral thrush is characterized by sore, white, raised patches in the mouth. In the diaper area or skin folds, it takes the form of an itchy red rash with a white top.

Conventional treatment

Antifungal drugs, such as Nystan.

NATURAL TREATMENTS

- Homeopathic treatment will be constitutional, but the following remedies may be useful for oral thrush:
  - Borax, at the first sign of an outbreak
  - Mercurius, when there is more saliva than usual, and your child's tongue trembles
  - Capsicum, for sore, hot patches
  - Arsenicum, for burning pains, mouth ulcers and feeling worn out
- For vaginal thrush in girls, try
  - Pulsatilla, for cloudy or watery discharge that causes smarting and soreness
  - Graphites, if the vagina is sore, with small ulcers on the labia
  - Calcarea, if there is vaginal itching, yellow or milky discharge and increased itchiness around periods
- Echinacea, to boost the immune system, will help to prevent chronic thrush and help the body to fight infection. It can also be applied directly to affected areas (in the mouth, or on your child's bottom).
- Oral thrush may be helped by preparing a mouthwash solution with lavender, lemon and peppermint essential oils (1 drop of each in 2 cups [(500 ml) of spring water)]. Rinse your baby's mouth, or dab a few drops on the affected areas.
- Use tea tree oil in a vaporizer in your child's room to boost the immune system and act as an antifungal agent.
- Very, very dilute lavender oil or tea tree oil can be dabbed onto patches in the mouth, and on the bottom. Avoid the genitals.
- Apply a little Bach Rescue Remedy cream (see page 260) to the affected area (externally) and a few drops of stock remedy to sores in the mouth.
- Olive can be useful if outbreaks are linked to exhaustion and stress.
- Give children older than 1 year frequent spoonfuls of live yogurt between meals, and apply to sore spots on the bottom.
- Offer acidophilus pills to restore the healthy bacteria in the body and fight the infection.

Useful therapies

Homeopathy, acupuncture, herbalism, aromatherapy, nutritional therapies, traditional Chinese medicine.

TONSILLITIS

Tonsillitis is an inflammation of the tonsils located at the back of the throat. It is generally due to either viral or bacterial infection (often by the streptococcal bacteria), and causes swelling and redness of the tonsils, possibly with white or yellow spots of pus. The adenoids may also become inflamed and infected. Tonsillitis can occur at any time, but is particularly common during childhood. In rare cases complications such as quinsy (an abscess behind the tonsil), kidney inflammation or rheumatic fever may develop.

Your child may have swollen glands (lymph nodes), a sore throat with pain on swallowing, a headache, ear pain and general weakness. Most cases are accompanied by fever at some point, and you may notice that your child's breath is bad.

Conventional treatment

Chronic tonsillitis may lead to the surgical removal of the tonsils. In most cases, however, antibiotics are prescribed.

NATURAL TREATMENTS

- Chronic tonsillitis must be treated constitutionally by a homeopath, but for acute conditions, try:
  - Belladonna, for a sore, tender throat, with shooting pains and a stiff neck
  - Hepar sulf., for a feeling that there is a fishbone caught in the throat, and if pain is alleviated by warm drinks. Breath is foul, and there is yellow pus.
  - Lycopodium, for a throat sore on the right-

hand side, when the tongue is dry and puffy but not coated. Better after cold drinks, and worse between 4 and 8 A.M. or P.M.

- Mercurius, when throat is dark red, swollen and sore, worse on the right-hand side. Breath is smelly and there are hot sweats.
- Phytolacca, for a rough, constricted hot throat, with red swollen tonsils and pain extending to the ears. Worse on the right-hand side and with heat.
- Thyme oil is a powerful antiseptic and has a local anesthetic effect to reduce the discomfort. Use in a vaporizer, and add one drop to a light carrier oil and massage into the neck.
- One drop of lavender oil can be added to a cup of cooled, boiled water, and gargled.
- Tea tree oil, on the end of a cotton swab, can be applied neat to the tonsils themselves to fight infection and reduce discomfort.
- A red sage gargle will address infection and reduce symptoms.
- Herbs to boost the immune system include echinacea, garlic, myrrh, sage and wild indigo (see page 207 for other remedies to boost immunity).
- Herbs to induce sweating and reduce fever include chamomile, elderflowers, yarrow and lime flowers.
- Agrimony, elderflowers, plantain and raspberry leaves will tone the mucous membranes and clear the catarrh and inflammation.
- Herbs to soothe painful tonsils include comfrey, mullein and marshmallow.
- Blackcurrant tea or juice (hand hot) will help to treat infection and relieve the sore throat.

Useful therapies

Cranial osteopathy, herbalism, homeopathy, aromatherapy, Ayurveda, reflexology (to boost immunity), nutritional therapies, acupuncture, traditional Chinese medicine.

TOOTHACHE

Aching or pain in a tooth is generally a result of tooth decay (or "caries"). When the hard enamel of the tooth is damaged, infecting organisms can enter the tooth, resulting in inflammation and pain. Other causes of toothache include sinusitis, a broken or damaged tooth, mouth ulcers, a dental abscess or gum disease. Occasionally an ear infection can lead a child to believe that his teeth hurt, and the reverse is also true.

Conventional treatment

A dentist will assess whether there is tooth decay and treat accordingly. A doctor would investigate any underlying cause (mouth ulcers or sinusitis, for example) and treat accordingly.

NATURAL TREATMENTS

- Homeopathic remedies can help. Try
  - Chamomilla, when there is unbearable pain, made worse by cold air, or warm food and drinks
  - Apis, when gums feel tight and swollen, and the toothache burns and stings
  - Staphisagria, for severe toothache made worse by cold air, food and pressure. Cheeks are red and swollen.
  - Plantago, for nervy teeth, aggravated by cold air and pressure, but better for eating
  - Belladonna, for throbbing pain and a dry mouth
  - Aconite, when pain comes on quickly
  - Arnica, for pain after a filling or an extraction
- One drop of peppermint or clove oil, diluted in 1 teaspoon (5 ml) of olive oil, can be applied directly to the affected area to act as a natural analgesic.
- Rub a drop of lavender oil, diluted in some olive oil, into the face and jaw to ease pain and distress.
- A herbalist might recommend tinctures of echinacea or myrrh to encourage healing and reduce the risk of infection.
- Bach Rescue Remedy (see page 260) can be applied to the affected area, and taken internally to reduce pain and encourage healing.

Useful therapies

Acupuncture, herbalism, homeopathy, aromatherapy, reflexology, cranial osteopathy if toothache is common or it hurts to chew when there is no decay present.

> **CAUTION**
> Toothache is an indication of an underlying problem that should be investigated by a dentist immediately.

TRAUMA

Trauma includes emotional as well as physical experiences and injuries. Emotional injury is essentially a normal response to an extreme event. It involves the creation of emotional memories that arise through a long-lasting effect on structures deep within the brain. The more direct the exposure to the traumatic event, the higher the risk for emotional harm. In this section we'll focus on emotional trauma, which can have a dramatic effect on health.

At different ages, children react differently to trauma, and some children appear to be more affected than others, for reasons that are not clearly understood. Even something like hearing the news of murders at schools (they have taken place in the U.K., Canada and the U.S.) can shock some children and make them irrationally (or perhaps not so irrationally) fearful. The horrific events in New York and Washington, as well as the threat of global violence, will also undoubtedly affect your child, even if she is unable to verbalize it. What you need to do is to get to the bottom of your child's fear, and help her to work through it.

Reactions to trauma may appear immediately after the traumatic event, or days and even weeks later. Loss of trust in adults and fear of the event occurring again are responses seen in many children and adolescents who have been exposed to traumatic events. According to the National Center for Post-Traumatic Stress Disorder of the Department of Veterans Affairs, other reactions vary according to age:

- **For children 5 years of age and younger**, typical reactions include a fear of being separated from a parent, crying, whimpering, screaming, immobility and/or aimless motion, trembling, frightened facial expressions and excessive clinging. Parents may also notice children returning to behaviors exhibited at earlier ages (these are called regressive behaviors), such as thumb-sucking, bedwetting and fear of darkness. These behaviors can lead to problems at school.

- **Children 6 to 11 years old** may show extreme withdrawal, disruptive behavior and/or inability to pay attention. Regressive behaviors, nightmares, sleep problems, irrational fears, irritability, refusal to attend school, outbursts of anger and fighting are also common in traumatized children of this age. Also, the child may complain of stomach aches or other bodily symptoms that have no medical basis. Schoolwork often suffers. Depression, anxiety, feelings of guilt and emotional numbing are often present as well.

- **Adolescents 12 to 17 years old** are likely to exhibit responses similar to those of adults, including flashbacks, nightmares, emotional numbing, avoidance of any reminders of the traumatic event, depression, substance abuse, problems with peers and antisocial behavior. Also common are withdrawal and isolation, physical complaints, school avoidance, academic decline, sleep disturbances and confusion.

If this sounds extreme, and unlikely to affect your own child, remember that anything can traumatize a child, even if it appears innocuous to an adult. You may remember one event from your childhood that stands out clearly in your mind—being lost at a fun fair, being forgotten at school, being left alone in your crib, being physically or emotionally abused, or witnessing abuse of others. These sorts of traumatic events can affect children dramatically. On the other hand, a car accident, a death in the family, a parental divorce, the death of a pet or even a physical injury can cause emotional trauma. All children differ in the way they deal with trauma. What one child will brush off may affect another child for many months.

Conventional treatment

Depending on the type of trauma, most doctors will recommend counseling (particularly for posttraumatic stress) and possibly even mild tranquilizers or antidepressants.

NATURAL TREATMENTS

- Flower essences (see page 254) can be particularly useful, and you can create a blend of several types to best match your child's outlook. For example, Aspen and Mimulus can be blended for fears, Rock Rose is appropriate for shock or trauma of any sort, and Bach Rescue Remedy (see page 260) is ideal for all types of shock or trauma.
- Homeopathic treatment will be constitutional, but it can make a big difference to emotional health. Consider some of the following remedies in the meantime:
  - Aconite, after any trauma, with Arnica, if there is physical injury
  - Ignatia, if trauma follows a bereavement or when there is intense grief
  - Opium, if your child is frightened by the death of a loved one, and numb with grief
  - Pulsatilla, if there is sleeplessness, helpless weeping and catarrh
  - Nat. Mur., for a child who rejects sympathy and prefers to hide his feelings
- For other treatments, see stress, anxiety and sleep disorders (pages 386, 303 and 380).

Useful therapies

All therapies will help with emotional trauma on some level.

SELF-HELP

- According to the Center for Post-Traumatic Stress Disorder, there are many, many things that families and close carers can do to ease the burden. For example:

Encourage your child to express his feelings, and help younger children to use words that help them do so. Don't force discussion of a traumatic event if your child does not want to open up. Make sure your child knows that you are there when he wants to talk. It might help to express your own feelings, and to identify with feelings that he might be experiencing. He might feel better about opening up if he sees you doing so.

- Let children and adolescents know that it is normal to feel upset after something bad happens.
- Return to your normal household routine, which can be reassuring for children. They'll know that whatever goes on outside, they are safe at home.
- Be patient with extra needs. If your child needs a light on at bedtime for a short time, try to accept it. He may need someone with him when he falls asleep, or he may want someone in the room with him at all times. Try to meet his demands until he is able to heal.
- Never make a child feel guilty or childish for expressing feelings, or for crying. These are healthy emotional expressions.
- Some children blame themselves for events that occur around them. Reassure them that they are not to blame, even if you cannot see any reason why they should consider themselves the cause.
- Some children need more time to heal than others, and it is important to be patient throughout the course. It can take many months for some children to get over something as simple as the loss of a pet or a friend, but in order to do so they need your sympathy and constant reassurance.

TRAVEL SICKNESS (*see* Nausea and vomiting)

TUMMY ACHES

There are many causes of stomachache in children and babies. In infants, colic can be a problem (see page 316), or simply gas. In older children, a bowel movement may relieve any abdominal pain or discomfort. Overeating, tension, gastroenteritis and abdominal migraine are other causes. Some children suffer from abdominal pain after eating certain foods, so ruling out a food allergy is a good starting point, particularly if it occurs frequently. In periods of stress, and during adolescence, many children experience pain in the abdominal area. There is a theory that headaches manifest themselves as stomach pain in young children. If your child is under stress or suffering from any of the common causes of headache (see page 356), but appears to have abdominal pain rather than pain in the head or neck, this may well be the cause.

Chronic tummy ache should always be investigated by a doctor, particularly if it is accompanied by regular vomiting, fever or severe pain that causes him to double up. In the short term, any acute pain that cannot immediately be explained should be investigated.

NATURAL TREATMENTS

- A warm drink, a hot water bottle on the tummy and avoiding solid food should ease the pain. If stomachache is recurrent and eased by a bowel movement, constipation may be the problem. In those circumstances, increase your child's intake of fluids and fiber-rich foods, and cut down on refined and processed foods.
- Ensure that your child gets plenty of fresh, bottled or previously boiled water to flush the system of anything that may be causing the condition.
- Add a drop of chamomile oil to a little apricot kernel oil, and massage into the abdominal area to ease the symptoms.
- The homeopathic remedy Bryonia is useful if your child is very irritable and screams at the slightest movement, and Chamomilla is good if your child seems better for comforting, but otherwise almost impossible to please. If overindulgence is the problem, Nux Vom. is appropriate. See also remedies for stress and constipation.
- If indigestion is the problem, a warm cup of peppermint or chamomile tea may help.
- Consider emotional factors. If your child has recurrent tummy aches, there may be something causing it. Flower essences (see page 254) can be appropriate for nerves (Mimulus), or try Impatiens

if your child does everything in a hurry and seems impatient. Again, Mimulus is good for pain caused by fears. Walnut will help if your child is undergoing change of any sort (adolescence, exams, a new school, a new girlfriend, a new caregiver).
- Nervous tummy aches can be eased with chamomile tea or valerian at bedtime.

Useful therapies

Homeopathy, herbalism, nutritional therapy, flower essences, yoga, Ayurveda, aromatherapy, reflexology, massage.

SELF-HELP

It's important to establish the cause before undertaking treatment. Look at all aspects of your child's life, and ensure that his emotional and physical needs are being met. Make sure he has a good, healthy diet, lots of sleep and exercise, time for himself and that he is not under stress of any sort. Many children suffer from tummy aches during the school term, which miraculously disappear once the holidays arrive. Don't dismiss the symptoms, however. Anything that causes pain should be addressed, even if it is on an emotional basis. Be patient and try to get to the root of the problem, using the remedies that are most appropriate as backup. Show concern and understanding, even if you know that school may be the root of it all. If you are worried about what is happening at school, talk to your child's teacher to see if there is anything obviously wrong.

URINARY TRACT INFECTIONS

Infections rank as one of the most common urinary problems among children, and experts estimate that some 3 percent of girls and 1 percent of boys have had a urinary tract infection (UTI) by the age of 11. The symptoms are not always obvious to parents, and younger children are usually unable to describe how they feel. For this reason, many cases of UTI go undetected, so the figures may well be significantly higher. Recognizing and treating UTIs is important, largely because untreated infections in the urinary tract can lead to serious kidney problems.

Normal urine is sterile, which means that it contains no bacteria (germs). Bacteria may, at times, get into the urinary tract (and the urine) from the skin around the rectum and genitals by traveling up the urethra into the bladder. When this happens, bacteria can infect and inflame the bladder, resulting in swelling and pain in the lower abdomen and side. This condition is known as cystitis, although this term is less commonly used for children and males. If the bacteria travel further up through the ureters to the kidneys, a kidney infection can develop. The infection is usually accompanied by pain and fever. Kidney infections are much more serious than bladder infections, largely because of the role the kidneys play in the body.

Some children suffer from repeated infections, and in this case, there may be an abnormality in the urinary tract. Most doctors will recommend further tests in children who have had more than one infection in the space of a year. In other cases, children develop UTIs because they have a predisposition to that type of infection, in much the same way that some children are prone to ear infections or colds.

If your child is very young (toddler or younger), the signs of a UTI may not be clear, since children that young cannot tell you just how they feel. Your child may have a high fever, be irritable, or not eat. On the other hand, sometimes a child may have only a low-grade fever, experience nausea and vomiting, or just not seem healthy. His urine may have an unusual smell, and be darker in color than usual. If your child has a high temperature and appears sick for more than a day without signs of a runny nose or other obvious cause for discomfort, she may need to be checked for a bladder infection.

An older child with bladder irritation may complain of pain in the abdomen and pelvic area. It's likely that he will need to urinate more frequently, and he may experience some pain under his ribcage (at the side), or in his lower back, if one or both kidneys are infected. Urine may be cloudy, scant and smelly, and it will probably hurt to urinate. Your child may also wet the bed or have "accidents" in the daytime.

Conventional treatment

If you suspect a urinary tract infection, you'll need to take a urine sample to your doctor to have it analyzed. Find a very clean jar and wash it with very hot water and soap, or put it in the dishwasher. When it is clean, encourage your child to urinate into the jar by holding it in the toilet bowl. For babies, bring along a wet diaper. Refrigerate the urine until you can take it to the doctor. Urinary tract infections are treated with antibiotics.

CAUTION

If you suspect a urinary tract infection, or your child is suffering extreme pain, or an unexplained fever or other signs of being unwell, see your doctor. In rare cases, an untreated UTI can lead to complications such as kidney damage. Furthermore, some symptoms of UTIs mimic those of other conditions, so it's always worth having it checked by your doctor.

NATURAL TREATMENTS

- Chronic infections should be treated constitutionally by a homeopath, but the following remedies can be taken in an attack:
  - Cantharis, when the urine burns and urination is violently painful
  - Mercurius, for violent pain with blood in the urine
  - Apis, for stinging pain that is better for cold water
  - Sarsaparilla, for burning pain after urinating
- Herbs used to treat UTIs include urinary antiseptics and diuretics, and you can offer your child comfrey, coughgrass or marshmallow as an infusion to soothe and relieve the burning pains.
- Anti-inflammatory and antiseptic herbs for the urinary tract include uva ursi, chamomile and yarrow. All of these (and the above) can be sipped lukewarm every couple of hours, and they can added to your child's bathwater.
- For fever, offer chamomile or lime flowers sipped throughout the day.

- Lavender and sandalwood essential oils are soothing and antiseptic. Add one drop to the bath water every evening.
- Offer plenty of live yogurt, which can ease the symptoms and prevent recurrence by building up the natural flora of the gut (see page 284).
- Offer unsweetened cranberry juice to discourage bacteria from sticking to the walls of the bladder and urinary tract. It both treats and prevents the condition.
- Barley water, mixed with some lemon juice and honey, is a traditional remedy for UTIs and can help discourage infection while soothing.
- Your child will need to drink plenty of fresh water to flush the urinary system
- Offer a good vitamin C supplement, which acts as a natural diuretic and boosts the immune system. Recurrent UTIs may mean that your child's immune system is not working as effectively as it should be. Take steps to boost immunity (see page 207).

Useful therapies

Homeopathy, herbalism, Ayurveda, nutritional therapies, acupuncture, traditional Chinese medicine.

SELF-HELP

- Simple hygiene can help to prevent the condition. Ensure that your child has regular baths (easy in babies and children; less easy to convince some adolescents) and add a drop of tea tree oil to the water to discourage infection.
- Girls should have the vagina and bottom patted dry, never rubbed hard, which can irritate. Teach your child to wipe herself from front to back. All children should wash their hands carefully after going to the bathroom.
- Ensure that your child always has plenty to drink, which keeps the urinary tract flushed.

VOMITING (*see* Nausea and vomiting)

WARTS

A wart is a small, hard growth, usually brown or flesh-colored, on the skin. It may be caused by any one of 30 strains of the human papilloma virus. Warts are highly contagious, but not dangerous, and can occur more frequently when the immune system is compromised. Some children seem to be prone to warts, for inexplicable reasons. Many children who suffer from atopic conditions (eczema, for example) seem to get them more often.

Conventional treatment

There are many solutions available to burn off the warts, or they may be surgically removed or burned off in your doctor's surgery. In most cases, they will be left to run their course.

NATURAL TREATMENTS

- Homeopathy can be very helpful, particularly if your child suffers from frequent warts. Try the following:
  - Thuja, for soft, fleshy warts that ooze and bleed
  - Causticum, for warts on the face or fingertips, and painful verrucas
  - Dulcamara, for hard, smooth, fleshy warts on the back of hands
  - Kali Mur., for warts on hands
  - Nat. carb., for weeping warts on the toes
- Rub fresh lemon into the wart daily, and keep moist (with a bandage), paring back any hardened skin.
- Rub fresh garlic into the wart to fight the fungal infection, and offer plenty of garlic in your child's diet to boost immunity.
- Apply a little lemon oil directly to the wart, and continue to do so until the wart disappears. When it has gone, add a few drops of lavender oil to vitamin E oil and apply to the area for a week, to encourage healing and prevent scarring and further infection.
- Milkwort can be mashed and applied directly to the wart.

- Some people claim to be able to charm away warts. If you should know such a person, it's always worth a try!

Useful therapies
Homeopathy, herbalism, Ayurveda.

SELF-HELP

Take steps to boost your child's immune system (see page 207). Add acidophilus to your child's diet to help ward off fungal conditions (among other things).

WHOOPING COUGH

Whooping cough (pertussis) is a bacterial infection that causes bouts of coughing and frequently vomiting, especially in younger children. It gets its name from the characteristic whoop when the child draws in his breath for the next bout of coughing, but the whoop may be absent in older children.

It starts with a runny or snuffly nose for about a week, together with the cough, which is always worse at night. There may be as many as 50 paroxysms of coughing, which can be so severe that the face goes red or blue and the eyes bulge. There may be some vomiting with the coughing spells. The cough improves slowly over many weeks, often taking months to settle completely.

Whooping cough is highly infectious. Children should not attend school or play with other children for 21 days from the onset of the cough. It's worth noting that many children who have been vaccinated come down with whooping cough, so don't rule out the diagnosis in the misguided belief that your child couldn't get it.

Conventional treatment
A vaccine is regularly offered to children (see page 213). Antibiotics are not particularly helpful, but may be indicated. If the illness is recognized early, however, erythromycin is often given, which appears to reduce your child's infectivity to others and reduce the length of the illness.

CAUTION
There is a risk of secondary infection, in particular, pneumonia and bronchitis. All cases of whooping cough should be seen by a doctor. If the cough is accompanied by vomiting, make sure there is adequate intake of fluid to prevent dehydration. Call your doctor immediately if your child becomes blue around the lips.

NATURAL TREATMENTS

- A few drops of tincture of thyme in a little fruit juice, available in health food stores, can be taken to loosen and expel the mucus .
- Elecampane is commonly used for children's coughs, and can be purchased in easy-to-use syrup form.
- After the bath, massage a little comfrey ointment into the chest and back to relax and expand the lungs.
- The following homeopathic remedies may be useful:
  - Aconite can be taken during an attack, or at the beginning of the illness
  - Antimonium tart. is particularly good when there is a rattling cough with gasping
  - Try Sanguinaria, for a harsh, dry cough
  - Drosera is useful when the cough is made worse by lying down, and there are pains below the ribs
  - Bryonia is suggested when there is a dry, painful cough and vomiting
  - Pertussin may be given in one dose toward the end of the disease to prevent an "echo" effect. This is particularly useful in the early stages of the condition if your child has been immunized against pertussis but fallen ill anyhow.
- Bach Rescue Remedy (see page 260) is excellent for calming a child who has difficulty drawing breath, and who is frightened by the condition. A few drops on pulse points, or sipped in a glass of cool water, will help. Take some yourself to stay calm. Cherry Plum will help if there is serious spasmodic coughing, and Mimulus and Olive are good in the later stages of the condition.
- Mix a few drops of lavender and chamomile oils in a

light carrier oil, and massage into the chest and back area to calm your child, and to relax tensed muscles.

- Tea tree, lavender, chamomile and eucalyptus can be used in a vaporizer to help open up the lungs and reduce spasm.
- Increase the intake of foods containing vitamin C and zinc, to aid the action of the immune system.
- Acidophilus should be taken after any illness to encourage the healthy bacteria in the gut.
- Try to avoid citrus fruits, which can cause vomiting.

Useful therapies

Homeopathy, herbalism, traditional Chinese medicine, Ayurveda, aromatherapy, flower essences (some of these will help your child to relax and recover more quickly).

WORMS

An infestation of worms in the digestive system is quite common, particularly in young children, who usually contract them at school. Worms can sometimes be seen around the anus, or in the feces, and they inflame the area of the bowel or rectum where they attach themselves. Threadworms are not dangerous, although they do tend to disturb sleep.

Conventional treatment

Over-the-counter preparations are available to stun or kill the worms, which are then excreted in the feces. These drugs are called anthelmintic drugs, and they will be chosen according to the type of worm present. Only one or two doses are normally required, but sometimes longer treatment is required. Laxatives may sometimes be offered to aid the expulsion of worms living in the intestines.

NATURAL TREATMENTS

- A teaspoon (5 ml) each of cayenne pepper and senna can be combined in a cup of live yogurt and taken by the teaspoon before meals. The former stuns the worms and the latter encourages them to be expelled. This treatment is safe for children over the age of three.
- Wormwood tea will stun the worms, but this

should be taken only under the supervision of a registered herbalist.

- Many herbs are toxic to worms. Garlic, for example, can be crushed and added to a tablespoon of honey and eaten before meals. This is an invaluable treatment, and almost instantaneous. We use it for our guinea pigs, too! Raw onions, carrots, apples and raw turnip will also kill worms.
- Laxative herbs, such as licorice and dandelion root, can be taken alongside the above to aid expulsion.
- Homeopathic remedies can be effective. Try:
  - Cina, which may alter the balance of the body so that the child expels threadworms naturally
  - Teucrium, for an itchy bottom and nose, worse in the evening and with restless sleep
  - Santoninum, when all else fails
- Rub a drop each of eucalyptus, lavender and tea tree oil into a bland ointment, such as petroleum jelly or chickweed. Rub around the anus to prevent itching, and to prevent eggs from being laid. This is particularly helpful at night.
- Bach Rescue Remedy (see page 260) is good for discomfort or distress. Rub into the pulse points, and around the anus to relieve itching. Crab Apple is excellent if your child feels unclean or polluted.
- Acidophilus pills should be taken for several weeks to improve the health of the bowel.

CAUTION
Conventional treatment is always necessary for roundworm or tapeworm infestations.

Useful therapies
Homeopathy, herbalism, aromatherapy, traditional Chinese medicine.

SELF-HELP

- Fastidious hygiene will prevent reinfection, and sugar (which worms thrive upon) should be removed from the diet.
- Whatever treatment you give, repeat it after two weeks to expel the worms that were embryos at the first treatment.

Appendix 1

Keeping Your Child Safe

ccidents happen. Even the most safety-conscious among us can find ourselves facing an emergency situation, and it's essential that all parents know how to treat an injured child. More importantly, however, we have a responsibility as parents to ensure that our children are as safe as possible. This involves more than putting locks on the medicine cabinet. All parents need to be aware of how accidents can happen and what we can do to prevent them—at home, at the swimming pool, in the playground, on the playing fields, in the car and at school.

Thousands of children die in accidents each year, and injuries run into the millions. The simple fact is that most accidents are preventable, and we can do a great deal to ensure that our children are safe.

As our children grow older we need to educate them about safety and explain how they can protect themselves. Most children are capable of learning their own addresses, and what to do if they are lost or in trouble. They can learn how to cross roads, buckle up seatbelts and take care by water. They can be taught not to put anything in their mouths that hasn't been checked by an adult, and they can understand the dangers of fire.

See the world through your child's eyes

It's difficult to see the world from a child's point of view. As adults we take risks that we do not want our children to take, and our higher (literally) perspective means that we often don't see the potential dangers that exist at a child's level. Many of us become rather blasé about safety, partly because it's become intrinsic to our behavior and partly because we are capable of weighing a situation and taking risks accordingly. As parents we need to re-educate ourselves before we take on the task of educating our children, and we need to get down on our hands and knees and look at the world through their eyes. The cord to the iron may prove to be an irresistible attraction to a child, as are a pack of matches, an open window, and a tantalizing array of bottles and sprays underneath the kitchen sink. We take these things for granted, but children do not. Children are intrepid investigators and they are infinitely curious. They learn by exploring and experimenting, and that process is crucial to their development. Equally, however, they need to learn early on what is safe and what poses a serious risk.

Many parents teach safety by scaremongering and this can have a detrimental effect on any child. First of all, this technique can encourage fears and even phobias. For example, if you are inordinately upset or fearful with your children at the roadside, they will pick up your feelings and become fearful themselves. While we do want to encourage a healthy fear of danger, it is important that children are not so frightened or shocked that they become immobile. If you have instilled an irrational fear of cars by shouting and holding your children back every time they reach a street corner, as they get older, they will need to learn to cross roads on their own, and the deep-rooted fear that they have developed may actually put them in more danger than if they had not learned safe crossing at all. Most children will look both ways before crossing a road. They've seen parents, crossing guards, and other children do the same thing. If your child panics, however, he may freeze when he sees a car, or find he is too frightened to cross.

The right approach is to teach and lead by example, remaining calm and reasonable. What we want is for our children to learn how to play safe by themselves, so that when they go into the world they can make reasonable judgments based on an understanding of risk. To do this successfully, they need to approach situations rationally and calmly. If we panic, we teach them to panic. If we overreact, they will too, Conversely, if we are cavalier about safety, our children will learn to take unacceptable risks. They are also more likely to be led into trouble, if they don't have the resources or the knowledge of what to do in a situation.

Empowerment is a message that runs throughout this book, and that holds true here too. We need to trust our children to make decisions, and it is our responsibility to give them the foundation upon which they can be made. All children need freedom. There is no question that a child kept indoors in a completely childproof house will have less chance of being injured, but one day that child will need to go out into the world and she will have no experience of correct behavior or have the strategies that will keep her safe. Giving a child some freedom, at an appropriate age, teaches them decision making and brings experience. It also encourages self-esteem and confidence. They will undoubtedly make some dubious decisions at times, but they will learn from their mistakes. Wrapping a child in cotton wool stifles her and puts her at risk in the future. In this chapter we'll look at some of the key areas in which we can teach our children about safety, and take steps to keep them safe. We'll also look at how to deal with emergency situations.

Making your home a safer place

Some children are naturally less curious than others, and you may not need to adopt all the suggestions listed here. But don't assume all children are as responsible as yours may be. If you regularly have your children's friends around to play, you'll need to do whatever you can to make your environment as child-friendly as possible.

Fire!

- Make sure that you have good fire or smoke detectors on each floor of your house—each room, if possible. Check the batteries regularly (at least twice a year).

- Keep a fire extinguisher on each floor, and learn how to use it. Teach older children how to use it as well, but make sure that they know not to play with it. Keep it out of reach of younger children.

- Plan two fire escapes, and get ladders if required. Put on a nightlight on each floor of your house, and at "exit" points, so that you can find your way out in the dark, or in a smoke-filled house.

- Keep all flammable liquids outside your home, in a shed or a locked metal box. Flammables include paint, thinners, kerosene, lamp fluid, lighter fluid and even oil for the fondue. If it sounds extreme, consider the effects if fire were to reach them.

- Keep lights and matches away from children, and teach them not to play with matches. If they see you using them with caution, they'll be more likely to do so themselves.

- Close bedroom doors while everyone is sleeping. Younger children who sleep alone can be heard with a baby monitor.

- In the U.S., more than 700 children die each year from fires and burns in the house. Of these children, two-thirds are under the age of four.

- In the U.K., the greatest cause of injury and death to children under the age of four is by fire.

Preventing burns

- Keep your hot water heater set below 120°F (48°C). Babies' and young children's bathwater should be no hotter than hand-hot. Check the temperature on your wrist before placing your child in the water. Swirl it first, to prevent "hotspots."

- Never carry your child and anything hot at the same time (hot drinks, an iron or even a hot water bottle, for example).

- Don't hold a child while you are cooking, and keep all pot handles facing toward the rear of the stove.

Child safety basics

- Teach road safety from toddlerhood onward. Make sure you practice what you preach.
- As soon as he's old enough, teach your child his telephone number and address. For younger children, put your telephone number in his coat pocket.
- From age five onward, teach your child how to telephone the emergency services. Explain the importance of using that number only for real emergencies (fire, injury, burns, for example— not when his sister has broken his favorite toy). Write it down beside the telephone.
- Keep your full address and telephone number on a pad beside the telephone. A child or a baby-sitter may need this information in an emergency.
- In the U.S., authorities recommend you finger-print and prepare a DNA pack for each child. Fingerprinting is easy—your local police station will undertake it for you, or you can do it at home with a stamp pad. Press your child's finger into the pad, turning it left and then right. Press it onto a piece of card, again, turning left and right without moving the finger. Do it for all fingers and both thumbs. For DNA information, use a clean cotton swab and run it inside your child's cheek. Let it air dry for 24 hours, in a clean, dry place. Once dry, place it in a plastic bag and seal carefully. Keep it in the freezer. This may sound extreme and possibly a little over the top, but if your child is injured or lost, it can help the authorities to trace or identify her.
- Keep an up-to-date information pack for each child, listing name, birthdate, address, emergency contact numbers, any allergies or medication, past injuries and inoculations, hair color, eye color, height and weight. Keep a photograph of your child with the pack. Chances are you may never need it, but if your child is lost or injured, you will have all the relevant information at hand to present to the authorities or medical practitioner.
- Plan a fire escape. Whether you live in an apartment or a mansion, you'll need to have two good escape routes in mind in the event of a fire. Teach your children the plan in case you aren't there, or you are injured.
- Don't quash your child's enthusiasm for life or instill unhealthy fears by being overprotective.
- Remember that knowledge is power. If you can provide it for your children, they'll have the tools they need to make the decisions that could change their lives.

- Turn off the burners when you have finished cooking, and use a knob guard to prevent children inadvertently turning them on.

- Use a fireguard or screen for young children, and never leave them alone in a room with a lit fire.

- Don't use the microwave to heat baby food or formula. They can heat unevenly and cause very hot spots.

- Keep cords for "hot" appliances well out of reach (irons, toasters or kettles, for example).

- Keep hot drinks well away from children.

Electricity

- Cover outlets with caps, to prevent shocks.

- Don't overload your outlets or extension cords, and keep all plugs safely out of reach of children (behind sofas or appliances, for example).

- Watch your electrical cords. Don't leave them hanging down, and make sure the cords are not frayed or broken.

- Don't be tempted to repair an electrical appliance yourself, unless you know what you are doing. Keep children away from faulty appliances.

- Never run extension cords under carpeting, as there is a risk of fire or electrocution if they become damaged.

- Unplug appliances that are not in use.

Poisoning

- Lock away harmful drugs, poisons and household products. Keep all medicines, including vitamins and herbs, securely locked in a medicine cabinet. Always replace child-resistant caps after use.

- Be scrupulous about following instructions for any medication prescribed to your child, and be equally vigilant with herbs and vitamins. Many products designed for children taste delicious, but all children should learn that they should be taken only under supervision, and that too much of any substance can make them ill.

- Try not to take your own medication in front of your children. Most children learn by imitation, and they might feel terribly grown-up popping a pill like you do. Similarly, don't let children play with empty medicine bottles. They'll be more likely to learn how to open the lids, and they may not distinguish between the "play" bottles and the real thing.

- Be careful when visiting other people's homes, particularly if they do not have small children. There may be unsafe products in easy reach of children's hands. Older people on medication may have bottles prominently displayed to remind themselves to take it!

- Keep the number of your local poison-control center by every telephone.

- Some experts recommend keeping a bottle of Ipecac syrup on hand, which will induce vomiting in the case of poisoning. Never use it, however, unless advised to do so by a poison-control center.

- Although some remedies may appear harmless (homeopathic remedies, for example), children should never be permitted to be in control of their own treatment. It may be tempting to send a bottle of remedies with your child to school, but until about the age of 12, they will not have the logic or reasoning ability to discern between acceptable remedies and unacceptable medication. It will also encourage other children to take medication on their own.

- Encourage honesty in your children, and try to ensure that they don't fear your reaction to confessions. Children who have knowingly taken something they should not have taken may feel frightened or guilty, withholding crucial information. This goes for young children and older children, who may have taken a recreational drug. Explain early on that lives can be saved only if doctors or other medical practitioners know all the relevant facts.

- Plants can be toxic. Make sure you don't keep anything poisonous in the backyard or the house, particularly when your children are young. Some of the most common poisonous plants include yew, privet and laurel berries, laburnum seeds, deadly nightshade (Belladonna) and many mushrooms.

- In the U.S. in 1997, more than 1.1 million unintentional poisonings among children aged five and under were reported to poison control centers. More than 100 children aged 14 and under, died from poisonings in the home.

- In the U.K., over 36,000 children receive treatment for poisoning, or suspected poisoning accidents every year.

- Lead poisoning is a common problem. Lead-based paint is the most obvious source (some children do put anything and everything into their mouths) but there are other causes. If your house was built prior to 1978, check paint for lead. Ask your water company to test your water supply for lead (many older pipes contain lead) or buy a testing kit from a home improvement store. Destroy all old batteries, including old car batteries, or take to the city's drop-off.

- Carbon monoxide poisoning is also on the increase, and many deaths are attributed to this type of poison. Always use a carbon monoxide detector in your home. Most plug into an outlet and are inexpensive. Have your chimney cleaned every year, and ensure that your furnace is inspected regularly. Make sure that all fires are properly vented (including those in stoves).

Preventing falls

- Falls remain the leading cause of unintentional injury for children, and those under the age of 14 account for more than 30 percent of all fall-related visits to emergency departments. The majority of falls are from furniture, stairs, baby walkers, playground equipment, windows and shopping carts.

- Falls are more common in the under-tens, as this coincides with natural curiosity, underdeveloped reasoning and risk assessment, and the development of motor skills.

- Never use a baby walker. As ridiculous as it may sound, some 80 percent of baby-walker injuries take place while the child is being supervised, and more than 50 percent of children who use a baby walker will suffer a fall that is severe enough to require emergency attention. Stationary activity centers are a much better bet.

- Teach children from an early age how to crawl up and down stairs. If you have a persistent escapee who hasn't yet mastered the stairs, you could consider stair gates, but as there is a chance they could be left open accidentally, and the homes of friends and family may not have them, it is more important that your child learn to negotiate the stairs with confidence.

- Move chairs and furniture away from windows. Bunkbeds are a common problem. Consider installing window guards or child locks on windows, or open the top (higher) half of the window rather than the lower half, if you have a choice. Always make sure that you have a key or other unlocking device to open windows in an emergency.

- Keep ladders away from children. Make sure ladders on bunkbeds are fixed to the bed.

- Ensure that the playground you visit has a soft surface (grass, sand or rubberized asphalt, for example).

- If you have an intrepid crib-escapee, consider moving him to a bed, or leave the side of the crib down, using pillows to cushion any falls.

- Never leave tripping hazards on the stairs.

- Stairs should be carefully maintained—damaged or worn carpet should be repaired or removed.

- Make sure balustrades are strong and do not have any footholds for climbing.

- Stairs should always be well lit.

- Keep floors free of toys and obstructions that can be tripped over.

- Always use a securely fitted safety harness in a stroller or highchair.

- Never leave babies unattended on raised surfaces. This goes for bouncing chairs as well. Most babies are capable of rocking a chair hard enough to move it from a surface.

Road safety

- According to research, children between the ages of five and nine are at the greatest risk from traffic-related pedestrian death and injury.

- Children are particularly vulnerable to pedestrian death because they are exposed to traffic threats that exceed their cognitive, developmental, behavioral, physical and sensory abilities. This is exacerbated by the fact that parents overestimate their children's pedestrian skills. Children are impulsive and have difficulty judging speed, spatial relations and distance. Auditory and visual acuity, depth perception and proper scanning ability develop gradually and do not fully mature until at least age ten. Don't assume that a mature child is ready to cross on her own. Play it safe.

- Make sure that you always practice correct pedestrian behavior. As tempting as it may be to nip across a busy road against the light, it will teach your children to take risks too.

- Encourage your child to make eye contact with drivers before crossing a road. Just because you can see the driver doesn't mean he's paying attention.

- In the U.S., children are encouraged to hold their arms out in front of them when they intend to cross a road. This is a good habit to assume, particularly for young children. Drivers are much more likely to be aware of your intentions if you make them obvious.

- Cross streets at a corner, using traffic signals and designated crossings whenever possible.

- Never run across a street with your child, no matter what the rush. Children are more likely to fall or to panic if they are encouraged to run.

- Get children to look left then right, then left again before they cross the road, and make sure that you do too.

- Teach children to walk facing traffic, as far away from the curb as possible. Adults should walk on the roadside of the pavement, children on their other side.

- If you walk or travel by bicycle in the evenings, wear reflective clothing or a light.

- Teach children never to run into the road, no matter what they have dropped or lost. Many children are killed running out for balls or other toys. Encourage them to find an adult if they lose something.

- Don't let young children play on driveways or unfenced yards, unless there is an adult present. Even older children should not be encouraged to play on the pavement in front of their homes. Children often lose all sense of their surroundings when they are excited, and it makes sense to prevent an accident before it happens.

In the car

- Car occupants form almost two-thirds of all road casualties, and children are at equal risk to adults.

- Seat belts are intended to reduce the severity of injuries suffered by car occupants in road accidents. No matter how much your child resists, make sure he is safely strapped into the car or car seat. Seat belts are a very effective safety measure. According to the American Academy of Pediatric Surgeons, ejection is the most important cause of death in automobile accidents and occurs ten times more often to unrestrained occupants. Seat belts also offer remarkable protection for occupants involved in frontal-impact collisions, reducing the chance of injury to the head or face by 60 percent. The Academy claims that there has been a decrease of 40 percent in fatalities in countries where seat belts are mandatory.

- Surveys have also shown that a substantial proportion of parents do not use child restraints when transporting their children, and many of the child seats that are used are incorrectly fitted. Not only is this dangerous, it's also against the law.

- Drivers and front-seat passengers in cars must wear a seat belt (all passengers in Canada), unless they have a medical exemption certificate.

- Forty-nine states (all except New Hampshire) and the District of Columbia have mandatory safety belt laws. In most states, these laws cover front-seat occupants only, although belt laws in 14 jurisdictions (Alaska, California, District of Columbia, Kentucky, Maine, Massachusetts, Montana, Nevada, Oregon, Rhode

Island, Utah, Vermont, Washington, and Wyoming) cover all rear seat occupants, too. People in passenger cars, pickups, utility vehicles, and vans are required to comply with belt laws in most jurisdictions, but in a few jurisdictions occupants of some kinds of vehicles (usually pickups) are exempt. All 50 states and the District of Columbia have child restraint laws, and all are standard except in Nebraska where the law is secondary only for those children who may be in safety belts and standard for those who must be in a child restraint device. These states require children to travel in approved child restraint devices, and some permit or require older children to use adult safety belts. The age at which belts can be used instead of child restraints differs among the states. Young children usually are covered by child restraint laws, while safety belt laws cover older children and adults. In Canada, no one can operate a motor vehicle in which there is a child under the age of six unless the driver ensures that the child is securely fastened by a properly utilized and adjusted restraint system that complies with the MVA.

- Concern has been expressed at the use of lap belts, which are generally located in the center of the backseat in most cars. Although three-point seat belts are best, wearing a lap belt is far better than wearing no seat belt at all, because the greatest risk of injury to car occupants in an accident comes from being thrown about inside the vehicle or being ejected from it.

- The lap belt should go over the top of the thighs (not the soft stomach area) and fit as tightly as possible.

- Child restraints are divided into categories, according to the weight of the children for which they are suitable. These correspond broadly to different age groups, but it is the weight of the child that is most important when deciding what type of child restraint to use. The rear-facing child seat should always go in the backseat for babies less than one year of age or less than 20 pounds in weight. Children over 20 pounds and over one year of age should ride facing forward. At about 40 pounds or four years of age, your child may no longer fit in the safety seat. Once your child has outgrown a child safety seat, he should use a lap and a shoulder belt restraint. If no shoulder restraint belt is available, then just a lap belt should be used. The middle of the rear seat is the safest position for children. Booster seats should be used for children between the age of four and eleven (or up to about 80 pounds).

- Children under the age of 12 should sit in the backseat of the car, and should be facing forward (unless the seats are themselves facing backward). If you have airbags, no one under the age of 12 should sit in the front seat. Airbags are responsible for suffocating many young children.

- Keep doors child-locked, and discourage children from opening windows themselves, unless they are fitted with appropriate stops.

- Never let your child stand up in the car, reach out of a car window, or poke his head or anything else out of a sun roof, even when the car is not moving. Get into the habit of buckling up as soon as you get into the car, and discourage the idea that a car can be a plaything.

Keep them seated

Many children find it difficult to sit in any position for long periods of time, and wily toddlers soon become adept at releasing themselves from their car seats. For safety reasons, however, children obviously need to learn to stay put. Here are some ideas to keep escapees in place:

- Always buckle up your own seat belt when you enter the car, and tell your children what you are doing.

- When you buckle up little ones, point out that they are buckled up "just like Mommy or Daddy." They'll be less likely to resist if they feel they are being "grown-up."

- Buy a car seat with a buckle cover, which prevents children from undoing the belts themselves.

- Make a star chart and keep it in the car—taped to the back of the front seat, for example. For every successful journey, offer plenty of praise and a star.

- If your child does escape, calmly pull over and wait until she returns to her seat. Don't make too much of a fuss. If she learns that this type of behavior attracts attention, she'll do it more often. Don't move on until she is fastened in, no matter how late you are. This is particularly useful when you are heading off to an activity that your child enjoys.

- If you do see a traffic accident, calmly mention that you hope the occupants were wearing seat belts. If there is an ambulance present, suggest that perhaps someone wasn't wearing a belt. You don't need to frighten your child, simply bring to her attention the fact that wearing belts can save lives.

- Many children hate being left on their own in the back of the car, and undo their belts to be closer to their parents or caregiver. Make sure they don't feel isolated in the back. Supply books or small toys and talk to them while you are driving to make them feel involved.

Cycling

More than 70 percent of children aged 5 to 14 ride bicycles, and despite the fact that injuries have declined a great deal since the advent of the cycling helmet, bicycles are still associated with more childhood injuries than any other vehicle except cars.

Cycling is an excellent form of exercise, and certainly no one should discourage a child from riding on safety grounds. It is relatively easy to ensure that your child is safe. Here are some of the best ways:

- Riding without a bicycle helmet significantly increases the risk of sustaining a head injury in the event of a crash. Nonhelmeted riders are 14 times more likely to be involved in a fatal crash than bicyclists wearing a helmet.

- Bicycle helmets have been shown to reduce the risk of head injury by as much as 85 percent and the risk of brain injury by as much as 88 percent. Bicycle helmets have also been shown to offer substantial protection to the forehead and mid-face. It is estimated that 75 percent of bicycle-related fatalities among children could be prevented with a bicycle helmet.

- Studies show that children are more likely to wear a bicycle helmet if riding with others (peers or adults) who are also wearing one, and less likely to wear one if their companions are not. If your child rides with children who do not wear helmets, talk to their parents and ensure that everyone become involved. Buy a helmet that looks trendy, or suggest that your child cover his with stickers (Barbie, football, Pokémon, bands—whatever appeals). As long as he wears it, it doesn't matter what it looks like.

- Make sure your child understands that a bicycle helmet is a necessity, not an accessory. It should be worn every time she rides. The majority of accidents occur less than a mile from home, so it's important that she understand that even short distances (around the block, for example) can be dangerous.

- Wear a bicycle helmet correctly. A bicycle helmet should fit comfortably and snugly, but not too tightly. It should sit on top of your child's head in a level position, and it should not rock forward and back or from side to side. The helmet straps must always be buckled.

- Encourage your child to learn the rules of the road and obey all traffic laws.

- Ride on the left side of the road, with traffic, not against.

- Investigate local cycling proficiency courses, and make sure your child has passed the course before he is allowed to ride alone. These courses teach appropriate hand signals, traffic signals and emergency measures, among other things.

- Cycling should be restricted to pavements and paths until a child is about ten years of age and able to show how well she rides and observes the basic rules of the road.

- Parental and adult supervision is essential until your child is old enough to understand the rules of the road, and to assess risks.

Sports injuries

- Children are more likely to be injured in organized sports outside school than in physical education classes, possibly because the supervision and training is not undertaken professionally. This is, obviously, no reason to prevent your child from enjoying sports. Sports are crucial to health and well-being on many levels, and they will benefit from a variety of organized activities. The majority of injuries take place during training, so it's important that your child learn to warm up and wind down before and after any form of exercise. A recent study indicates that these types of exercises do not prevent injuries, but if you have ever played an impromptu game of football in the park, or taken a long bike ride after a long period of inactivity, you'll know that muscle strains and sprains are much more common if you go in cold. Simple stretching exercises and a quick run will be enough for most children.

- Make sure that you investigate any club or center where your child intends to play sports. Staff should deal with the physical and emotional needs of children appropriate for their individual developmental stages, and provide appropriate safety equipment, a safe playing environment, adult supervision and a set of safety rules that are taught and enforced.

- Many accidents occur when children play with older or fitter children. Make sure you match and group children according to developmentally appropriate skill level, weight and physical maturity, especially for contact sports. Children are more prone than adults to sports and recreational injuries since they are unable to assess the risks involved and have less coordination, slower reaction times and less accuracy. Children develop at different rates, both physically and psychologically. A less developed child competing against a more mature child of the same age and weight is at a disadvantage and may be at greater risk of injury.

- Children aged 5 to 14 account for nearly 40 percent of sports-related injuries for all ages. The rate and severity of sports-related injury increases with a child's age. Prior to the onset of puberty, the risk of sports-related injury between boys and girls is the same, as they are approximately the same size and weight. During puberty, boys are injured more frequently and severely than girls. Among children aged 5 to 14, boys account for nearly 75 percent of all sports-related injuries. In addition, boys are more likely than girls to suffer from multiple injuries.

- Children should always wear appropriate safety gear when participating in sports and recreational activities. That means mouthguards, protective pads or helmets where appropriate. Even if equipment is expensive, it is worth the investment. Inappropriately protected children are over 80 percent more likely to suffer injury.

- Ensure that children drink an adequate amount of liquids while engaging in athletic activities, and offer snacks to keep blood sugar levels stable. Overexertion is a major cause of injury, particularly for older children, and they should never be pushed—or encouraged to push themselves—to a point where they are in any discomfort.

- No child should be encouraged to play on after sustaining an injury. Children may become embarrassed, or they may not want to let down team members, but injuries must be reported and dealt with.

- Make sure your children get proper training and skills building when they are learning a new sport.

The playground

Play is an essential component of healthy development in children, and playgrounds provide an opportunity for children to develop motor, cognitive, perceptual and social skills. All too often, however, playgrounds are the site of unintentional injuries. Playground equipment can be great fun, but it makes sense to choose your playground carefully and to keep a close eye on children of all ages.

- Don't be tempted to curtail activities if you are frightened, and try not to overreact if a child climbs or swings too high. Most children will not take unacceptable risks unless they are encouraged by older children. Talk to your child first about which equipment is most appropriate, and show him how to get on and off, and to climb up and down. Suggest that he hold on tightly, and make sure he knows what to do when he gets stuck. Natural curiosity will undoubtedly be stifled if you stand too close and watch, or cringe every time he slips. Give him a little freedom on appropriate equipment, and if he hurts himself, suggest he try it again another day. Children learn by experimentation, and although safety is extremely important, they must all learn through some trial and error.

- Always supervise children unobtrusively when using playground equipment. Prevent unsafe behaviors like pushing, shoving, crowding and inappropriate use of equipment.

- Ensure that children play on age-appropriate equipment.

- If you have a wildcat on your hands, who swings too high and climbs beyond what you consider safe, consider investing in a helmet, which will prevent the risk of head injuries. If you suggest a bike ride first, you can just conveniently forget to take it off!

- Watch out for drawstrings, neckties and any other dangling bits of clothing that can cause strangulation or trap a child. Keep everything carefully tied and tucked in. Never allow children to wear necklaces, purses or scarves at the playground.

Fun and games?

Billions of toys and games are sold every year, and it is the ultimate irony that something designed to provide hours of excitement is all too often linked to common injury. Children under the age of four are at the highest risk. Falls and choking cause the majority of deaths and injuries, but children can also suffer from strangulation, burns, drowning and poisoning while playing with toys. What's the answer? Take care!

- The leading cause of toy-related death is choking, mostly on latex balloons. In 1997, 85 percent of toy-related deaths in the U.S. were due to choking, and more than half of these involved latex balloons. Children should not, under any circumstances, play with balloons that have not been inflated. Discard broken or deflated balloons immediately.

- Children under age three are at greater risk than older children for choking on toys, mostly because they tend to experiment more by putting things in their mouths. There are now obligatory warnings on toys that are not suitable for children under the age of three, and the risk of choking is the main cause for these warnings. Don't be tempted to give your child an unsuitable toy, no matter how "advanced" you may think he is.

- When selecting toys, consider the child's age, interests and skill level. Always choose good-quality design from a reputable maker. Always follow age and safety recommendations from the manufacturers.

- Ensure that toys are used in a safe environment. Riding toys should not be used near stairs, areas of traffic or swimming pools.

- Always supervise children at play. Play is even more valuable when adults become involved and interact with children during play, rather than supervising from a distance.

- Teach your children to put toys away safely after playing. Ensure that toys intended for younger children are stored separately from those for older children.

- Consider purchasing a small parts tester to determine whether small toys may present a choking hazard to children under age three.

- Inspect old and new toys regularly for damage and potential hazards. Old and broken toys should be kept out of children's reach, or discarded.

- Keep toys clean, particularly if they are used by small children who put them in their mouths.

- Toy chests should have safety supports to prevent the lid from falling on a child's head or fingers. Toy chests should also contain a locking hasp. If a child does climb into a chest, he should be able to get out.

- Never store toys on top of furniture or on shelves in a closet. Children may fall while climbing to reach these toys.

- If you can't be there, use a baby monitor to listen for children while they are playing.

Water play

Children can get hours of enjoyment from a bucket of water or a few inches of water in a bath, but it is essential that any play that involves water—no matter how little—is supervised by an adult. Drowning is the cause of a horrific number of deaths, and the majority of cases occur in children under the age of four. More than half of drownings among infants (under age one) occur in baths. Drownings in this age group also occur in toilets and buckets.

- Children can drown in as little as 1 in (2.5 cm) of water, and that makes bathtubs, wading pools, diaper buckets, toilets, hot tubs and washing bowls potentially dangerous.

- Drowning usually occurs quickly and silently. Many children are, in fact, in the presence of a parent or other caregiver who left them unattended for just a few moments.

- Empty all containers immediately after use and store out of reach.

- Never leave a child unsupervised in or around a swimming pool or spa, even for a moment.

- Don't assume that water wings or a float will protect your child. Similarly, swimming lessons will encourage good water habits and confidence, but young children can still drown in less than two minutes. It doesn't take long for a child to panic, or to slip under the water after tripping or banging a head.

- Swimming pools should be surrounded on all sides by a fence that it is at least 5 ft (1.5 m) high, with a self-closing and self-latching gate.

- Children should wear a life jacket when on a boat or near open bodies of water. Parents and caregivers should do the same.

- Do not encourage children to dive into the water until they are at least eight, and then only when there is at least 6 ft (1.8 m) depth of water.

- Encourage your children to take swimming lessons and, when they are older, water survival courses. This will never be a replacement for adult supervision, but it can help to prevent an accident.

- Never leave a child unsupervised in the bath, even with an older child. Children should not be encouraged to bathe or shower alone until at least eight years of age.

If you have to leave an older child alone for a few seconds, continue to talk to him and ensure that he is talking back.

Out and about

It's a sad fact that we can no longer feel confident about letting our children play outside alone. Most parents have justifiable concerns about traffic and the risk of abduction, and it can be difficult to assess what level of freedom to offer as our children get older. In the U.K., the NSPCC (National Society for the Prevention of Cruelty to Children) outlined ten points that parents should consider to keep their children safe outdoors:

1. In most situations, children under about eight years old shouldn't be out alone, especially in busy towns. Even when out playing with other children, they need to be kept in the care and sight of an adult or a much older child who is mature and trustworthy.

2. Never leave young children in unsupervised play areas in shops or parks. And don't leave them alone in the car or outside a shop, even for a few minutes.

3. If you're in a crowded place, keep children in a stroller or shopping cart, hold hands tightly, or use a harness. Don't walk far ahead of small children who can't keep up.

4. As soon as children are able to understand, teach them their full name, address, and telephone number.

5. You can start teaching children simple rules about personal safety from as young as two or three. Tell them clearly that they must never go off with anyone, not even someone they know, without first asking you or the adult who is looking after them.

6. Teach older children safe ways of crossing roads, going shopping and asking adults for directions, and let them practice these with you until you are sure that they have understood. When they are mature enough to be out alone, make sure they tell you who they're going out with, where they're going, and when they'll be back.

7. In busy public places, arrange somewhere safe to meet in case you get separated. Make sure that children know what to do if they get lost and who is safest to ask for help—a police officer, a cashier or someone with a young child.

8. Help to build your child's self-esteem with lots of love, praise and attention. Bullies and dangerous adults may tend to pick out less confident children or those who are neglected and often left alone.

9. Let children know they never have to do anything they don't like with an adult or older child—even if it's someone they know. Practice this at home by never making them kiss or hug an adult if they don't want to.

10. Listen to your children, especially when they are trying to tell you about things that worry them. Is there a bully at school or a baby-sitter they don't like? Let children know that you will always take them seriously and do whatever you can to keep them safe.

At what age can they . . . ?

- Children need to be supervised while crossing the road, and playing, until the age of nine or ten.
- They can be left alone in a room in a house with a caregiver nearby (but not in the same room) for short periods from the age of five.
- They can be allowed out to play on their own from the age of ten, but they should be taught road safety and emergency measures for a variety of situations, including injuries, becoming lost or being harassed.

The safety pact

Talking to children about safety can make a big difference to the way they view the outside world. We don't want to raise children who see their surroundings as in hostile. Instead, we need to equip them with the information and knowledge they need to deal with any situation that confronts them. If children are confident, they'll be much more likely to make rational decisions and appropriate judgments.

Make a pact with your child. Sit down and analyze what freedom you can allow, and at what age. Discuss what you expect from your child, once he is given this freedom. For example, at nine it might be appropriate to allow your child to walk to the corner store with a friend. He'll need to know that he is expected to leave and return at appointed times, and he'll need to be talked through road safety. In return for following a few simple rules, your child will be given privileges. These can be increased or withdrawn according to how well a few trials go.

Any child given her first taste of freedom needs to learn a few basic points. She should be able to answer questions on any of these points upon demand (that doesn't mean constant quizzing—just reassure yourself that she knows them!). It's also worth instilling a few positive statements that can be printed out and placed on a bulletin board or the refrigerator.

For example, children can learn the following rules, which will ensure that they remain confident in difficult or unknown situations:

- I will always tell my parents where I am going and when I'll be home, and return before dark.

- I will always play or go to places with at least one other person. If I go somewhere alone, I must stay on the route agreed with my parents.

- I do not have to do anything I do not want to do for strangers. I can say no and run away from any situation that is uncomfortable.

- Unless I know the person driving or in the passenger seat, I will not get into any car. Even if I do know them, I will check with another adult to make sure that it's safe.

- There are certain kinds of strangers who can assist me when I need help. For instance, mothers with children, other children, police in uniform or store assistants behind counters.

- I will walk and play only where my parents have agreed I can. I will not take short-cuts, or go down alleys, or play by water if I am not with an adult.

- I will not allow adults to trick or force me into going to places or doing things like help find pets, carry packages, take pictures, play games, eat candies or ice cream, or take drugs with them. I will always check with my parents first.

- I will not accept candies, money, gifts or rides from any adult without my parent's permission.

- I will always lock my home and car doors. I will not tell anyone that I am home alone.

- I will learn to dial 911.

- I will learn how to make a reverse-charges call from a pay telephone by dialing the operator and asking for the charges to be reversed to my family.

- I will learn my own address and telephone number, but I will not supply it to strangers unless I am lost or in danger.

Around the house

Many of the potential dangers have already been addressed, but it is practical to look at the various rooms of a typical home, to work out where safety measures can be undertaken.

The kitchen and dining room

- Use the back burners of the stove when young children are in the kitchen.
- Always turn off the electricity or gas when you have finished cooking.
- Keep children away from the front of the oven while it's on. It can be dangerously hot.

- Consider installing a stove guard to prevent curious little fingers from turning on the knobs or reaching for hot pots and pans.

- Turn pot handles toward the rear of the stove.

- Place the microwave oven out of the reach of young children so they can't open it or push the buttons. Never permit your child to use the microwave oven, unless supervised by an adult.

- Keep all sharp utensils in a childproofed drawer or cabinet.

- Install childproof locks on drawers and cabinets that are within a child's reach.

- Unplug appliances when not in use.

- If you have a waste disposal, use a switch blocker to prevent children from turning on the appliance.

- Install appliance latches to prevent children from playing with your appliances. It's not unheard of for children to trap themselves in the dryer.

- Watch out for sharp edges on tables and cabinets. Buy covers if they seem sharp or jagged.

- Keep high chairs far enough away from the table or work surfaces to prevent children from pushing them over.

- Secure booster seats firmly to chairs to prevent children from slipping and sliding.

- Place hot food items in the center of the table to prevent children from pulling them off the table.

The playroom

- Install window catches and sliding glass door locks. Windows and doors should not be opened more than 4 in (10 cm). Keep the keys at hand for emergencies!

- Ensure all carpets are firmly tacked or taped in place.

- Remove tables with glass inserts. Save them for when your children are older.

- Install corner cushions on your tables to protect your children when they fall.

- Use fireguards for any open fires, and never leave your child unsupervised if a fire is lit.

- Remove small and breakable objects from lower shelves.

- Wind up blind or curtain cords so that children can't reach them.

- If furniture is unsteady, consider bolting it to the wall, or remove the lower shelves to prevent climbing.

Stairways

- Keep stairs clear of clutter. Don't collect items on the stairway, and don't place things on the stairs that need to be taken upstairs.

- Keep stairways properly illuminated.

- Use gates to prevent children from playing on stairs.

- Banister rails should be no more than 4 in (10 cm) apart. Larger openings permit children to place their head between the rails. All banisters and hand rails should be secure.

- Discourage sliding down the banisters! It may seem like great fun, but it can be dangerous.

Bedrooms

- Take time to assemble your child's furniture properly, and make sure that it is made by a reputable manufacturer. Cheap children's furniture may be cost-effective, but if it doesn't meet safety standards, it can be dangerous.

- Always keep the side rail up when your child or toddler is in the crib, unless he is a determined climber, in which case it may be safer to leave the side down for safer departures!

- Use bed rails to prevent the child from falling out of bed.

- Do not place furniture under windows. Children love to climb.

- Be sure that your children's bedroom doors cannot be locked. Either install a door knob without a lock or use tape to prevent the door from being locked.

- Watch out for picture frames within reach of children, particularly if they contain glass.

- Use safety toy chests. Make sure they will lock open and not fall on a child's head.

- When emptying your pockets at night, put items in a childproof container. Small items pose a choking hazard to young children.

- Remove dry-cleaned clothes from their plastic bag and throw the bag away. If you must keep the clothes in their bags, tie a knot at the bottom to prevent children from getting into the bag.

- Put all toys away at the end of the day, and use a night light. Children may trip when trying to get to the bathroom or to you!

The bathroom

- Always empty sinks and baths after use.

- Keep one hand on younger children at all times, and never leave a child under the age of eight in the tub alone.

- Set water temperatures (see page 402) to avoid burns.

- Install spout covers on taps to protect from burns and falling accidents.

- Use a nonslip mat or stickers in the bath to prevent falls.

- Remove any potentially dangerous products or items from around the bath (shampoo, essential oils, razors, etc.).

- Keep lid down and install toilet lock to prevent child from playing in the toilet.

- Install cabinet locks to prevent children from getting into the medicine cabinet. Purchase only child-resistant products.

- Ensure that the bathroom door doesn't lock. If you want privacy, put a latch on at an adult's eye level.

The garage

- Use only garage door openers with automatic stopping devices. These doors will automatically reopen if they sense an obstruction.

- Empty all buckets, and turn off hoses at the source.

- Keep hazardous chemicals out of the reach of children.

In the backyard

- Store tools in their proper place after using them. Many children imitate their parents. My son found a power trimmer in the backyard shed and, at age seven, decided he'd help me out. In 30 seconds he had cut the cord! A lesson learned.

- Never use electrical equipment close to swimming pools, sprinklers or other water sources.

- Always empty portable pools and turn them upside down to prevent rain from collecting.

Important safety tips

- Watch out for strange or overzealous dogs both at home and out-of-doors.

- Don't leave a dog and a child alone together.

- Keep sewing materials out of reach.

- Replace plate glass windows and French doors with safety glass or film.

- Keep electrically powered appliances out of reach.

- Beware of swing doors and those with automatic closures.

- Avoid using paraffin heaters if you can.

- Avoid using hot water bottles for small children. Use only hand-hot water for older children.

- Never leave a child or baby alone with food or a bottle.

- Don't give nuts to preschool children.

- Don't give grapes or cherries to small children unless they are cut up.

- Don't give a child an electric blanket.

- Make sure all of your appliances are grounded.

- Avoid trailing cords.

- Never leave a child in a room with an iron.

- Take care around balconies.

- Beware of rugs on polished floors.

- Safety-check all bicycles.

- Keep children away from plastic bags and empty trunks or boxes.

- Do not give a baby a pillow when he is sleeping.

- Use a high SPF (15–25) sunscreen if your child is in the sun. Babies should not be exposed to sun at all.

- Put a wide-brimmed sunhat on children and avoid midday sun.

- Sterilize all your baby's feeding equipment.

- Always use a safety harness in a high chair and stroller.

- Never leave your front door open.

- Buy toys that have an approved safety mark.

- Buy only nontoxic paints and writing materials.

- When your child begins to climb out of her crib, move her to a bed.

- Use rail nettings or other protection to prevent children from squeezing through deck or porch railings.

- Use safety gates to protect children from steps.

- Put a fence around, or a mesh cover over, ponds or fountains.

Basic first aid

By their nature, children are prone to accidents and mishaps. The likelihood of an emergency situation arising is greater than for any other age group, and above all it is important for parents and caregivers to be prepared to deal with these emergencies. Many emergency situations are handled differently for children, and you should, therefore, never assume that your child should be treated as an adult. Children are not always able to describe their symptoms and it is all the more important to be familiar with the features of a condition or situation so that you can act swiftly.

Remember not to panic. Children are sensitive and they will pick up on anxiety.

What to do in an emergency

There are four steps to remember in any emergency. Above all, stay calm.

1. Assess the situation. Do so quickly. Think of the following:
  - The nature of the accident and how it happened.
  - Who is injured and how badly.
  - Is there any existing or continuing danger or is the child causing danger to anyone else?
  - Should the doctor or emergency services be called?
  - Do I need help?

2. Assess the safety aspect. Do so quickly. Think of the following:
  - Will you or anyone else be injured by treating the child?
  - Can you remove the source of danger from the child easily and safely?
  - Should you move the child—bearing in mind that you should not move a casualty unless absolutely necessary?

3. Phone for help. Call the emergency services or a doctor.

4. Stay with the child and provide constant reassurance. If she is seriously injured, check her pulse and breathing constantly.

What to do where there is a casualty.

1. Check the airway.
- Tilt the head back and lift the chin.
- Check that the airway is clear.
- If the airway is blocked, see page 428. Try to swipe your fingers into the throat to clear any obstruction.

2. Check breathing. Is the child obviously breathing? For example:
- Is the chest rising and falling?
- Place your hand across the mouth and nose—can you feel any air movement? Can you hear any sounds of breathing?
- Place your head against the child's chest—can you hear any breathing? If he is not breathing, begin artificial respiration.

3. Check circulation.

To check for a pulse in a baby:
- Place two fingers in the inner arm, halfway between the shoulder and the elbow.
- Press into the bone.
- If you do not feel a pulse in five seconds, begin external cardiac compression and artificial respiration.

Remember ABC: Airways, Breathing, Circulation.

Emergency remedies

There's a good natural first aid kit outlined on page 228, but most parents will benefit from keeping the following either in the car glove compartment, a handbag or within easy reach for most emergencies:

- Arnica 30—a homeopathic remedy that can be given for bumps, bruises, blows or, in fact, virtually any injury to the body.

- Aconite 30—a homeopathic remedy for shock. Give it to any child who has been hurt or traumatized in any way. Even unconscious children can have homeopathic powders sprinkled around their mouths (unconscious children should never have anything put in their mouths).

- Bach Rescue Remedy—a flower remedy designed for shock and trauma (see page 260). Offer by mouth, or for young or seriously injured children, rub it into the pulse points (wrists and neck).

Granules or drops are the easiest way of administering homeopathic remedies in emergencies because they can be put directly on the tongue and dissolve very quickly. If you have only pills, crush them between two clean spoons and dissolve in a teaspoon of warm water. If your child is unconscious, place the remedy between the lip and gum. Never give more than six doses in any emergency.

To check for a pulse in a child:

- Tilt back the head and find the carotid artery in the neck that runs up either side of the Adam's apple. You'll find the pulse in the hollow between the Adam's apple and the neck muscle.
- Press lightly into the hollow.
- If you do not feel a pulse in five seconds, begin external cardiac compression and artificial respiration.

Artificial respiration

Phone for help immediately.

Babies

When a baby is unconscious and not breathing, but has a good pulse, resuscitation should be done through the nose and mouth. This is called mouth-to-mouth-and-nose ventilation.

1. Tilt the baby's head back and ensure the airway is clear.

2. Seal your lips around the baby's mouth and nose and breathe until the chest rises.

3. Remove your mouth and allow the baby to exhale as the chest falls.

4. Continue for one minute, breathing in once every three seconds.

5. Check the pulse every ten breaths.

Children

Children should be ventilated through the mouth, unless there is a mouth injury. Breathe in every three seconds (about 20 per minute), a little less if the child is older.

CPR (Cardiopulmonary Resuscitation)

Phone for help immediately.

Babies

1. If there is no pulse in the baby, put her on a firm surface and place two fingers a half inch (one centimeter) or so below the point on the chest between her nipples.

2. Press at a rate of about a hundred compressions per minute—nearly two per second—about 1 inch (2 cm) into the chest.

3. Artificial respiration must be combined with this action in order for oxygen to reach the brain and other parts of the body.

4. Compress five times for every breath of air.

Children under five

1. If there is no pulse in the child, lay him on a flat surface and find the point of compression as you would with an adult.

2. Using the heel of one hand only, press into this area at a rate of a hundred compressions per minute—almost two per second—about 1 to 2 inches (2.5 to 4 cm) into the chest.

3. Artificial respiration must be combined with this action in order for oxygen to reach the brain and other parts of the body.

4. Compress five times for every breath of air.

Children over the age of five

1. While compressing the heart as above, breathe into the mouth or nose of the child twice for every 15 compressions of the heart.

2. Continue compressing the heart, alternating with 2 breaths of artificial respiration every 15 compressions, until there is some evidence of circulation. Check for a pulse (see page 423) every two minutes.

3. If you feel a pulse, stop compression immediately, but continue with artificial respiration until the child is breathing on his own.

4. Place the child in the recovery position when breathing is restored, but check every three or four minutes that breathing and circulation (see page 423) are maintained.

Treating shock

Medical shock exists when the blood circulation has failed. There are many causes for this, including a weakened heart that cannot manage to pump the blood effectively, a reduced amount of blood in the body, perhaps from a wound, or a loss of body fluid from, for example, vomiting or dehydration.

Your child may be in shock if

- she is very pale and blue or gray-colored

- her skin is cold and moist

- there is shallow breathing and rapid, weak circulation

- she is very thirsty and appears very tired

- she experiences nausea and perhaps some vomiting

- there is possible loss of consciousness

- she feels extreme fatigue, causing yawning

Caution: If your child is in shock, never offer anything to eat or drink, no matter how thirsty she appears. Never leave her, and reassure her constantly. Panic will make the condition much worse.

Treatment

Telephone for help as soon as you suspect shock—or ask someone else to do so.

1. Lay your child down and raise her feet above the level of her head—on some folded clothing, a car tire or some books perhaps. This encourages the flow of blood to the major organs instead of the legs.

2. Treat any obvious wounds.

3. Loosen any tight clothing and ensure that the child does not move. All movement requires blood, so it is essential that the circulation be concentrated mainly in the areas that need it most.

4. Cover her with a single coat or blanket—never allow her to overheat or get too cold.

5. Continue to check pulse and breathing every two or three minutes.

Some common emergency situations

Bites and stings

Bites and stings should always be treated immediately. Stings from a bee, wasp or hornet are not usually dangerous unless your child suffers from an allergy. Bites may be more serious, partly because germs from the animal's mouth can be injected deep into the flesh, causing infection, and partly because a bite may break bones and damage tissue.

▶ *Top tips for bites and stings*

- Always remove a sting before beginning treatment. Animal bites should be carefully washed with soap and warm water.

- Prevent insect bites by diluting essential oils of eucalyptus or citronella in half a mug of water, and then gently applying to exposed areas, avoiding the eyes and mouth. Use cider vinegar in the same way.

- Witch hazel is useful on mosquito bites.

- Apply a paste of bicarbonate of soda and water to a bee sting to relieve pain.

- Apply garlic and onion to ant bites, and use cucumber juice to ease the discomfort.

- Make a compress from a pad of cotton wadding soaked in lemon juice and apply to a wasp sting.

- Bathe any wounds with Hypericum and Calendula solution.

- For jellyfish or bee stings, take the homeopathic remedy Apis every five minutes for up to ten doses.

- Arnica is useful for any bites that cause swelling, bruising or pain.

- Take Cantharis when there is redness and burning, or Hypericum when there are shooting pains in the affected limb.

> **Caution:** Multiple stings, or stings to the eyes, ears or mouth should be treated in thehospital. Animal bites that cause bleeding should be seen by a doctor—particularly if there is any possibility of contracting rabies.

Minor burns

Minor burns are those that do not cover more than 9 percent of the body. They will be superficial (not deep).

▶ *Top tips for minor burns*

1. Cool the affected area with cold running water for at least ten minutes.

2. Remove all constrictive clothing.

3. Dress the burn with a sterile burn sheet, or any sterile (or very clean) fabric that is not fluffy.

4. If you are concerned about the extent or severity of the burn, call your doctor immediately.

5. Offer Bach Rescue Remedy (orally) (see page 260) and the homeopathic remedy Aconite, for shock. When burns have been cooled, offer Arnica 30 (three doses) followed by Cantharis 30 (up to six doses). If there is still stinging, follow with Urtica 6 every 30 minutes for up to 6 doses.

6. Give your child 300 mg of vitamin C daily following the burn to encourage healing.

Choking

Choking occurs when a foreign body, such as a piece of food, becomes lodged in the airway, preventing air from reaching the lungs. Without an air supply, the body becomes starved of oxygen. A blocked airway is a serious medical emergency, and should be treated immediately.

Signs of choking include:

- clutching at the throat

- turning blue or very pale

- breathing with difficulty or sometimes not at all

- becoming unconscious within a few minutes

What to do
Babies
A baby who is choking may turn blue and breathe noisily or not at all. Call for help immediately.

1. Lay the baby face down along your lower arm with her head supported in your hand.

2. With the heel of your other hand, slap her back sharply, four or five times, just between the shoulder blades.

3. With your fingers, try to clear her airways.

4. If she is still choking, turn her on her back along your other arm and support her head with your hand.

5. With two fingers placed at the line where the ribs meet, just below the breastbone, thrust upward four or five times. Make sure her head is below the level of her lungs, but do not hang her upside down.

6. Continue this process: slap four or five times; clear the airways with your fingers; thrust four or five times, until the obstruction is cleared or help arrives.

Children

A child who is choking will probably be able to cough to eject the obstruction. If this does not work, call for help immediately and follow these steps.

1. Lay a small child across your lap face down and slap her sharply, four or five times, between the shoulder blades, or until the obstruction clears.

2. Turn her onto her back and, with the heel of your hand placed below the ribs, between the chest and abdomen, thrust four or five times upward, until the obstruction is cleared.

3. If the obstruction does not move, try clearing the airway with your fingers, and then begin to slap her back again.

Work as quickly as you can; if you cannot clear the obstruction within 30 seconds, you should call for an ambulance immediately and continue to try to clear it.

When the obstruction has cleared, offer Bach Rescue Remedy (see page 260) to calm her.

Cuts and bruises

Children acquire a huge variety of bruises and cuts, and if they are not serious, you can easily treat them at home. If there is extensive bleeding, or any other unusual symptoms, such as dizziness, difficulty breathing, or head injury, take your child to the hospital for emergency treatment. Otherwise, call for help immediately and take the following steps.

What to do

For minor cuts

1. Carefully clean the wound with soap and water, and cover with a sterilized piece of gauze or a bandage. Apply gentle pressure to stop bleeding.

2. For bruises, soak a clean cloth in witch hazel, and apply to the affected area. A cold compress will also help.

For serious cuts

1. Remove clothing in order to treat the wound. Don't try to remove any objects in the wound and be careful that you do not wound yourself trying to perform treatment.

2. Squeeze the sides of the wound together; apply direct pressure to the wound with your fingers, hand, or preferably a pad made from a clean bandage or a handkerchief. An article of clean clothing will do.

3. An injured limb should be raised and supported above the level of the heart. This may be easiest if the casualty is lying down.

> **Caution:** Do not move a child if there is a risk of fracture to the head, neck or spine.

4. Firmly bandage the original pad in place, but take care not to cut off the circulation to the area. If there is an object still protruding from the wound, pad either side until a bandage can be wrapped around it without pressing it further into the wound.

5. Watch carefully for signs of shock and call for emergency help immediately.

▶ *Top tips for cuts and bruises*

- Give your child an Arnica pill, to help disperse the bleeding and encourage healing.

- If she has lost a lot of blood, and feels restless and chilly, offer Arsenicum.

- If the bleeding is difficult to stop, and it flows in fits and starts, offer Phosphorus.

- Bach Rescue Remedy (see page 260) will help to calm.

Febrile convulsions

Febrile convulsions are the result of a high fever, which interferes with the activity of the brain. All cases of high fever accompanied by convulsions in small children require immediate medical treatment; treated immediately, they should not cause any damage.

The priorities are to:

- Call for emergency help.

- Protect the baby or child from anything that may cause injury; for instance, place him on the center of the bed and watch him carefully.

- Take steps to cool him in order to reduce the fever.

What to do

1. Remove any constrictive clothing and place the baby somewhere safe.

2. Sponge him with lukewarm water. Take care not to overcool.

3. Place him on his side, if possible, and call for help.

4. If he becomes unconscious, watch that his breathing doesn't stop. If it does, prepare to resuscitate (see page 424).

If the fever remains high and your child is red-faced, offer Belladonna 30. See also page 341 for fever remedies.

Nosebleeds

The lining of the nose is very thin, and even heavy blowing or a minor jolt can rupture a capillary and cause bleeding. Unless there is an accompanying blow to the head, or intense pain, nosebleeds are not usually serious.

▶ *Top tips for nosebleeds*

- During a nosebleed, gently pinch together the nostrils, and lean forward. Hold for several minutes, until the bleeding stops. Avoid blowing the nose for several hours after a nosebleed.

- A cold compress of witch hazel can be applied to the nose (externally).

- The homeopathic remedy Arnica should be taken, particularly if there has been a blow to the nose.

- If bleeding is brought on by violent nose-blowing, offer Phosphorus.

- Nosebleed that is accompanied by a headache, which feels worse when he bends his head forward, calls for Hamamelis.

- Apply lemon juice to a cotton wool swab to dab inside the nose and staunch the bleeding.

Poisoning

Each year hundreds of children attend emergency departments, having swallowed a drug or chemical that may cause poisoning. Most of these poisonings are preventable.

What to do

- If you suspect that your child has swallowed something, phone the hospital or your local poison control center immediately for instructions on what to do, and if necessary, get him to hospital as soon as possible. Take evidence of what was swallowed with you to the hospital.

■ Offer Bach Rescue Remedy (see page 260) to calm. If your child is unconscious, call for emergency assistance then apply it to pulse points.

Sunburn

Sunburn is the result of overexposure to the ultraviolet (UV) rays of the sun, or a sun lamp. Sunburn is normally superficial, characterized by redness, some swelling and pain. More severe cases will blister and may be accompanied by heatstroke. Children are much more sensitive to the sun than adults, and you should take every precaution to keep them covered up, applying a good sunscreen with a high sun protection factor, and ensuring that they do not go out into the sun during the middle hours of the day.

What to do

1. Cool the skin by pouring cold water over the affected areas, or by very gently sponging the skin. A cool bath might be helpful, but avoid a sudden very cold bath for fear of hypothermia.

2. Offer sips of cold water and dress the skin with a soothing lotion like aloe or calamine.

3. Watch for signs of blistering, which should be brought to the attention of a doctor.

▶ *Top tips for sunburn*

■ Superficial burns can be soothed by applying aloe vera gel, Bach Rescue Remedy cream (see page 260) or Urtica Urens cream on the affected area. If there is blistering, see your doctor.

■ Sol. 30 (a homeopathic remedy) should be taken every four hours as a preventative measure, especially in children who are fair or particularly sensitive to sunlight (most of them!).

Travel sickness

Although the exact cause is not known, it is believed that travel sickness occurs because of a disturbance of the balancing mechanisms of the inner ear. Common symptoms are nausea, dizziness, fatigue, pale and clammy skin, and vomiting. Travel sickness is very common in children, which can make car journeys very difficult.

▶ *Top tips for travel sickness*

- It may be helpful to offer small sips of ginger ale, or offer some candied ginger root, to ease the nausea.

- If you are traveling by car, hang some fresh angelica leaves on the mirror. This is a remarkably effective traditional remedy for travel sickness.

- Ensure that your child has lots of fresh air while traveling. Make sure she eats a light meal before you travel, and take care to avoid sugary or greasy foods.

- There are acupressure points on the wrist that are said to prevent the symptoms of travel sickness when stimulated. You can now purchase slim wristbands to do this.

- Good homeopathic remedies include Tabacum, when your child becomes nauseous, giddy, faint, pale and is in a cold sweat. He may complain about a tight band around his head.

  - Rhus Tox. is suitable if your child is fidgety but feels better lying down

  - Cocculus is indicated if the sight of food makes him sick, and he feels giddy and tired, wanting to lie down

  - Nux Vom. may help if she feels queasy and has a headache at the back of her head or over one eye

- See also Nausea and vomiting, page 373.

Appendix 2

Vitamins and Minerals

Understanding nutrition

Vitamins

Vitamins have many roles in the body (see pages 435–436), but they are crucial for energy production, balanced hormones and a healthy heart, nervous system, brain, immune system and, of course, teeth, bones, nails, hair and virtually every other part of the body. Major deficiencies cause diseases like scurvy and rickets. Minor deficiencies can cause behavioral problems, poor growth, reduced immunity, fatigue, headaches, sleep and skin problems and a host of other conditions that seem to have no obvious cause.

Vitamins are fat soluble (A, D, E and K), which means that they are stored in our bodies to a certain extent. Or they are water soluble (Bs and C), which means that they cannot be easily stored. Foods containing vitamins B and C must, therefore, be eaten daily to ensure that adequate levels are maintained.

Minerals

Some minerals, including calcium, magnesium, iron and phosphorus are required by the body in relatively large quantities. These are called "macro-minerals." Others, including chromium, selenium, manganese and zinc are required in smaller amounts and are known as "trace elements." All of the above fall under the umbrella term "minerals." Minerals are required for the body to function, and are involved in all body processes. Once again, minor deficiencies are common, and symptoms can include insomnia, hyperactivity, constipation, irritability, fatigue, excessive thirst, cravings for sweet foods, poor appetite, nausea and intellectual impairment, among other things.

All vitamins and minerals are important for children and adults alike, and chances are that most of us are not getting enough.

Breaking them down

You don't need to be a nutritionist to grasp the basics of vitamins and minerals. A healthy diet based around whole, unrefined, fresh foods ideally offers a variety of nutrients. It is, however, helpful to know which foods contain which vitamins and minerals. This helps you to pinpoint, at a glance, where your child's diet is weakest, and explains why variety is important!

The following table presents the main vitamins and minerals, their sources and their primary roles in the body. Where appropriate, cautions and any research into links with the treatment of diseases are noted. For more information, see page 283.

VITAMINS

A (retinol in animal foods and beta-carotene in plant foods)

Good sources: Beta-carotene—brightly colored fruits and vegetables, including apricots, carrots, leafy green vegetables, squash and melon. Retinol—liver, oily fish, eggs, butter and cheese.

Function: Needed for strong bones, good vision and healthy skin.

Special notes: Research shows that low vitamin A levels in children are linked with growth problems related to a lack of growth hormone.

B1 (Thiamin)

Good sources: Liver, whole grains, potatoes, nuts, legumes and liver.

Function: Converts blood sugar into energy, and is involved in key metabolism. Promotes growth and is a tonic for the nerves.

Special notes: There is some evidence that vitamin B1 may help to improve IQ and memory, and it may help to control diabetes.

Caution: In very high doses, vitamin B1 can be toxic.

B2 (Riboflavin)

Good sources: Milk and dairy produce (particularly yogurt), green leafy vegetables, poultry, eggs, fish and wheatgerm.

Function: Essential for the production of energy, and is an antioxidant (see page 284). Aids in cell respiration, growth and reproduction.

Caution: May be toxic in very high doses.

B3 (Niacin)

Good sources: Lean meats, legumes, potatoes, poultry, whole grains, nuts and yeast extracts.

Function: Essential for sex hormones, increases energy, aids nervous system, helps digestion.

Caution: Toxic in high doses.

B5 (Pantothenic acid)

Good sources: All meats and vegetables, especially dried fruits and nuts.

Function: Aids in healing wounds, fights infection, strengthens immune system, builds cells.

Special notes: B5 has been shown to increase immune activity in children, so if you have a chronically ill child, it might be worth considering whether or not her diet is adequate.

B6 (Pyridoxine)

Good sources: Poultry, fish, eggs, game, whole grains, nuts, yeast extract, soy products and bananas.

Function: Required for the functioning of more than 60 enzymes, aids the nervous system and the production of cells. Crucial for a healthy immune system.

Special notes: Promising research indicates that this vitamin can help protect against some types of cancer, and it has been used successfully in the prevention of some skin diseases and nervous disorders.

B12 (Cyanocobalamin)

Good sources: Fish, dairy produce, organ meats, eggs.

Function: Forms and regenerates red blood cells, increases energy, improves concentration, maintains nervous system.

Special notes: There is evidence that vitamin B12 protects against some toxins and allergens.

Caution: Toxic in high doses.

Folic acid

Good sources: Fresh leafy green vegetables, wheatgerm and legumes.

Function: For red blood cell formation in bone marrow; metabolism of sugar; and amino acids; manufacture of antibodies; crucial to normal functioning of the nervous systems and for the normal production of DNA and RNA, which determines hereditary patterns.

Caution: Toxic in large doses.

C (ascorbic acid)

Good sources: Fresh fruit and vegetables, potatoes, leafy herbs and berries.

Function: Vital for healthy skin, bones, muscles, healing and protection from viruses, toxins, drugs, and allergies. Necessary for cholesterol metabolism. An effective antioxidant (see page 284).

Special notes: There is plenty of evidence to suggest that vitamin C has a major role in our bodies. We know that it boosts immunity against infection, lowers cholesterol, speeds healing of wounds, help maintains good vision and may even counteract asthma.

Caution: May cause kidney stones, gout, diarrhea and cramps in excess.

D (calciferols)

Good sources: Milk products, eggs, oily fish, fish oil. Synthesized in the skin from sunlight.

Function: Vital for normal calcium formation and growth, and health of bones and teeth. Increases absorption of calcium from diet.

Caution: Toxic in high doses.

E (tocopherols)

Good sources: Nuts, seeds, eggs, milk, whole grains, unrefined oils, leafy vegetables, avocados and soy.

Function: Essential for absorption of iron and metabolism of essential fatty acids; protects the circulatory system and cells; slows the aging process and is an antioxidant (see page 284).

Special notes: Vitamin E has been used successfully in the treatment of a number of skin problems, and, as an antioxidant, it has been proved to reduce the risk of cancer.

Caution: Toxic in very high doses, and may elevate blood pressure.

K

Good sources: Green vegetables, milk products, molasses, apricots, whole grains, cod liver oil. Synthesized in the intestines.

Function: Produces blood clotting factors.

Caution: Toxic in very high doses.

MINERALS
Calcium

Good sources: Milk, cheese and dairy products, leafy green vegetables, tinned salmon and sardines, nuts, root vegetables, broccoli and tofu.

Function: Necessary for the action of a number of hormones; necessary for action of muscles; required for release of neurotransmitters in the brain, and aids nervous system; necessary for blood clotting and blood pressure regulation; maintains strong bones and teeth; helps to metabolize iron; necessary to keep heart beating; necessary for cell structure; helps the body to absorb vitamin B12.

Special notes: Calcium has been used successfully to ease growing pains in children, and can help to prevent osteoporosis and possibly some allergies. Insomnia and other sleep problems may be eased by increasing calcium in the diet.

Chromium

Good sources: Liver, whole grain cereals, meat and cheese, brewer's yeast, molasses, mushrooms, and egg yolk.

Function: Chromium works in the body as the GTF (glucose tolerance factor), which governs blood sugar levels.

Iron

Good sources: Liver, poultry, dark chocolate, sardines, molasses, dark green leafy vegetables.

Function: Necessary for production of hemoglobin (the part of the blood that carries oxygen) and certain enzymes; necessary for immune activity; protects against some free radicals (see page 7).

Special notes: Iron has been used successfully in the treatment of anemia, growth problems, poor resistance to infection and fatigue.

Caution: Excess iron can cause constipation.

Magnesium

Good sources: Brown rice, soy beans, nuts, brewer's yeast, whole grains, bitter chocolate and legumes.

Function: Repairs and maintains body cells; required for hormonal activity; required for most body processes, including energy production, and the action of our muscles. Also important for bone development and growth.

Special notes: Magnesium deficiency has been linked to asthma, and used successfully in its treatment.

Caution: Magnesium can be toxic to children with kidney problems.

Manganese

Good sources: Whole grains, nuts, root vegetables, brown rice and legumes.

Functions: Necessary for the functioning of the brain; required for metabolism of energy; important for bone structure and normal functioning of the thyroid gland.

Potassium

Good sources: Avocados, leafy green vegetables, bananas, dried fruits, fruit and vegetable juices, nuts, soy flour, potatoes, nuts and molasses.

Function: Necessary for transportation of carbon dioxide by the red blood cells; required for water balance, the proper synthesis of protein and nerve and muscle function.

Caution: Excessive potassium may cause ulceration of the small intestine.

Selenium

Good sources: Whole grains, nuts, brown rice and legumes.

Function: Antioxidant (see page 284); required by the immune system; improves liver function; maintains healthy eyes and eyesight; maintains healthy skin and hair; protects against heart and circulatory diseases; may impede the aging process.

Caution: Toxic in small doses.

Zinc

Good sources: Seafood, poultry, lean red meats, sunflower seeds, peanuts, whole grains.

Function: Required for male fertility, hormones, immunity, growth and energy metabolism; antioxidant (see page 284).

Special notes: Zinc is an excellent immune booster, and has been used therapeutically with some success. Growth problems and allergies have also responded to zinc.

Resources

NUTRITION

American Nutraceutical Association
5120 Selkirk Drive, Suite 100
Birmingham, Alabama 35242
Tel: (205) 980-5710
Fax: (205) 991-9302
For products and membership: (800) 566-3622
Email: info@ana-jana.org
Website: www.americanutra.com/index.html
The American Nutraceutical Association was established in February 1997 with a straightforward mission: to develop and provide educational materials and program on nutraceuticals and nutrition for health care professionals, consumers and sales associates from nutraceutical companies. The association provides up-to-date information on all health matters relating to nutrition, including recent studies. They produce the *Journal on Nutraceuticals and Nutrition*, which also appears online.

American Society for Nutritional Sciences
9650 Rockville Pike
Bethesda, Maryland 20814
Tel: (301) 530-7050
Fax: (301)571-1892
Email: jnutrition@asns.faseb.org
Website: www.asns.org
The American Society for Nutritional Sciences is the premier research society dedicated to improving the quality of life through the science of nutrition. The society produces the *Journal of Nutrition*, which also appears online on their website. Great source of up-to-date information.

Center for Food Safety and Applied Nutrition
200 C Street SW
Washington, DC 20204
Tel: (888)-SAFEFOOD
Website: www.cfsan.fda.gov

CFSAN, in conjunction with the FDA, is responsible for promoting and protecting the public's health by ensuring that the nation's food supply is safe, sanitary, wholesome, and honestly labeled, and that cosmetic products are safe and properly labeled. Their website and telephone service offer consumer advice on a broad range of subjects, including food allergies, food-borne illnesses, nutritional content of food, health claims by manufacturers, pesticides, product labeling and more.

Office of Dietary Supplements National Institutes of Health
Building 31, Room 1B29
31 Center Drive, MSC 2086
Bethesda, Maryland 20892-2086
Tel: (301) 435-2920
Fax: (301) 480-1845
Email: ods@nih.gov
Website: ods.od.nih.gov
The ODS supports research and disseminates research results in the area of dietary supplements. The ODS also provides advice to other federal agencies regarding research results related to dietary supplements. Plenty of information on the role of supplements in health, and research.

Organic Consumers Association (OCA)
6101 Cliff Estate Road
Little Marais, Minnesota 55614
Tel: (218) 226-4164
Fax: (218) 353-7652
Website: www.organicconsumers.org
OCA is a U.S. consumer advocacy organization promoting organic food and fiber production and affiliated with the Campaign for Food Safety. The web page provides book reviews (mainly on food safety), lists of U.S. and Canadian food co-operatives and community-supported agriculture farms (by state), green pages, an eco-directory, sources of organic fertilizers,

list of events, links and facts about organic agriculture, food safety and organic standards, OCA projects and other information.

Organic Crop Improvement Association (OCIA)
International Office
1001 Y Street, Suite B
Lincoln, Nebraska 68508-1172
Tel: (402) 477-2323
Email: info@ocia.org
Website: www.ocia.org
The Organic Crop Improvement Association is an international program of certification to strict organic standards. With thousands of certified members in seventeen countries, OCIA is a respected voice in the international organic community. They offer help and advice to farmers and consumers, and their website provides a wealth of literature on the subject of organic living. State chapters are listed by region.

Vegan Action
P.O. Box 4288
Richmond, Virginia 23220
Tel: (804) 254-8346
Email: info@vegan.org
Website: www.vegan.org
A non-profit organization that educates the public about becoming a vegan and adopting a vegan lifestyle. Plenty of recipes, advice and news reports.

The Vegetarian Resource Group (VRG)
P.O. Box 1463, Dept. IN
Baltimore, Maryland 21203
Tel: (410) 366-VEGE
Email: vrg@vrg.org
Website: www.vrg.org
A fantastic organization involved in all levels of government, consumer, business and research into vegetarianism. They have numerous publications and offer advice on all aspects of nutrition,

including fun meal plans, recipes, research, journals, an advice service and games. Great for kids, too.

Websites

Nutrition for kids

www.nutritionforkids.com
A very useful website aimed at parents, teachers and professionals, explaining how best to teach children to understand the importance of healthy eating. They have newsletters, games, action packs, recipes, books, stickers and much, much more.

Eatsmart

www.eatsmart.org
A great website run by the Washington Dairy Council. Plenty of advice, news and games for children to test their eating habits and knowledge.

Nutrition Sleuth

exhibits.pacsci.org/nutrition/sleuth/sleuth
Another website aimed at nutrition for kids, with a series of exciting games that will teach them about healthy eating as they play.

Think Fast

www.thinkfast.co.uk
Website for young people giving fast food facts and a quiz show.

Why do I have to eat this stuff?

www.pbs.org/kids/fungames
A website with great games for kids, teaching them the importance of healthy eating in a fun way.

EXERCISE

American Council on Exercise (ACE)
4851 Paramount Drive
San Diego, California 92123
Tel: (858) 279-8227 or (800) 825-3636
Fax: (858) 279-8064
Website: www.acefitness.org
ACE advocates healthy, active lifestyles for all segments of society. They are the leading provider of certification and education to the professional, commercial and retail fitness markets. They protect the public against unsafe and ineffective fitness products and instruction, and support individuals, services, and products that achieve ACE's standards of excellence. ACE now supports Operation FitKids® as its youth outreach program. Operation FitKids is dedicated to enriching the lives of America's youth with enhanced education for healthy lifestyles and increased opportunities for physical activity. Check out their website for details of programs, instructors and loads of fun games and "fit facts."

Electrikids

P.O. Box 6063
San Pedro, California 90734
Email: electrikids@hotmail.com
Website: www.electrikids.com
ElectriKids is a company that inspires kids to lead a healthy, active lifestyle, by creating fun, innovative and energizing "stuff" for 21st-century kids. In their own words, they "electrify the future!" Their website offers fun information and facts designed to inspire kids, and they provide classes across the U.S.

Fun-Attic, Inc.
3719 Jasmine NE
Grand Rapids, Michigan 49525
Tel: (616) 559-3642
Website: www.funattic.com
A company specializing in unique toys, games and outdoor sporting goods for virtually any child's interests and talents. Free games and ideas for sports and activities to keep kids active.

National Association for Sport and Physical Education (NASPE)
1900 Association Drive
Reston, Virginia 20191
Tel: (703) 476-3410
Email: naspe@aahperd.org.
The National Association for Sport and Physical Education seeks to enhance knowledge and professional practice in sport and physical activity through scientific study and dissemination of research-based and experiential knowledge to members and the public. They have plenty of resources and information available for parents who want to improve their children's fitness.

President's Council on Physical Fitness and Sports (Kidfit)
701 Pennsylvania Avenue, NW
Suite 250
Washington DC 20004
Website: www.kidfit-usa.com
Great exercises and fitness plans for kids between the ages of five and 12, designed to encourage them to start and stay being active.

Websites

Active for Life

www.active.org.uk
Great site with a self-assessment quiz (for kids, too), excuse "busters" and ideas for keeping fit by analyzing your current lifestyle.

Shape up America!

www.shapeup.org
Shape Up America! is a high profile national initiative to promote healthy weight and increased physical activity in America, involving a broad-based coalition of industry, medical/health, nutrition, physical fitness and related organizations and experts. Their website offers tips for keeping fit and staying healthy, games, quizzes, details of forthcoming events and much more.

SLEEP

National Sleep Foundation
1522 K Street, NW, Suite 500
Washington, DC 20005
Tel: (202) 347-3471
Fax: (202) 347-3472
Website: www.sleepfoundation.org
The National Sleep Foundation (NSF) is an independent non-profit organization dedicated to improving public health and safety by achieving understanding of sleep and sleep disorders, and by supporting education, sleep-related research and advocacy. They have a variety of programs, including National Sleep Awareness week, and provide educational materials, a helpline and *Sleepmatters*, an

award-winning magazine, for the public. They also offer publications and a wealth of information on their website.

Talk about Sleep
P.O. Box 382276
Germantown, Tennessee 38183
Tel: (901) 482-2025
Fax: (901) 757-2828
Website: www.talkaboutsleep.com
This site is dedicated to providing information, education and support for all your sleep needs. Their goal is to be the center of sleep information and discussion on the Internet. Loads of advice, facts, figures and information on sleep disorders and general problems with kids and sleep.

Websites

American Academy of Sleep Medicine
www.aasmnet.org
A great website with information, quizzes, fact sheets, details of publications, recommendations for sleep centers and much more.

British Sleep Society
www.british-sleep-society.org.uk
The British Sleep Society is a registered British charity that aims to improve public health by promoting education and research into sleep and its disorders. Plenty of advice and information on this website.

Sleepnet
www.sleepnet.com
Sleepnet has loads of ideas for getting to sleep and for dealing with sleep disorders in children of all ages.

ENVIRONMENT

Absolute Environmental Allergy Store
3504 South University Drive
Davie, Florida 33328
Tel: (954) 472-3773
Fax: (954) 474-0133
Email: allergy@allergystore.com
Website: www.allergystore.com
Although this is primarily a store pro-viding allergen control products (allergy, asthma and dust mite control products including: HEPA air cleaners, air purifiers, odor removal products, vacuum cleaners, dust mite mattress encasings, water purification, household cleaning products and many more items), there is a great deal of information on environment and the impact on children's health. Well worth a visit.

American Academy of Environmental Medicine
7701 East Kellogg, Suite 625
Wichita, Kansas 67207
Tel: (316) 684-5500
Fax: (316) 684-5709
Email: administrator@aaem.com
Website: www.aaem.com
A group of clinicians from various specialties banded together in the 1965 and formed a medical society that has evolved into the American Academy of Environmental Medicine. Environmental medicine is the comprehensive, proactive and preventive strategic approach to medical care dedicated to the evaluation, management, and prevention of the adverse consequences resulting from environmentally triggered illnesses. Their website offers a list of physicians, as well as plenty of advice and information.

Center for Occupational and Environmental Medicine
7510 Northforest Drive
North Charleston, South Carolina 29420
Tel: (843)572-1600
Fax: (843) 572-1795
Website: www.coem.com
The Center for Occupational and Environmental Medicine specializes in treating patients with environmentally triggered health problems, including injuries sustained as a result of exposure to chemicals in the environment. Good site for information on the impact of your child's environment on his heath.

Children's Environmental Health Institute
P.O. Box 50342

Austin, Texas: 787-63-0342
Tel: 512-657-7405
Website: www.cehi.org
The Children's Environmental Health Institute (CEHI) was established to identify, validate, and develop solutions to adverse health effects to children, occurring as a consequence of exposure to hazardous environmental substances. Plenty of advice and information for parents.

Environmental Health Watch
4115 Bridge Avenue, #104
Cleveland, Ohio 44113
Tel: (216) 961-4646
Fax: (216) 961-7179
Email: e-h-w@ehw.org
Website: www.ehw.org
Environmental Health Watch is a non-profit public interest organization that provides information, assistance and advocacy to protect and sustain human health, and the health of the environment. Plenty of advice and information on creating a healthy home, including up-to-date news articles, as well as community and global environmental health issues.

Feng Shui U.S.A.
4201 Ohio Avenue
Tampa, Florida 33616
Tel: (813) 835-0053
Email: Tigerchi@aol.com
Website: www.fengshuiusa.com
A feng shui organization that offers books, advice and classes on changing your environment to promote good health.

The Healthy House Institute
430 North Sewell Road
Bloomington, Indiana 47408
Phone/fax: (812) 332-5073
Email: healthy@bloomington.in.us
Website: www.hhinst.com
The Healthy House Institute offers help and advice in creating a healthy interior environment for your family. They have books, videos, news releases, articles, links, a "healthy house" quiz and lots more.

Parents of Allergic Children
P.O. Box 1808
Midlothian, Virginia 23113

Website: www.parentsofallergic
children.org
This website will provide you with
information on how to get help and
support for yourself and your children. Includes help for children suffering from ADHD, a Parents of
Allergic Children Support Group,
information about and details of treatment for autism, ear infections, candida, hay fever, eczema, food
sensitivities, as well as diet and environment. Loads of information and
advice.

TV-Turnoff Network
1601 Connecticut Avenue NW
Suite 303
Washington, DC 20009
Tel: (202) 518-5556
Fax: (202) 518-5560
Website: www.tvfa.org
TV-Turnoff Network, formerly TV-
Free America, is a non-profit organiza-
tion that encourages children and
adults to watch much less television in
order to promote healthier lives and
communities.

Websites

Agency for Toxic Substances and Disease Registry (ATSDR)
www.atsdr.cdc.gov
The mission of the Agency for Toxic
Substances and Disease Registry
(ATSDR), as an agency of the U.S.
Department of Health and Human
Services, is to serve the public by
using the best science, taking respon-
sive public health actions, and providing trusted health information to
prevent harmful exposures and disease
related to toxic substances. ATSDR's
Child Health Program emphasizes the
ongoing examination of relevant child
health issues in all of the agency's
activities, and stimulates new projects
to benefit children. Plenty of resources
and information for parents.

Birth Defect Research for Children
www.birthdefects.org
This organization provides comprehensive fact sheets about birth defects,
as well as other information. If your
child was born with a birth defect,

they provide parent matching opportunities and information resources,
including books and links. If you are
researching birth defects, they have a
location on their site to get you
started.

Children's Environmental Health and Safety Inventory of Research (CHEHSIR)
www.epa.gov/chehsir
CHEHSIR is a publicly accessible
database created and maintained in
response to United States Presidential
Executive Order 13045 on the protection of children. It was created to
ensure that researchers and federal
research agencies have access to information on all research conducted or
funded by the federal government that
is related to adverse health risks in
children, resulting from exposure to
environmental health risks or safety
risks. This information is available to
the public, scientific, and academic
communities, as well as all federal
agencies.

Children's Environmental Health Network
www.cehn.org
The Children's Environmental
Health Network is a national, multi-
disciplinary organization, whose mission is to protect the fetus and child
from environmental health hazards
and promote a healthy environment.
This website provides information
about the network, children's environmental health, and links to sources of
information and resources.

Environmental Defense
www.environmentaldefense.org
Through various program areas,
Environmental Defense brings
together experts in science, law and
economics to tackle complex environmental issues that affect our oceans,
air, natural resources, the livability of
our man-made environment, and the
species with whom we share our
world. In addition to publishing
reports on its program activities,
Environmental Defense produces
print and email newsletters, fact sheets
and educational materials on "green"

behavior and business practices that
can help sustain and improve our
environment.

Institute for Children's Environmental Health
www.iceh.org
The Institute for Children's
Environmental Health (ICEH),
founded in 1999, is a non-profit educational organization working to
ensure a healthy, just and sustainable
future for children and the planet.
The primary mission of ICEH is to
reduce and ultimately eliminate environmental exposures that can undermine the health and well-being of
children, and to detoxify environments wherever children spend time.
ICEH accomplishes this mission by
educating and mobilizing diverse,
affected constituencies, and by foster-
ing collaborative initiatives to mitigate
environmental exposures that can
undermine the health of current and
future generations. Their website has
plenty of information and links for
parents wishing to make the right
decisions toward health and well-
being.

IMMUNIZATION

Centers for Disease Control and Prevention
1600 Clifton Road
Atlanta, Georgia 30333
Tel: (404) 639-3311
National Immunization Hotline:
English (800) 232-2522; Spanish
(800) 232-0233
Website: www.cdc.gov
A government agency with a great
deal of information about immunization. Tends to be pro-immunization,
but they outline many of the pros and
cons, and provide immunization
schedules.

Immunization Resource Kit Children's Hospital Medical Center of Cincinnati
3333 Burnet Avenue
Cincinnati, Ohio 45229-3039
Tel: (513) 636-4200, 1-800-344-2462
Website: www.cincinnatichildrens.org
Excellent and fairly unbiased informa-

tion on vaccination. Also a great resource for parenting articles and virtually every health condition affecting babies and children. Worth a visit.

Websites

Dispelling vaccination myths

www.sumeria.net/health/myth2.html
An excellent resource for parents who want to know the truth about vaccination and the links to various illnesses.

Sunderland University Autism Unit

osiris.sunderland.ac.uk/autism/vaccine.htm
Information exploring the problems associated with immunization, and the link between MMR and autism and bowel disease. Very user friendly and accurate.

Vaccination resources

www.whale.to/vaccine/articles1.html
Whale.to is a website dedicated to making articles available on a variety of health issues affecting adults, children, and animals. The vaccination link provides plenty of anti- and pro-vaccination discussions, articles, research and facts to help parents decide the best course of action for their children. Some of the statistics are shocking!

EMOTIONS and SPIRIT

American Psychological Association Healthy Adolescents Project and EMSC

Public Interest Initiatives Office
American Psychological Association
750 First Street, NE
Washington, DC 20002-4242
Tel: (202) 336-6031
Fax: (202) 336-6040
Website: www.apa.org
Email: healthyadolescent@apa.org
Great articles about teaching children to cope in an increasingly violent world and to adopt "gentleness." Includes facts, information and advice on emotional problems in children. They also run the "healthy adolescents project," which focuses on helping

adolescents to be healthy and happy.

The Children's Health Fund

317 East 64th Street
New York, New York 10021
Tel: (800) 535-7448
Website: www.childrenshealthfund.org
Kids First, Kids Now! is a national, non-partisan public awareness and education campaign to build support for the establishment of a health-care safety net for all of America's children. Launched in 1994 with the help of Doonesbury cartoonist Gary Trudeau, Kids First, Kids Now! works to increase awareness of child health issues and to ensure that the impact of policy decisions on these matters is demonstrated to government policymakers and the public alike. Excellent information for parents and caregivers on the importance of looking after the emotional health of children.

The Federation of Families for Children's Mental Health

1101 King Street, Suite 420
Alexandria, Virginia 22314
Tel: (703) 684-7710
Fax: (703) 836-1040
Website: www.ffcmh.org
Email: ffcmh@ffcmh.org
A national parent-run non-profit organization focused on the needs of children and youth with emotional, behavioral or mental disorders and their families. They provide details of local chapters that can arrange training and support groups for parents, and they offer a wealth of information, resources, publications, fact sheets and meetings.

Websites

Connect for Kids

www.connectforkids.org
Connect for Kids, an award-winning multimedia project, helps adults make their communities better places for families and children. The website offers a place on the internet for adults—parents, grandparents, educators, policymakers and others—who want to become more active citizens, from volunteering to voting with kids in mind. Loads of news, information on subjects as diverse as adoption,

diversity and awareness, out of school time, media and television, health, children and politics, and much more. Details of state-by-state resources.

Familycommunications.com

www.familycommunications.com
A website by families for families. Their purpose at familycommunications.com is to help families stay connected, have fun together, and to help make family life a little easier in this busy world we live in. Plenty of diverse information including resources for parents, special sections for "mom to mom" and "just for dads," kid-safe internet surfing sites, homework help, and more.

Parenting magazine's website

www.parenting.com
Good website with time-savers for busy parents and sound advice on dealing with emotional problems in kids, discipline issues and improving the family dynamic.

ACUPUNCTURE

Acupuncture and Oriental Medicine Alliance

14637 Starr Road SE
Olalla, Washington 98359
Tel: (253) 851-6896
Fax: (253) 851-6883
Website: www.AOMalliance.org
Provides details of practitioners, as well as up-to-date information and news on Oriental medicine and acupuncture in the United States.

American Association of Oriental Medicine

433 Front Street
Catasauqua, Pennsylvania 18032
Tel: (610) 266-1433, 1(888) 500-7999
Fax: (610) 264-2768
Website: www.aaom.org
Email: aaom1@aol.com
The American Association of Acupuncture and Oriental Medicine (AAAOM) was formed in 1981 to be the unifying force for American acupuncturists who are committed to high ethical and educational standards, and a well-regulated profession

to ensure the safety of the public. As the umbrella organization representing the acupuncture profession in the United States, the AAAOM assisted in the formation of both the National Commission for the Certification of Acupuncturists (NCCA, now NCCAOM) and the National Council of Acupuncture Schools and Colleges (NCASC, now CCAOM) in 1982. Will refer you to a practitioner and provide details of treatment.

AROMATHERAPY

American Alliance of Aromatherapy
P.O. Box 309
Depoe Bay, Oregon 97341
Tel: (800) 809-9850
Fax: (800) 809-9808
A resource center for aromatherapy practitioners and educators to share knowledge.

Aromatherapy Registration Council (ARC)
Professional Testing Corporation
1350 Broadway 17th floor
New York, New York 10018
Tel: (212) 356-0660
Email: info@aromatherapycouncil.org or at
Website: www.aromatherapycouncil.org
The Aromatherapy Registration Council is independent from any membership body, organization, or educational facility. This assures an impartial and unbiased body distinct from a body where members pay to belong to it and from one that accredits or endorses specific schools. They supply details of registered practitioners, and information and news about aromatherapy in general.

The National Association for Holistic Aromatherapy
2000 2nd Avenue, Suite 206
Seattle, Washington 98121
Tel: 888-ASK-NAHA, (206) 256-0741
Fax: (206) 770-5915
Email: info@naha.org
Website: www.naha.org
The National Association for Holistic Aromatherapy (NAHA) is an educational, non-profit organization dedicated to enhancing public awareness of the benefits of aromatherapy. NAHA is actively involved with promoting and elevating academic standards in aromatherapy education and practice for the profession. NAHA is also involved in furthering the public's perception and knowledge of true aromatherapy, and its safe and effective application in everyday life. They publish *Aromatherapy Journal* and can provide advice on finding practitioners and resources.

AYURVEDA

The Ayurvedic Institute
11311 Menaul NE
Albuquerque, New Mexico 87112
Phone: (505) 291-9698
Fax: (505) 294-7572
Email: info@ayurveda.com
Website: www.ayurveda.com
The Ayurvedic Institute is a non-profit organization that teaches the principles and practices of Ayurveda, the ancient science of life. They provide authentic education in a supportive environment that encourages the integration of Ayurveda by individuals into their daily living and by health care professionals into their clinical practices. They offer advice on Ayurvedic practice, online resources, publications and products.

Maharishi Ayurveda Products International
P.O. Box 49667
Colorado Springs, Colorado 80949
Tel: (800) 255-8332
Fax: (719) 260-7400
Email: info@all-veda.com
Website: www.mapi.com
Maharishi Ayurveda Products International, Inc. (MAPI) is a leading research, manufacturing and global distribution firm specializing in Ayurvedic herbal supplements, teas, gourmet food products and beauty care. Although this is an unabashedly commercial site, there is a great deal of good information on self-care, the practice of Ayurveda, news, research and links. Good for a beginner!

BUTEYKO

Buteyko Breathing Studio
867 Gravenstein Highway South
Sebastopol, California 95472
Tel: (707) 823-3712
Email: dor@buteykobreathworks.org
Information on the Buteyko method, including how to find a practitioner or implement the method at home.

Buteyko U.S.A.
Tel: (Toll-free) (877) ASTHMA-3 ((877) 278-4623)
Email: buteyko@buteyko-usa.com
A great resource for anyone who wants to know about the Buteyko method and the way it works to treat asthma and hyperventilation. Details of practitioners, advice on treatment, quizzes, resources, news and research.

CHINESE HERBALISM

American Association of Acupuncture and Oriental Medicine
433 Front Street
Catasauqua, Pennsylvania 18032
Phone: (610) 266-1433
Toll-free: (888) 500-7999
Fax: (610) 264-2768
Email: aaom@aol.com
Website: www.aaom.org
See Acupuncture, above.

Institute of Traditional Medicine
2017 SE Hawthorne Boulevard
Portland, Oregon 97214
Tel: (503) 233-4907
Fax: (503) 233-1017
Email: general questions or comments itm@itmonline.org
Offers advice on Oriental medicine, including research, online journals and articles, a list of practitioners, and general information about the subject.

Rocky Mountain Herbal Institute (RMHI)
P.O. Box 579
Hot Springs, Montana 59845
Tel: (406) 741-3811
RMHI, a private educational and research organization, has offered professional training in Chinese herbal sciences since 1987 (since 1992 in Hot Springs, Montana). The herbal sci-

ences program has been accredited by the American Association of Drugless Practitioners. They offer herbs for sale online, as well as advice on finding a practitioner, using herbal medicine, research, news and resources.

CHIROPRACTIC

Council on Chiropractic Education
8049 North 85th Way
Scottsdale, Arizona 85258-4321
Telephone: (480) 443-8877
Fax: (480) 483-7333
Email: cce@cce-usa.org
Website: www.cce-usa.org
The Council on Chiropractic Education (CCE) is the agency recognized by the U.S. Secretary of Education for accreditation of programs and institutions offering the doctor of chiropractic degree. CCE seeks to insure the quality of chiropractic education in the U.S. by means of accreditation, educational improvement and public information. CCE develops accreditation criteria to assess how effectively programs or institutions plan, implement and evaluate their mission and goals, program objectives, inputs, resources and outcomes of their chiropractic programs. They provide advice on finding a registered practitioner.

Federation of Chiropractic Licensing Boards
901 54th Avenue
Suite 101
Greeley, Colorado 80634-4400
Tel: (970) 356-3500
Fax: (970) 356-3599
Email: fclb@fclb.org
Website: www.fclb.org
Offers consumer information, a register of chiropractics, news, research and resources.

Website

Chiropractic America
www.chirousa.com
A wide variety of resources, including information, standards, what to expect from and look for in a chiropractor, research, and the basics of treatment.

FLOWER ESSENCES

Bach Flower Essences International Education Program
100 Research Drive
Wilmington, Massachusetts 01887
Phone: (800) 334-0843
Fax: (978) 988-0233
Email: education@nelsonbach.com
Website: www.nelsonbach.com
For information on the use and purchase of Bach Flower Remedies, and Nelson's Homeopathic remedies.

Ellon (Bach U.S.A.) Inc.
P.O. Box 320
Woodmere, New York 11598
Tel: (516) 825-2229
Headquarters for Bach Flower Remedies in the United States. Will offer advice on practitioners, as well as details of how to use the remedies and where they can be purchased.

Flower Essence Society
P.O. Box 459
Nevada City, California 95959
Tel: (800) 736-9222 (U.S and Canada), (530) 265-9163
Fax: (530) 265-0584
Email: mail@flowersociety.org
Website: www.flowersociety.org
The Flower Essence Society was founded in 1979 to promote plant research and empirical clinical research on the therapeutic effects of flower essences. They offer plenty of research, case histories, advice, articles, classes and news.

HERBALISM

American Botanical Council
P.O. Box 144345
Austin, Texas 78714-4345
Tel: (512) 926-4900
Website: www.herbalgram.org
The American Botanical Council is the leading non-profit education and research organization disseminating science-based information promoting the safe and effective use of medicinal plants and phytomedicines. Founded in 1988, ABC works to educate the public, healthcare practitioners, media, and government agencies on the safe and effective use of medicinal plants and phytomedicines. Good *materia medica* of herbs online, a news archive and educational resources.

American Herbalists Guild
1931 Gaddis Road
Canton, Georgia 30115
Phone: (770) 751-6021
Fax: (770) 751-7472
Email: ahgoffice@earthlink.net
Website: www.americanherbalists
guild.com
The American Herbalists Guild was founded in 1989 as a non-profit, educational organization to represent the goals and voices of herbalists. It is the only peer-review organization in the United States for professional herbalists specializing in the medicinal use of plants. AHG membership consists of professionals, general members (including students) and benefactors. They sell books and publications online, and can help you to find a registered herbalist in your area.

American Herbal Products Association
8484 Georgia Ave.
Suite 370
Silver Spring, Maryland 20910
Tel: (301) 588-1171
Fax: (301) 588-1174
Email: ahpa@ahpa.org
Website: www.ahpa.org
The American Herbal Products Association (AHPA) is the national trade association and voice of the herbal supplement industry. The website has a good frequently-asked-questions section on using herbs, a bookshop, plenty of up-to-date information on the use of herbs in medicine, and a useful links section. The site is well worth a visit if you're new to the subject.

Herb Research Foundation
1007 Pearl Street, Suite 200
Boulder, Colorado 80302
Tel: (303) 449-2265, (800) 748-2617
Fax: (303) 449-7849
Email: info@www.herbs.org
Website: www.herbs.org
The Herb Research Foundation claims to be the world's first and foremost source of accurate, science-based

information on the health benefits and safety of herbs—and expertise in sustainable botanical resource development. What sets HRF's work apart is their vast storehouse of information resources, including a specialty research library containing more than 300,000 scientific articles on thousands of herbs. They also have extensive field experience in sustainable development of botanical resources. They offer lots of information and resources on various herbs, including research, appropriate use and safety notes.

International Herb Association
910 Charles Street
Fredricksburg, Virginia 22401
Phone: (540) 368-0590
Fax: (540) 370-0015
Email: members@iherb.org
Website: www.iherb.org
A great resource for information about herbs. Publishes a newsletter and provides plenty of applications for herbs, including health, crafts and diet.

HOMEOPATHY

American Association of Homeopathic Pharmacists (AAHP)
33 Fairfax St.
Berkeley Springs, West Virginia 25422
Tel and Fax: (800) 478-0421
Email: info@homeopathyresource.org
Website: www.homeopathyresource.org
This organization works as an alliance between homeopathic manufacturers and pharmacists. They offer good advice on choosing quality products and provide a wealth of information in the form of books, press releases, journals and articles on their website.

Council for Homeopathic Certification (CHC)
1199 Sanchez Street
San Francisco, California 94114
Tel : (866)242-3399 (Toll free)
Fax: (415) 869-2867
Email: chcinfo@homeopathicdirectory.com
Website: www.homeopathicdirectory.com
The CHC has established the largest professional certification standard in North America and is open to all professional homeopaths, including both

licensed and non-licensed practitioners. It offers a list of qualified and registered practitioners.

National Center for Homeopathy
801 North Fairfax Street, Suite 306
Alexandria, Virginia 22314
Tel: (877) 624-0613, (703) 548-7790
Fax: (703) 548-7792
Website: www.homeopathic.org
The National Center for Homeopathy was set up to promote health through homeopathy. By providing general education to the public about homeopathy, and specific education to homeopaths, they help to make homeopathy available throughout the U.S. They have a monthly magazine called *Homeopathy Today*, can help with finding a practitioner and a homoeopathic pharmacy, and offer advice and information on taking homeopathic remedies. They also offer a variety of different classes throughout the United States. Their site is well worth a visit for the research alone!

Florida Homeopathic Medical Society
668 Lake Villas Drive
Altamonte Springs, Florida 32701
Tel: (407) 628-9708
Email: prswan@aol.com
Dedicated to classical homeopathic medicine, FHMS consists of licensed medical professionals and associate members (laypeople who have taken 150 hours of NCH approved coursework). They encourage the recognition and acceptance of homeopathic medicine, offer fellowship for practitioners and plan to act as a representational voice for homeopathy in Florida.

Foundation for Homeopathic Education
356 Middle Street
Amherst, Massachusetts 01002
Tel: (413) 256-5949
Fax: (413) 256-6223
Email: fhe@nesh.com
Publishes the biannual, peer-reviewed *New England Journal* and educational materials.

Homeopathic Pharmacopoeia Convention of the United States (HPCUS)
P.O. Box 2221
Southeastern, Pennsylvania 19399-2221
Tel: (610) 783-0987
Fax: (610) 783-5180
Email: hpus@aol.com
Website: www.HPCUS.com
The Homeopathic Pharmacopoeia Convention of the United States (HPCUS) investigates substances for inclusion, sets standards for identification, testing, and preparation of homeopathic remedies. The HPUS is recognized in the Food and Drug Act as the source of regulation of homeopathic drugs in the U.S.

Homeopaths Without Borders—North America
P.O. Box 1550
Basalt, Colorado 81621
Fax: (970) 927-9550
Email: hwb@igc.org
Member of the International Federation of Homeopaths Without Borders. Provides homeopathic education, clinical training and treatment to communities in need. Ongoing Cuban project: training medical doctors, veterinarians and pharmacists; supplying books, computers and software.

National Integrative Medicine Council
5151 East Broadway, Suite 1095
Tucson, Arizona 85711
Tel: (520) 571-1110
Fax: (520) 571-1177
Website: www.nimc.org
Founded by Dr. Andrew Weil, this non-profit membership-based education and advocacy organization promotes a healing-oriented approach to health care.

North American Society of Homeopaths (NASH)
1122 East Pike Street, #1122
Seattle, Washington 98122
Tel: (206) 720-7000
Fax: (208) 248-1942
Email: NashInfo@aol.com
Website: www.homeopathy.org

NASH is the association that certifies professional homeopaths in the United States and Canada. Registered members are entitled to use the designation RSHom(NA). Associate or Student memberships in NASH are open to everyone. Members receive *The American Homeopath* (NASH's annual journal), *NASH News* (quarterly newsletter) and discounts on NASH's annual conference and seminars.

Ohio State Homeopathic Medical Society (OSHMS)

5779 Wooster Pike
Medina, Ohio 44256
Tel: (330) 784-4493
A group of medical professionals supporting the advancement of homeopathic education and practice.

Texas Society of Homeopathy

4200 Westheimer, Suite 100
Houston, Texas 77027
Tel: (713) 621-3184
Fax: (713) 877-8035
Email: info@txsoho.com
Website: www.txsoho.com
The Texas Society of Homeopathy is a non-profit professional and lay homeopathic organization formed to promote homeopathic education in Texas and the surrounding areas. The September annual conference features a special speaker and provides the availability of earning continuing educational and CCH credits.

HYPNOTHERAPY

American Society of Clinical Hypnosis

2200 East Devon Avenue, Suite 291
Des Plaines, Illinois 60018-4534
Tel: (708) 297-3317
Fax: (708) 297-7309
Website: www.asch.net
The American Society of Clinical Hypnosis is the largest U.S. organization for health and mental health care professionals using clinical hypnosis. Founded by Milton H. Erickson, M.D., in 1957, ASCH promotes greater acceptance of hypnosis as a clinical tool with broad applications. Today, ASCH offers

workshops, certification, and networking opportunities that can enhance both professional and personal lives. They have a member referral database, they publish the *American Journal of Clinical Hypnosis*, and offer courses, workshops and advice to the public.

International Society of Hypnosis

Level 1, South Wing
Austin and Repatriation Medical Centre
Repatriation Campus
300 Waterdale Road
Heidelberg Heights, Victoria 3081
Australia
Tel: (613) 9496-4105
Tel: (613) 9496-4107
Website: www.ish.unimelb.edu.au
This society moved recently from the U.S. to Australia. It's an excellent resource for anyone interested in hypnosis, and has a great deal of advice and information available for hypnosis worldwide. As a governing body, they can recommend a practitioner or the appropriate body in your local area. Great resources.

Society for Clinical and Experimental Hypnosis

SCEH Central Office
Washington State University
P.O. Box 642114
Pullman, Washington 99164-2114
Phone: (509) 335-7504
Fax: (509) 335-2097
Email: sceh@wsu.edu
Website: www.sunsite.utk.edu/IJCEH
Founded in 1949, the Society for Clinical and Experimental Hypnosis (SCEH) is an international organization of nurses, social workers, dentists, psychologists, psychiatrists and other physicians who are dedicated to the highest level of scientific inquiry and the conscientious application of hypnosis in the clinical setting. They have a research database, a list of recognized practitioners, a journal, and will offer advice on finding the right practitioner for you and your child.

Website

Society of Clinical and Experimental Hypnosis

www.hypnosis-research.org
Run by the Society of Clinical and Experimental Hypnosis, this is a free interactive database with 11,744 references to hypnosis-related material in scholarly journals and books, as well as presentations at professional meetings.

MASSAGE

Nurse Healers–Professional Associates International (The Official Organization of Therapeutic Touch)

3740 South Highland Drive, Suite 429
Salt Lake City, Utah 84106
Tel: (801) 273-3399
Fax: (801) 273-3352
Email: NH-PAI@Therapeutic Touch.org
Website: www.therapeutic-touch.org
Nurse Healers–Professional Associates International, Inc., the official organization of Therapeutic Touch, serves as the expert resource for information on Therapeutic Touch. NH-PAI sets the standards for the practice and teaching of Therapeutic Touch. They have a directory of reputable schools and practitioners, details of research, merchandise, advice and much more.

NATUROPATHY

American Association of Naturopathic Physicians

8201 Greensboro Drive, Suite 300
Mclean, Virginia 22102
Tel: (703) 610-9037 (referrals)
Fax: (703) 610-9005
Website: www.naturopathic.org
Founded in 1985, the American Association of Naturopathic Physicians (AANP) is the national professional society representing naturopathic physicians who are licensed or eligible for licensing as primary care providers. They can provide you with details of a practitioner near to you, and advice and information about naturopathy.

Homeopathic Academy of Naturopathic Physicians
12132 S.E. Foster Place
Portland, Oregon 97266
Phone: (503) 761-3298
Fax: (503) 762-1929
Email: hanp@igc.apc.org
Website: www.healthy.net/hanp
The Homeopathic Academy of Naturopathic Physicians (HANP) is a specialty society within the profession of naturopathic medicine, and is affiliated with the American Association of Naturopathic Physicians. Their purpose is to further excellence and success in the practice of homeopathy by naturopathic physicians. They publish a newsletter and have many naturopathic resources on their website.

OSTEOPATHY

American Academy of Osteopathy
3500 De Pauw Boulevard, Suite 1080
Indianapolis, Indiana 46268-1136
Tel: (317) 879-1881
Fax: (317) 879-0563
Website: www.academyofosteopathy.org
The American Academy of Osteopathy is an osteopathic medical society with a focused educational mission. Members are predominantly osteopathic physicians (Doctors of Osteopathy, or D.O.s) and osteopathic medical school students who have a high degree of interest in osteopathic principles and practice, including the art and science of osteopathic manipulative treatment (OMT). They can provide you with details of D.O.s in your area or training colleges, and plenty of information on the practice of osteopathy. Send $5 plus an SAE for their member register.

American Osteopathic Association (AOA)
142 East Ontario Street
Chicago, Illinois 60611
Tel: (800) 621-1773, (312) 202-8000
Fax: (312) 202-8200
Email: info@aoa-net.org.
Website: www.aoa-net.org
The AOA is the national organization for the advancement of osteopathic medicine in the United States, and the professional association for over

48,000 physicians. The AOA accredits the Colleges of Osteopathic Medicine, osteopathic internship and residency programs, and healthcare facilities. They can help you find a D.O. online, by state, supply fact sheets and details of treatments, safety codes and an understanding of osteopathy in general. They have news updates regularly on their website.

REFLEXOLOGY

International Institute of Reflexology
5650 First Avenue North
P.O. Box 12642
St. Petersburg, Florida 33733-2642
Tel: (727) 343-4811
Fax: (727) 381-2807
Email: iir@tampabay.rr.com
Website: www.reflexology-usa.net
Offers training, a list of registered practitioners to members (the public can join), workshops, information on the practice of reflexology, as well as a list of branches.

Reflexology Association of America
4012 Rainbow Street, K-PMB#585
Las Vegas, Nevada 89103-2059
Tel/Fax: (702) 871-9522
Website: www.reflexology-usa.org
The Reflexology Association of America is a non-profit organization that promotes the scientific and professional advancement of reflexology. Their mission is to elevate and standardize the quality of reflexology services available to the public. The Reflexology Association of America works to unify and support state reflexology associations in order to create one national movement toward greater excellence, integrity, research and public safety. They will help you to find a registered reflexologist in your area, can provide details of legislation as well as safety, and have hundreds of articles and fact sheets available to the public.

YOGA

International Association of Yoga Therapists
2400A County Center Drive
Santa Rosa, California 95403
Tel: (707) 566-9000
Email: mail@iayt.org
Website: www.iayt.org
The International Association of Yoga Therapists holds annual conferences, publishes an annual journal, and a newsletter. They have many articles on their website, and are a good source of general information about the benefits of yoga. They can also put you in touch with a reputable teacher from their membership.

Mid-Atlantic Yoga Association (MAYA)
P.O. Box 10658
Silver Spring, Maryland 20914
Website: www.mayayoga.org
Maya is a non-profit corporation that provides its members with a forum to encourage the study and practice of yoga. Members of MAYA include professionals who have written articles and books about yoga and who teach nationally and internationally, instructors who have studied with some of the best-known teachers in the world, and students who simply want to bring peace and good health into their lives. They offer a wealth of information about yoga and can put you in touch with a teacher in your area.

Yoga in Daily Life Center
2402 Mount Vernon Avenue
Alexandria, Virginia 22301
Tel: (703) 299-8946 (local and international calls)
Toll-free in the U.S.: (866) 293-0723
Fax: (703) 299-9051
Email: alexandria@yoga-in-daily-life-usa.com
Web Page: www.yoga-in-daily-life-usa.com
The Yoga in Daily Life system of Mahamandaleshwar Paramhans Swami Maheshwarananda is a science of health based on ancient teaching of yoga adapted for today. They can provide you with details of classes, a basic understanding of yoga, merchandise, books and *Yoga News Online*.

Websites

Interactive yoga instruction online
www.yogaclass.com
A great site with instructions (free) online for yoga, relaxation, meditation and breathing.

Yoga Directory
www.yogadirectory.com
Just what it says: A directory of teachers in your area, and links to other yoga sites. Lots of teachers who specialize in teaching yoga to children.

SAFETY

American Red Cross
P.O. Box 37243
Washington, DC 20013.
Website: www.redcross.org
Contact for details of your local chapter, who will provide training, advice, first-aid information and classes, news and up-to-date information on safety in the community and at home, resources, community and youth services and much more.

Children's Safety Network
National Injury and Violence Prevention Resource Center
Education Development Center, Inc.
55 Chapel Street
Newton, Massachusetts 02458-1060
Telephone: (617) 969-7100, ext. 2207
Fax: (617) 969-9186
Website: www.edc.org/HHD/csn
The resource center for child and adolescent injury and violence prevention. Plenty of online resources, links and advice.

International Center for Injury Prevention
5009 Coye Drive
Stevens Point, Wisconsin 54481-5078
Tel: (715) 344-7583, (800) 344-7580
Fax: (715) 341-8400
A wealth of information on preventing injuries both in the home and in the community.

National Safety Council
A Membership Organization Dedicated to Protecting Life and Promoting Health
1121 Spring Lake Drive
Itasca, Illinois 60143-3201
Tel: (630) 285-1121
Fax: (630) 285-1315
Website: www.nsc.org
The National Safety Council is the nation's leading advocate for safety and health. They offer advice, information, fact sheets, links, news, statistics, research and much more to help Americans stay and play safe. The National Safety Council library is one of the most complete safety and health information resources anywhere. Together with its nationwide network of local chapters, community volunteers and members representing business, labor, industry, and government, the Council provides information that gives clear, practical guidance on injury prevention.

SafeUSA
P.O. Box 8189
Silver Springs, Maryland 20907-8189
Website: www.safeusa.org
SafeUSA is a working alliance of major public and private partners dedicated to significantly reducing the high rates of injuries and deaths related to injuries in the United States and increasing the levels of safety in the nation's homes, schools, work sites, transportation areas, and communities. Their fine website offers newsletters, fact sheets, information on safety in the playground, at home, when traveling, at school and more.

Websites

SAFE KIDS
www.safekids.org
The National SAFE KIDS Campaign is the first and only national non-profit organization dedicated solely to the prevention of unintentional childhood injury—the number one killer of children ages 14 and under. More than 300 state and local SAFE KIDS coalitions in all 50 states, the District of Columbia and Puerto Rico comprise the Campaign. The website is a valuable resource for information on all aspects of child safety, including an e-newsletter, details of produce recalls, safety information and prevention tips, and laws and regulations.

SOURCES

The Apothecary
5415 Cedar Lane
Bethesda, Maryland 20814
Orders and information: (800) 869-9159
Fax: (301) 493-4671
Email: APOTH123@aol.com
Website: www.the-apothecary.com
This shop (offering online, catalog and personal shopping) stocks the most reputable brands of nutritional supplements and dozens of hard-to-find items. Some time ago, they developed their own line of "super-quality" nutritional supplements under the PATHWAY label. You should be able to find any remedy listed in this book in their catalog. If you phone them, they'll often be able to source unusual items.

Homeopathy Overnight
929 Shelburne Avenue
Absecon, New Jersey 08201
Orders: (800) ARNICA30 ((800) 276-4223)
Information: (609) 407-9245
Website: www.homeopathy overnight.com
Homeopathy Overnight has over 3,500 different homeopathic remedies, books on homeopathy, kits and much more. A good source for any homeopathic requirements.

GENERAL

National Institute of Child Health and Human Development
P.O. Box 3006
Rockville, Maryland 20847
Toll-free number: (800) 370-2943
Fax: 301-984-1473
Email:NICHDClearinghouse@mail.nih.gov
Website: www.nichd.nih.gov
The National Institute of Child Health and Human Development (NICHD) is part of the National

Institutes of Health, the biomedical research arm of the U.S. Department of Health and Human Services. The mission of the NICHD is to ensure that every person is born healthy and wanted, that women suffer no harmful effects from the reproductive process, and that all children have the chance to fulfill their potential for a healthy and productive life, free of disease or disability. They offer information, advice, resources, helplines, research, news and prevention on their website.

National Institutes of Mental Health

NIMH Public Inquiries
6001 Executive Boulevard, Room 8184, MSC 9663
Bethesda, Maryland 20892-9663
Tel: (301) 443-4513
Fax: (301) 443-4279
Email: nimhinfo@nih.gov
Website: www.nimh.nih.gov
A good source of information on emotional health problems for people of all ages, with research, statistics, links and advice.

National Center for Complementary and Alternative Medicine

NCCAM Clearinghouse
P.O. Box 7923
Gaithersburg, Maryland 20898
Tel: (301) 519-3153
(888) 644-6226 (Toll-free, and fax-on-demand)
(866) 464-3615 (Toll-free, TTY)
Fax: (866) 464-3616 (Toll-free)
Email: info@nccam.nih.gov
Website: nccam.nih.gov
The National Center for Complementary and Alternative Medicine (NCCAM) is one of the 27 institutes and centers that make up the National Institutes of Health (NIH). The NIH is one of eight agencies under the Public Health Service (PHS) in the Department of Health and Human Services (DHHS). Their mission is to support rigorous research on complementary and alternative medicine (CAM), to train researchers in CAM, and to disseminate information to the public and professionals on which CAM modalities work, which do not, and why.

They are a virtual fount of information on every complementary and alternative therapy and the first place to go for up-to-date research, advice and information.

United Nations Children's Fund (UNICEF)

3 UN Plaza
44th Street
New York, New York 10017
Tel: (212) 824-6369
Fax: (212) 824-6464
Email: dalnwick@unicef.org
Website: www.unicef.org
Their mission is to protect children around the world, and they offer many programs and research initiatives for children in the U.S. as well. Worth a look, as there are games, facts, statistics, "voice of the children" commentaries, and much more.

The U.S. Department of Health and Human Services

200 Independence Avenue, SW
Washington, DC 20201
Tel: (202) 619-0257, Toll-free: (877) 696-6775
Email: hhsmail@os.dhhs.gov
Website: www.hhs.gov/contacts
A great resource with online information on all aspects of health and safety for children, and in fact sheets, which can be ordered at the above number. They offer a list of websites for kids, and information on everything from nutrition and exercise to adoption.

American Holistic Medical Association

4101 Lake Boone Trail, Suite 201
Raleigh, North Carolina 27607
Tel: (919) 787-5181
Website: holisticmedicine.org
AHMA was founded in 1978 to unite licensed physicians who practice holistic medicine. Their mission is to transform health care so that it addresses physical, environmental, mental, emotional, spiritual and social health, thereby contributing to the healing of the planet. They will provide details of a holistic doctor near you, as well as information on resources, publications and other organizations.

Child Welfare League of America

440 First Street, Suite 310
Washington, DC 20001
Tel: (202) 638-2952
Fax: (2020 638-4004
Website: www.cwla.org
The Child Welfare League of America is the nation's oldest and largest membership-based child welfare organization. They are committed to engaging people everywhere in promoting the well-being of children, youth, and their families, and protecting every child from harm. They offer a broad range of publications, a newsletter, parenting tips, community services, programs and training.

American Holistic Health Association

P.O. Box 17400
Anaheim, California 92817-7400
Tel: (714) 779-6152
Email: mail@ahha.org
Website: www.ahha.org
The American Holistic Health Association (AHHA) encourages you to actively participate in enhancing your health and well-being. Information can assist you to do this confidently and effectively. For over a decade the volunteers of AHHA have collected potential sources for this type of information, in response to requests from people all across the U.S. These resources are offered here as a free public service, so that you have a variety of options to explore. Plenty of information on treatments, articles, a database of practitioners and lists of compatible organizations.

Holistic Dental Association

Complementary/Alternative Dentistry
P.O. Box 5007
Durango, Colorado 81301
Tel: (970) 259-1091
Email: hda@frontier.net
Website: www.holisticdental.org
This association believes that dentistry should also be "holistic"—that is, aimed at the health and well-being of the entire person rather than just a set of teeth. They have a great online journal, as well as links and referrals to members.

Notes

Chapter 1: Natural Nutrition

1. Patrick Holford, *Optimum Nutrition Bible* (Berkely, CA: Crossing Press, 1999).
2. Ibid.

Chapter 5: Fit for Life

1. From "Ten Things You Should Know about Youth Sports and Exercise," *Sports Trend*, April 2000.

Chapter 6: And So to Bed

1. *New York Times*, December 27, 1995.
2. Ibid.

Chapter 7: A Natural Environment

1. This information is based on a 1998 study, undertaken by a team at Bristol University in the United Kingdom, led by Professor Denis Henshaw. This was the second study they performed showing the same outcome. The Bristol conference closely followed a finding by the prestigious U.S. National Institutes of Health that electromagnetic fields from power lines should be considered possible causes of human cancer.
2. From John Ashton and Ron Laura, *The Perils of Progress* (London: Zed Books/UCT Press, 1998). All of the studies are listed in *Electromagnetics Forum*, (August–December 1996).
3. Ibid., and B. W. Wilson, E. K. Chess and L. E. Anderson, "60 Hz electric field effects on pineal melatonin rhythms: Time course and onset of recovery," *Bioelectro-magnetics* 7: 239–242 (1986).
4. From *The Stewart Report*, published in May 2000 in the United Kingdom. Information on damage to white blood cells was presented by Roger Coghill at a mobile phone safety meeting in Florida in June 1999. Another study in 2002 by Dr. Fiorenzo Marinelli, at the National Research Council in Bologna, Italy, published in *New Scientist* (November 2000), confirms these findings.
5. Ibid., and from research by Dr. George Carlo, commissioned by the mobile telephone industry, reported in *New Scientist* in October 1999. A study commissioned by the BBC's television show *Panorama* in May 1999 found large differences between the amount of microwave radiation absorbed by the brain from different makes of phone.

Chapter 8: The Key to Happiness: Emotional Health

1. This survey was carried out by the Office for National Statistics in the United Kingdom, in partnership with a team at the Institute of Psychiatry and the Maudsley Hospital, in London. The results were published in 1999 in "The Development and Well-Being of Children and Adolescents in Great Britain," *British Medical Journal*: 319:1456 (1999).

In March 2002 the World Health Organization and the United Nations Children's Fund issued the "Report of the Global Consultation on Child and Adolescent Health and Development: A Healthy Start in Life," in which they warned that up to one in five of the world's children is suffering mental or behavioral problems. Among other things, they found depressive disorders are the fourth leading cause of disease and disability, and are expected to rise to second place by 2020.

2. The study I am referring to here was Sainsbury's Supermarket in the U.K. in 2001, but there are two other studies that confirm these findings, including one by the British Dietetic Association (2000) and the Institute of Grocery Distribution (IGD) (2002).

Chapter 9: Understanding Illness

1. E. A. Shalabi, "Acetaminophen inhibits the polymorphonuclear leukocyte function in vitro." *Immunopharmacology* 24(1):37–45 (July–August 1992); and N. M. Graham, C. J. Burrell, "Adverse effects of aspirin, acetaminophen, and ibuprofen on immune function, viral shedding and clinical status in rhino virus infected volunteers," *Journal of Infectious Diseases* 162(6):1277–82 (January 1990).

2. The idea that echinacea can prolong illness (in particular, the common cold) was published in B. P. Barrett, R. L. Brown, K. Locken, R. Maberry, J. A. Bobula, and D. D'Alessio, "Treatment of the Common Cold with Unrefined Echinacea. A Randomized, Double-Blind, Placebo-Controlled Trial," *Annals of Internal Medicine* 137, no. 12 (December 17, 2002), and represents the findings of a study by the University of Wisconsin. However, the research was found to be flawed by several reputable scientists; even the chief researcher of the study admitted that the results could be due to the specific preparation of echinacea they used, which could be different from other versions of the herbal remedy. In my own experience, echinacea works best on an on-off basis, and there is plenty of other evidence that it reduces the duration of illnesses when offered in the presence of acute symptoms. Two good studies showing this are T. Jefferson, "Advances in the diagnosis and management of influenza," *Current Infectious Disease Report* 4(3):206–210 (June 2002); and L. S. Kim, R. F. Walters, and P. M. Burkholder, "Immunological activity of larch arabinogalactan and echinacea: A preliminary, randomized, double-blind, placebo-controlled trial," *Alternative Medicine Review* 7(2):138–49 (April 2000).

3. There are literally dozens of studies showing that garlic has a role in preventing cancer, and even in the treatment of tumors. The study I refer to here was undertaken by the University of North Carolina at Chapel Hill, and published in A. T. Fleischauer, C. Poole, L. Arab, "Garlic consumption and cancer prevention: meta-analyses of colorectal and stomach cancers," *American Journal of Clinical Nutrition* 72:1047–1052 (October 2000).

4. The studies I've used to write this chapter and to which I refer throughout include the following: T. Ronne, "Measles virus infection without rash in childhood is related to disease in adult life," *The Lancet* 1–5 (January 1985); H. Niedermeyer, W. Arnold, W. J. Neubert, H. Hofler, "Evidence of measles virus RNA in otosclerosic tissue, ORL" *Journal for Oto-Rhino-Laryngology and its related specialities* 56 (3):130–132 (1994); M. H. Helfrich, R. P. Hobson, P. S. Grabowski, A. Zurbriggen, S. L. Cosby, G. R. Dickson, W. D. Fraser, C. G. Ooi, P. L. Selby, A. J. Crisp, R. G. Wallace, S. Kahn, S. H. Ralston, "A negative search for a paramyxoviral etiology of Paget's disease of bone: Molecular, immunological, and ultrastructural studies in U.K. patients," *Journal of Bone and Mineral Research: The Official Journal of the American Society for Bone and Mineral Research,* 15(12): 2315–2329 (December 2000) Y. Chen, P. C. Wu, J. H. Lang, W. J. Ge, P. Hartge, L. A. Brinton, "Mumps: Risk factors for epithelial ovarian cancer in Beijing, China," *International Journal of Epidemiology,* 21(1): 23–29 (February 1992): "Inves-

tigative report on the vaccine adverse event reporting system," National Vaccine Information Center (NVIC), 512 Maple Ave. W. #206, Vienna, VA 22180; W. C. Torch, "Diptheria-pertussis-tetanus (DPT) immunization: A potential cause of the sudden infant death syndrome (SIDS)," (American Academy of Neurology, 34th Annual Meeting, April 25 – May 1, 1982), *Neurology* 32(4), pt. 2; P. E. Fine, R. T. Chen, "Confounding in studies of adverse reactions to vaccines," (Review article: 38 references) Comment in: *American Journal of Epidemiology* 139(2):229–30 (January 15, 1994); C. L. Cody, L. J. Baraff, J. D. Cherry, S. M. Marcy, C. R. Manclark, "Nature and rates of adverse reactions associated with DTP and DT immunizations in infants and children," *Pediatrics*, 68(5): 650-60 (November 1981); B. Trollfors, E. Rabo, "Whooping cough in adults," *British Medical Journal* 696–97 (September 12, 1981); M. L. Cohn, E. D. Robinson, M. Faerber, D. Thomas, S. Geyer, S. Peters, M. Martin, A. Martin, D. Sobel, R. Jones, et al. "Measles vaccine failures: Lack of sustained measles specific immunoglobulin G responses in revaccinated adolescents and young adults," *Pediatric Infectious Disease Journal* 13(1):34–8 (January 1994); L. Yuan, "Measles outbreak in 31 schools: Risk factors for vaccine failure and evaluation of a selective revaccination strategy," *Canadian Medical Association Journal* 150(7):1093–8 (April 1, 1994); C. E. Frasch, E. E. Hiner, T. P. Gross, "Haemophilus b disease after vaccination with Haemophilus b polysaccharide or conjugate vaccine," *American Journal of Diseases of Children* 145(12):1379–82 (December 1991); P. A. Briss, L. J. Fehrs, R. A. Parker, P. F. Wright, E.C. Sannella, R. H. Hutcheson, W. Schaffner, "Sustained transmission of mumps in a highly vaccinated population: Assessment of primary vaccine failure and waning vaccine-induced immunity," *Journal of Infectious Diseases* 169(1):77–82 (January 1, 1994); L. K. Ammari, L. M. Bell, R. L. Hodinka, "Secondary measles vaccine failure in healthcare workers exposed to infected patients," *Infection Control & Hospital Epidemiolog* 14(2):81–6 (February 1993); "Measles Prevention," *Morbidity and Mortality Weekly Report* 38:8–9 (December 29, 1989); "Measles—United States, First 26 Weeks," *Morbidity and Mortality Weekly Report* 23:38 (50):863-6, 871-2 (December 22, 1989); "Measles outbreak among vaccinated high school students—Illinois," *Morbidity and Mortality Weekly Report* 33:24 (June 22, 1984); G. A. Poland, R. M. Jacobson, "Failure to reach the goal of measles elimination. Apparent paradox of measles infections in immunized persons" (Review article: 50 references), *Archives of Internal Medicine* 154(16):1815–20 (August 22, 1994); P. G. Auwaerter, G. D. Hussey, E. A. Goddard, J. Hughes, J. J. Ryon, P. M. Strebel, D. Beatty, D. E. Griffin. "Related Articles, Links Abstract Changes within T cell receptor V beta subsets in infants following measles vaccination." *Clinical Immunology and Immunopathology,* 79(2): 163–170 (May 1996); Trevor Gunn, "Mass Immunization: A Point in Question," p. 15 (from E. D. Hume, *Pasteur Exposed: The False Foundations of Modern Medicine,* Sydney, Australia: Bookreal, 1989.); Hoffman Buttram, M.D., "The Dangers of Immunization," *Mothering Magazine,* 30 (Winter 1985); Drs. Kalokerinos and Dettman, "A Supportive Submission," *The Dangers of Immunisation* (Warburton, Victoria, Australia: Biological Research Institute, 1979), p.49.

The FDA's VAERS (Vaccine Adverse Effects Reporting System) receives about 11,000 reports of serious adverse reactions to vaccination annually, some 1% (112+) of which are deaths from vaccine reactions. Source: National Technical Information Service, Springfield, VA 22161.

The FDA estimates that only about 10% of adverse reactions are reported, says K. M. Severyn, R.Ph.,Ph.D., a spokesperson for the Ohio Parents for Vaccine Safety, in the *Dayton Daily*

News, May 28, 1993 (Ohio Parents for Vaccine Safety, 251 Ridgeway Dr., Dayton, OH 45459).

The U.S. Federal Government's National Vaccine Injury Compensation Program (NVICP) has paid out over $724.4 million to parents of vaccine injured and killed children, in taxpayer dollars. The NVICP has received over 5,000 petitions since 1988, including over 700 for vaccine-related deaths, and there are still over 2,800 total death and injury cases pending that may take years to resolve. Source: National Vaccine Injury Compensation Program (NVICP), Health Resources and Services Administration, Parklawn Building, Room 7-90, 5600 Fishers Lane, Rockville, MD 20857.

Chapter 10: Natural Therapies for Children

1. David M. Eisenberg; Roger B. Davis; Susan L. Ettner; Scott Appel; Sonja Wilkey; Maria Van Rompay; Ronald C. Kessler, "Trends in Alternative Medicine Use in the United States, 1990-1997: Results of a Follow-up National Survey," *Journal of the American Medical Association* 280(18): 1569–1575 (November 11, 1998).

2. AMEDNEWS.com, March 27, 2000.

3. Dr. David Stretch, a researcher at the University of Leicester in the U. K., found that the aroma of lavender oil worked as effectively as sleeping tablets in a study of elderly insomniacs. He also speculated that lavender may have an even more powerful effect on young insomniacs because people tend to lose their sense of smell with age.

   A project run by the University of Liverpool in the U.K. is providing stress-therapy units for two Merseyside primary schools, which offer intensive six-week courses in tackling anxiety among children aged between five and eleven. Aromatherapy is part of the program, and parents claim that their children are calmer after this therapy and find it easier to talk about their problems.

4. This research was done by Dr. Viola Frymann, the director of the Osteopathic Center for Children in San Diego, California. She details her findings on her website, www.osteopathiccenter.org. The American Academy of Osteopathy has published her collected works, *The Collected Papers of Viola M. Frymann, D.O.: Legacy of Osteopathy to Children*, edited by Hollis H. King, 1998.

5. The BBC News website reported on Tuesday, August 25, 1998, that a 1998 study in Manchester, U.K., showed that two-thirds of babies with disturbed sleep were remarkably improved by cranial osteopathy. The babies went from just a couple of hours of rest a night before treatment to up to thirteen hours of unbroken sleep after. And for most babies, the change was fast and permanent.

6. E. Kyo, N. Uda, S. Kasuga, Y Itakura, "Immunomodulatory effects of aged garlic extract," *Journal of Nutrition* 131(3):1075S–9S (September 2001); D. Lamm and D. Riggs, "Enhanced immunocompetence by garlic: role in bladder cancer and other malignancies," *Journal of Nutrition*, 131(3):1067S–1070S (September 2001); D. Lamm and D. Riggs, "Enhanced immunocompetence by garlic. Recent Advances on the Nutritional Benefits Accompanying the Use of Garlic As a Supplement," The Pennsylvania State University and the National Cancer Institute, Newport Beach, CA. November 15–17, 1998.

7. J. P. Ferley, D. Zmirou, D. D'Admehar, et al., "A Controlled evaluation of a homoeopathic preparation in the treatment of influenza-like syndrome," *British Journal of Clinical Pharmacology* 27:329–35 (March 1989).

8. There are numerous studies on the benefits of massaging premature infants. The one I refer to here is: J. Dieter, T. Field, M. Hernandez-Reif, and E. Emory, "Preterm infants gain more

weight following 5 days of massage therapy, *Journal of Pediatric Psychology.* Other good studies include: T. Field, N. Grizzle, F. Scafidi, S. Abrams, and S. Richardson, "Massage therapy for infants of depressed mothers," *Infant Behavior and Development* 19:109–114 (1986); T. Field, "Interventions for premature infants," *Journal of Pediatrics* 109:183–191 (1986); T. Field, "Alleviating stress in newborn infants in the intensive care unit," *Perinatology* 17:1–9 (1990).

9. Wringing strokes are those that mimic the action of wringing a washcloth or something similar—gently twisting the skin/muscle in opposite directions with both hands.

10. J. Simu'th, J. Trnovsky, and J. Jeloskova', "Inhibition of bacterial DNA-dependent RNA polymerases and restriction endonuclease by UV-absorbing components from propolis," *Pharmazie,* 41(2): 131–132 (1986); P. B. Ross, *"The effects of propolis fractions on cells in tissue culture,"* M.Phil. Thesis, University of Wales College of Cardiff, U.K. xii, 193 (1990); Z. H. Karimova and E. I. Rodionova, "Propolis in the treatment of lung tuberculosis," *Apimondia,* Edition Apimondia, Bucharest, Romania (1975); J. M. Grange and R. W. Davey. "Antibacterial lproperties of propolis (bee glue)," *Journal of the Royal Society of Medicine,* London, U.K. 83(3): 159–160 (1990); L. Meresta and T. Meresta, "Antibacterial activity of flavonoid compounds of propolis, occurring in flora in Poland," *Bulletin of the Veterinary Institute in Pulawy,* 28–29(1–4): 61–63 (1985–1986); V. Maksimova-Todorova, et al. "Antiviral effects of some fractions isolated from propolis." *Acta Microbiologica Bulgarica* 17: 79–85 (1985); S. Scheller, et al. "The ability of ethanolic extract of propolis EEP to protect mice against gamma irradiation," *Zeitschrift fur Naturforschung,* C, 44:1049–1052 (1989); S. Scheller, et al. "Trials of immunoregulation in patients with chronic bronchitis," *Immunologia Polska* 14(3/4): 204–305 (1989); S. Scheller, et al. "Immunization trials in two cases of alveolitis fibroticans with decreasing conductivity of the immune system: effect of ethanol extract of propolis (EEP), Esberitox N. and a calcium-magnesium preparation," *Heilkunst,* 102(6): 249–255 (1989); S. Scheller, et al. "Trace elements in propolis and in its ethanolic extract (EEP) as determined by neutron activation analysis," *Zeitschrift fur Naturforschung,* 44:170–172 (1989); S. Scheller, et al. "Antitumoral property of ethanolic extract of propolis in mice-bearing Ehrlich carcinoma, as compared to bleomycin." *Zeitschrift fur Naturforschung,* C. 44:1063–1065 (1989).

11. Many children suffer from abdominal migraine. It is characterized by episodes of midline abdominal pain, often accompanied by nausea, anorexia and sometimes vomiting. Some children also experience dizziness and sensitivity to sound and light. The episodes last between one and 72 hours, and resolve spontaneously. Children who suffer this condition often go on to have migraine headaches in later childhood/adulthood.

Chapter 11: Natural Treatments for Common Ailments

1. The figures came from the National Center for Environmental Health in the United States.

2. C. K. Buffington, G. Pourmotabbed, A. E. Kitabchi, "Amelioration of insulin resistance in diabetes with dehydroepiandrosterone," *American Journal of Medical Science* 306:320–4 (1993); R. Bergman, J. Beard, M. Chen, "The minimal modeling method assessment of insulin sensitivity and B-cell function in vivo," in W. Clarke, J. Larner, S. Pohl, eds., *Methods in Diabetes Research* (New York: Wiley, 1986, 15–34); J. E. Nestler, "DHEA: A coming of age," *Annual Report of the New York Academy of Science* 774:ix–xi (1995); J. E. Nestler, "Regulation of human dehydroepiandrosterone metabolism by insulin," *Annual Report of the New York Academy of Science* 774:73–81 (1995).

3. *New Scientist* (April 24, 1999).

4. This study was reported on *BBC News* on January 20, 2000. The research was done at the University of Essex in the U.K., and was funded by the U.K. departments of health and education.

5. M. M. Candela i Agusti, "Anorexia nervosa and zinc," *Rev Enferm.* Jul–Aug: 8(84–85):18–9 (1985); "Anorexia, depression, and zinc deficiency," *Lancet* 2(8412):1162–3 (November 17, 1984); "Anorexia and zinc," *Lancet* 2(8407):874 (October 13, 1984); R. Bakan, "The role of zinc in anorexia nervosa: etiology and treatment," *Medical Hypotheses* 5(7):731–6 (July 1979); P. P. Tannhauser "Anorexia nervosa: a multifactorial disease of nutritional origin?" *International Journal of Adolescent Medical Health* 14(3):185–91 (July–September 2002); H. Yamaguchi, Y. Arita, Y. Hara, T. Kimura, H. Nawata, "Anorexia nervosa responding to zinc supplementation: a case report," *Gastroenterolgy Japan* 27(4):554–8 (August 1992).

6. I refer to a number of studies here, including the following: S. M. Hill, et al. "Colitis caused by food allergy in infants," *Journal of the Archives of Disease in Childhood* 65:1 (January 1990); J. A. Anderson, "Milk, eggs and peanuts: Food allergies in children," *American Family Physician* 56:5 (October 1997); M. Boris et al., "Foods and additives are common causes of the attention deficit hyperactive disorder," *Annals of Allergy, Asthma, and Immunology* 72:5 (1994); H. J. F. Hodgson, "Inflammatory bowel disease and food intolerance," *Journal of the Royal College Physicians* 20:1 (1986); E. Novembre et al., "Foods and respiratory allergy," *Journal of Allergy and Clinical Immunology* 81 (1988); F. Conleth, "Coeliac disease," *British Medical Journal Clinical Review* 319 (1999); R. F. Lemanske et al., "Adverse reactions to foods and their relationships to T. Ahmed et al., "Gastrointestinal allergy to food: A review," *Journal of Diarrhoeal Diseases Research* 15:4 (1997).

7. E. S. Johnson et al. "Efficacy of feverfew as prophylactic treatment of migraine," *British Medical Journal* 291: 569–573 (1985). J. J. Murphy, S. Heptinstall, and J. R. A. Mitchell. "Randomized double-blind placebo-controlled trial of feverfew in migraine prevention," *Lancet* ii: 189–192 (1988).

8. L. A. Joe, L. L. Hart, "Evening primrose oil in rheumatoid arthritis," [review] *Annals of Pharmacotherapy* 27:1475–7 (1993).

9. G. Snyder and J. Kalinowski (submitted). "An analysis of stuttering treatment measurements and therapy efficacy: Implications for a new stuttering therapy paradigm." *Perceptual and Motor Skills.*

Index

abscesses, 300
accidents, 98, 117, 137, 139, 166, 399
acidophilus, 147, 209, 284
acne, 300–301
Aconite, 229, 274
activity levels, 60–61, 63, 98, 99, 110
acupressure, 240
acupuncture, 235, 239–241
additives, food, 4, 5, 20, 40, 73–75
adolescents, 89–92, 110–12
    colors (bedroom), 152–55
    fitness, 162–63
    obese, 5, 55
    rebellion, 89–90, 110
    sleep, 110, 114, 116–17, 122, 137–39
affection, physical, 178–79
alcohol, 110–11, 115
Alexander Technique, 293
allergens, 10, 30, 33, 40, 69, 74, 75, 83, 124, 142, 301–2, 344–49
allowance, 110, 181, 198
amino acids, 14, 285
anaphylactic shock, 302
anemia, 302–3
anorexia nervosa, 334–35
antibiotics, 28–29, 40, 41, 211–12, 233
antioxidants, 7, 24, 42, 74, 154, 211, 284, 285–86
anxiety, 40, 114, 116, 124, 172, 303–4
aromatherapy, 133, 229, 235, 242–47
art therapy, 247–48
artificial colors (food), 153
artificial respiration, 424
artificial sweeteners, 49, 55, 56, 154
aspartame, 7, 154
asthma, 7, 12, 30, 37, 40, 74, 75, 124, 219, 304–5
athlete's foot, 305–6
attention, 176, 179, 184, 189, 197, 226, 227, 415
attention deficit disorder (ADD), 219, 306–8. See also hyperactivity

attention deficit and hyperactivity disorder (ADHD), 306–8
aura reading, 163, 237
authority, 183–84, 189
autism, 216, 219, 308–10
Ayurvedic medicine, 211, 235, 292–93

babies
    active, 106,
    diet, 11, 15, 83–84
    eating habits, 68–69
    ill, warning signs, 225
    learning the difference between night and day, 128–29
    massage, 276, 277–80
    serving sizes, 22–23
    sleep, 118, 119–20, 121, 125–28, 133, 134
    unattended, 406
    weaning, 82–83
    See also newborns
baby blue syndrome, 31
baby food, 41–42, 74, 154
babysitters, 137, 402
baby walkers, 405
Bach, Edward, 256
Bach flower remedies, 208, 234, 256–62. See also flower remedies
back pain, 124
bacteria
    friendly, 149, 208, 209, 212, 284
    harmful, 140, 141, 208, 209
    resistant strains. See superbugs
balance
    diet, 10, 16, 17, 44, 62, 76–77, 85, 90, 96, 282 (see also food pyramid)
    family life, 193–95
    [physical] home environment, 163–66, 167
balanitis, 310
barbecues, 31
baths, 121, 243, 265, 414–15
bedrooms, 123–25, 161–65
bedtime routine, 116, 119–22
bedtime stories, 121, 122, 123
bedtime struggles, 114, 119, 123, 130–32

bedtimes, 127, 129
bedwetting, 310–11
bee propolis, 284
behavior
    encouraging good, 184
    messages about, 174–76
    modeling appropriate, 184 (see also parents, modeling after)
    ignoring negative, 286
    parent controlling child's, 179–80
behavioral disorders, 172
Belladonna, 229–30, 274
benzoin oil, 246
bergamot oil, 246
beta-carotene, 7, 94, 284
bicarbonate of soda, 143
bicycle helmets, 410
Birch, Leann, 61
bioflavonoids, 285–86
birth defects, 7, 24, 37, 39
birth trauma, 253
bite problems, 71–72
bites, 426–27
bleach, 143, 150
bleeding gums, 6
blindness, 123
blood sugar, 16, 38, 85, 86, 412
body clock, 128, 138
body image, 62, 178, 179
body mass index (BMI), 60, 64
body rocking, 357–58
body shape, 97
boils, 311–12
bone mass, 6, 98
bone strength, 98. See also fractures
bottle-feeding, 82–83, 135, 136, 282
bottled water, 20
botulism, 74
boundaries, 190. See also discipline
brain cancer, 154, 156
brain diseases, 25
brain function, 7, 11, 85, 98–99, 110, 117
bread, alternatives, 54
breakfast, 16, 19, 60, 85–86, 90
breast cancer, 6, 27, 28, 37

breastfeeding, 11, 80–81, 125, 128, 136, 208, 282
breastmilk, 15, 80–81, 208
bronchitis, 312
bruises, 274, 429, 430
BSE (bovine spongiform encephalopathy), 25–26, 27, 32
BST (bovine spongiform somatotropin), 29, 30
bug sprays, 144. See also pesticides
bulimia nervosa, 335
burns, 58, 402–3, 427–28
Buteyko, Konstantin, 250
Buteyko method, 250–251
B vitamins, 6, 16, 210, 283–284

caffeine, 7, 153
calcium, 6, 7, 16, 30, 55, 58, 92, 93, 284, 436
cancer
    environmental pollutants, 155, 157
    link to nutrition, 3, 6, 7, 12, 14, 24, 31, 32, 33, 37, 41, 42, 43, 56
    and natural medicine, 233
    See also free radicals; names of specific cancers
carbohydrates, 10, 15–17, 23
carbon monoxide poisoning, 405
carbonated drinks, 6, 55–56
carcinogens, 24, 31, 73, 74
carotenoids, 24, 94
carpets, 143, 150, 406
cars, 108, 407–9
catarrh, 312–13
cell phones, 155–56
cereals, 16, 17, 19, 44, 52, 86
cerebral metabolic rate, 117
chamomile
    oil, 246
    tea, 58, 133
Chamomilla, 230, 274
change
    child's fear of, 173
    developmental landmarks (age), 198
cheese, and dental health, 92
chemicals. See additives, food; household chemicals; pesticides

chi, 158, 163, 239–40, 287. *See also* energy; energy medicine; vital force
chicken pox, 215, 224, 313–14
childhood obesity, 5, 11, 12, 55, 59–65, 81, 97, 100
Chinese medicine, 30, 235, 239–40, 291
chiropractic, 235, 293
choice
    behavior, 182–83, 184
    exercise, 109
    food, 24, 61, 70, 87, 93
    See also empowering child
choices and consequences technique, 131, 183
choking, 428–29
cholera, 216
chores, 109
chromium, 16, 436
chronic fatigue syndrome (CFS), 314–15
chronic wasting disease, 26–27
circadian clock, 137
clapping away old energy, 165–66
cleaning products, 143, 149–50
clutter, clearing, 164–65
cocoa (recipe), 57–58
cod liver oil, 13, 283
coenzyme Q10 (CoQ10), 285
coffee, 57, 138, 153, 154
cold sores, 315–16
colds, 30, 116, 200, 245, 317–18
colic, 133, 245, 316–17
colon cancer, 6, 98
color, 159–61
    additives, 73
    bedroom, 123, 161–63
    food, 153
    fruits and vegetables, 24
color therapy, 160, 163, 293
colostrum, 80
communication, 185–88
complementary therapies, 233, 234. *See also* natural therapies
complex carbohydrates, 15–16, 17
compresses, 244, 265
computers, 101, 121, 155, 156, 193
conjunctivitis, 318–19
constipation, 319
conventional medicine, 203, 233–34
coughs, 320–21
cow's milk, 29, 30, 80, 81, 82
CPR (cardiopulmonary resuscitation), 424–25

cradle cap, 321
cranial osteopathy, 251–54
creams, 243–44, 265
creativity, 196
Creitzfeldt-Jakob disease (CJD), 25
crib death, 127
cribs, 406, 419
Crohn's disease, 30
croup, 274, 321–22
crythrosien, 73
crying, 125, 134, 322–23
cure, laws of, 273
cuts, 429–30
cycling, 106, 409–10

dancing, 106, 107, 112, 249
deadlocks, breaking, 189–90
decoctions, 264
dehydration, 56, 103, 226, 412
dental health, 71–72, 92, 126
depression, 6, 37, 137, 155, 172, 323–24
desserts, healthy, 94–95
detoxification, 141, 142, 145–48, 238–39. *See also* postvaccination cleansing
diabetes, 14, 31, 38, 99, 124, 324–25
diaper rash, 325–26
diarrhea, 202, 326–27
diet, analyzing, 77–79
diets, 62, 63, 77, 81, 348–49
diets, special, 91–93
diphtheria, 213, 214, 215, 216, 223
discipline, 179–85
diverticulosis, 24
diving, 414
DNA pack, 402
doctors, 211, 234
dog walking, 107–8
dowsing, 237
drinking
    during illness, 226
    healthy, 55–58, 67
drug resistance, 212
DTaP (vaccine), 223
DTP vaccine, 223
dust mites, 150–51
dyslexia, 124, 327–30
dyspraxia, 330–31

earache, 332–34
ear infections, 81, 332–34
eating disorders, 63, 334–37
    eating habits, 8, 59, 61–62, 65, 66–70, 93

eating plans, 76–77, 86
eating problems, 59–75
Echinacea, 209, 384
E-coli, 28
eczema, 12, 23, 37, 219, 337–39
EFAs. *See* essential fatty acids
electricity, 403
electromagnetic (EM) fields, 155. *See also* EM radiation
elimination diets, 347–49
EM radiation, 155–57, 158
emergencies, 422–24
emotional
    coaching, 169
    health, 168–91
    factors, illness, 202, 204–5
    outlets, 184–85, 190–91
    ups and downs, 175
    vocabulary, 187–88
emotions, negative, 204, 255–56, 258–60
empowering child, 61, 70, 86, 87, 89, 93, 109, 110, 130–31, 169, 183, 190, 400. *See also* personal freedom; praise
emulsifiers, 152
encephalitis, 215, 339–40
endorphins, 98
energy, 140, 141, 158, 163, 164–65, 191, 203
energy medicine, 204, 232, 268
epilepsy, 340–41
essential fatty acids (EFAs), 5, 12–13, 66, 209–10
essential oils, 144, 242–43, 265
    applications, 150, 245
    best, 246–47
    safety, 244–55
    using, 243–44
exercise, 96
    amount, 103
    associations with, 106–7, 108
    balanced, 68
    fun, 105, 107–8, 190
    importance of, 97–100
    statistics, 100
    time for, 100–2, 104–7
    type, 103–4
    video, 108
expectations (parental), 179–80, 181–82, 191, 193, 194, 197

facial cues, 185–86, 188
falling asleep, 118, 132–33
    during feeding, 125, 127
falls, 405–6
family bed, 126, 135, 136
fast food, 4, 89, 96, 115

fats, 10, 11–14, 23
fatty acid deficiency, 13–14
febrile convulsions, 430–31
feelings, expression, 185, 187–88, 208. *See also* emotional outlets; personal freedom
feng shui, 163–67
fertility, 6, 36, 37
fertilizers, 31, 40, 41
fevers, 227, 274, 341–43. *See also* febrile convulsions
fiber, 10, 17, 18–19, 67
fillers, 40, 88, 153
filtered water, 20–21
fingerprinting (child), 402
fire, 401–3
first aid, 422–33
fitness assessment, 111, 112–13
flavonoids, 285–86
flavor enhancers, 74, 155
flavors (additive), 48, 152
flaxseed oil, 13, 210, 283
fleas, 144
flexibility, 99, 103
flower remedies, 208, 228, 234, 235, 254–63
flu, 343–44
fluoride, 144, 148
folate, 24
folic acid, 435
food
    additives, 4, 7, 20, 40, 73–75, 152–55
    advertising, 3, 9, 63
    allergies, 10, 30, 33, 40, 69, 74, 83, 344–49
    alternatives, 50–54
    associations with, 61, 63, 84
    banned, 25, 28, 33
    barbecued, 31
    canned, 41, 54, 95
    dislikes, 68, 69
    first (babies), 83–84
    fortified, 16
    fresh, 95–96
    frozen, 95
    fun, 10, 90
    healthy-sounding, 38, 155
    for ill child, 225–26
    intolerance, 83, 84, 344, 347–49
    irradiation, 35, 36
    kids', 4, 6, 8, 38, 50–54
    nitrate-containing, 31–32
    obsessions, 62
    preservatives, 32, 40
    processed, 4, 7, 8, 12, 22
    raw, 19

unrefined, 14, 15–16, 17
variety, 4, 7, 10, 43, 44–45, 68, 69, 72, 94
See also baby food; diet; fast food; food pyramid; GM foods; junk food; meals; organic foods
food poisoning, 28, 149
food preparation, 71, 93
food pyramid, 22, 23, 61, 66, 85, 87
food scares, 25–39
formula milk, 30, 80, 82
fractures, 7, 55, 98
free radicals, 7, 35, 94, 284
friendships, 195
fructose, 38, 39
fruit drinks, 56
fruit juice, 57
fruits and vegetables
benefits of, 24
canned, 54
irradiated, 35–36
raw, 19
recommended intake, 5, 23
statistics, consumption, 4–6

games, 107, 108, 413–14
games consoles, 101, 105, 121, 138, 193. *See also* computers; video games
gamma-linolenic acid (GLA), 283, 285
gargles, 244
garlic, 210, 284–85
gastroenteritis, 350–51
genetically modified foods. *See* GM foods
geranium oil, 246
German chamomile oil, 246
German measles. See rubella
glandular fever, 352–53
glucose, 38, 85
glue ear, 30, 353–54
GM foods, 8, 32–34, 43, 82
grazers, 71
green movement, 140–41
greengrocers, 43, 95
grinding teeth, 354
grogginess, remedy, 245
growing pains, 354–55
growth and development, 14, 30, 66, 73, 99, 110, 117–18
growth hormone, 27–28, 99, 116
guidance, 180, 184, 193
guilt, 63, 71, 116, 134, 137, 174, 193

Gulf War Syndrome, 218
gyms, 105, 111

hair analysis, 238
hand-washing, 149, 209
hay fever, 355–56
head banging, 357–58
headaches, 356–57. *See also* migraine
healing power of illness, 205–206
heart disease, 5, 6, 11, 14, 38, 42, 65, 66–67, 98
heartbeat recordings, 124
help yourself policy, snacks, 62, 88
herbal teas, 58
herbalism, 262–67
herbs, 230–31, 265–67
hiccups, 358–59
high blood pressure, 65, 97
high-fiber products, 17
high-voltage power cables, 157–58
highly strung children, 173, 180
hives, 359
holidays, 108, 111
home environment, 140–67, 208
home improvement products, 142–143
home safety, 401–6, 417–22
homeopaths, 272–73
homeopathy, 234, 235, 238, 267–75
nosodes, 219, 225
remedies, 225–26, 229–30, 274–75
treatment, after immunization, 220, 224
homework, 99, 100–1, 121, 122, 183
homocysteine, 24
honesty, 185, 188, 404
hot drinks, 57–58
household chemicals, 142–44, 208
household rules, 180, 181
hunger, 24, 61, 69, 85, 88. *See also* satiety
hydrogenation, 12
hygiene products, 143, 144, 148
hyperactivity, 7, 38, 40, 73, 74
hyperventilation, 250
hypnotherapy, 290–91
hysterical children, 189, 228

illness
emotional factors, 202, 204–5

cure, laws of, 273
healing power of, 205–6
importance of, 201–2
warning signs, 225–26
imagination, 196
immune system, 6, 29, 35, 36, 38, 73, 116, 137, 141, 149, 205
boosting, 207, 208–11
weakened, 208
impetigo, 359–60
independence, 126, 134, 193, 198. *See also* empowering child; personal freedom
Indian medicine. *See* Ayurvedic medicine
indoor games, 104
infant mortality rate, 221
information pack, 402
infusions, 264
injuries, sports, 99, 411–12
insecticides, 37, 144
insecurity, 360–61
insomnia, 7, 40, 58, 124
insulin, 81, 99
intensive farming, 28, 40, 41, 42, 282
iridology, 238
iron, 16, 91, 436
iron-deficiency anemia, 5, 283, 299–300
irritable bowel syndrome (IBS), 37

junk food, 4, 10, 15, 44, 62, 66, 69–70, 89, 96
justice, child's sense of, 182, 184, 185
juvenile arthritis, 361–63

ketchup, 94
kids' food, 4, 6, 8, 9, 38, 50–54
Kirlian photography, 238

labels, 32, 33, 34, 35, 36, 38, 40, 65, 70, 73, 152, 155, 295
lactovegetarians, 91
lead poisoning, 405
leaky gut syndrome, 364–65
La Leche League International, 81
leukemia, 155
lice, 121, 245, 366
lifestyles, 8, 40, 63, 67–68, 96, 101, 115, 121
light, natural, 158–59, 165
lighting, sleep, 123–24, 161, 162
lost children, 402, 417
lotions, 243–44

love, 178, 191, 192, 227, 415
lullabies, 124
lunch, 86, 87

mad cow disease, 25–26
magnesium, 437
manganese, 437
margarine, 12
massage, 235, 243, 275–80
massage therapists, 277
materialism, 194–96, 198
meals
family, 8, 67, 72, 93–95, 193
preparation, 24, 61, 93
ready-prepared, 8
school, 63, 86
skipping [breakfast], 85
small, 71
measles, 213, 214, 215, 217, 219, 220, 222, 223, 225, 366–68
meat, 25–29
medications, 203, 233–34, 294–96
medicine kit, 228–31
meningitis, 81, 223–24, 368–69
menus, 24, 45–49, 61, 93
meridians, 240, 241
metabolic rate, 98. *See also* cerebral metabolic rate
metabolism, 24, 66, 67
migraine, 7, 37, 74, 124, 369–70
milk, 29–30, 42, 58, 71. *See also* cow's milk; formula milk; soy milk
mind-body relationship, 202, 204–5
minerals, 10, 22, 155, 434, 436–37
MMR vaccine, 213–25
moisture, in home, 151–52
molluscum contagiosum, 370–71
monounsaturates, 12
mood swings, 14, 16, 37, 137, 138
moody children, 173
Moskowitz, Richard, 216–18, 219
mouth ulcers, 371–72
mouthwashes, 244
MSG (monosodium glutamate), 49, 75, 154
multiple sclerosis, 14
mumps, 213, 214, 215, 218, 223, 372–73
muscles, strained, 274
music, 106, 107, 123, 124, 129
music therapy, 124, 248–50

myalgic encephalitis (ME), 314–15

naps, 118, 120, 127, 129, 136
natural light, 158–59, 165
natural home medicine kit, 228–31
natural medicine, 203, 232–33, 294
natural practitioners, 232–33, 235–38
natural remedies, 211, 234–35
natural sweeteners, 39
natural therapies, 232–93
natural treatments, common ailments, 297–398
natural world, 194
naturopathy, 293
nausea and vomiting, 373–74
negative energy, 165, 167, 182, 191
negative words, 174
neutraceutical industry, 22
newborns, 31, 80, 82, 118, 120
night and day, learning the difference, 128–29
nightlights, 123–24, 161, 419
night terrors, 382–83
night waking, 114, 123, 129, 132, 133–37
nightmares, 131, 383
nitrates, 31–32, 41, 74
NLP (neurolinguistic programming), 185–86
nosebleeds, 431
nosodes, 219, 225
Nutrasweet, 154
nutrients, 10–22, 434–37
nutrition, 3–7. See also balance, diet; diet; food pyramid
nutritional therapies, 280–87

obesity in children, 5, 11, 12, 55, 59–65, 81, 97, 374–75
oils, 12, 13, 14
ointments (herbal), 265
older children
    colors (bedroom), 162
    and fitness, 110–12
    night and day, learning difference, 129–30
    physical affection, 178
    sleeping, 121–22
omega-3 oils, 5, 12, 13, 210
omega-6 oils, 5, 12, 13
organic farming, 41, 42
organic foods, 7–8, 28, 29, 32, 33, 34, 36, 39–52, 95

organized sports, 104, 411
organophosphates, 36
osteopathy, 235, 251. See also cranial osteopathy
osteoporosis, 30, 65, 98
outdoor activities, 107–8
    playing alone, 102, 414–16
outer ear infection, 333
outlets, emotional, 184–85, 190–91
ovarian cancer, 27, 219
overenergy, 172, 173
overprotectiveness, 400
over-the-counter (OTC) drugs, 206, 294, 295
ovo-lactovegetarians, 91

pacifiers, 126–27
packed lunches, 87
paints, 142–43, 405
parental sleep, 134, 136
parental time, 189, 195
parents
    controlling type, 61, 68, 70, 179–80
    educating child (health/safety), 44–45, 70, 90, 137–38, 189, 397–98
    modeling after, 10, 21, 61, 63, 69, 72, 101, 105, 109, 115, 173–74, 184, 187, 191–92, 398
    rules for, 182
peace, 192, 193
peanuts (allergy), 344
peer pressure, 3, 9, 44, 62, 70, 86, 89, 98
penalties, 181–82
personal freedom, 102, 180, 183, 191, 196, 198, 398, 416
pesticides, 36–37, 40, 41–42, 143, 144
pests, 144
pets, 107–8, 144, 151, 198
pharmaceutical industry, 221–22
physical affection, 178–79
physical education programs, 63, 100, 101, 102
physical punishment, 182, 188–89
phytochemicals, 24
phytoestrogens, 82, 347
picky eaters, 3, 5, 8, 29, 48, 67, 68–72, 94, 210, 284
picrorrhiza, 211
pills (herbal), 265
play, 102, 103, 104, 407
playgrounds, 102, 405, 412

pneumonia, 375–76
poisoning, 403–5, 431–32
polio, 213, 215, 217, 223
polyphenols, 285–86
polyunsaturates, 12
positive energy, 191–92
positive language, 174–76. See also praise
postvaccination cleansing, 220, 224
potassium, 16, 24, 437
potassium nitrate, 74
poultices, 265. See also compresses
poverty, 195
powdered drinks, 56
powders (herbal), 264–65
power, 182–85, 189, 193
power lines, 157–58
praise, 62, 71, 89, 93, 109, 110, 121, 130, 132, 135, 176, 177, 178, 182, 184, 196, 415
prana, 292
preservatives, 32, 40, 73, 154
progesterone, 27
prostate cancer, 6, 27, 94
proteins, 10, 14–15, 23, 67, 91
punishment, 125, 181–82, 185
pyramid structure, diet, 22, 23–24

Qigong, 291

radionics, 237
rashes, 376–77
raw juices, 57
rebelliousness, 173, 189, 190
refined carbohydrates, 15, 16
reflexology, 238, 287–90
Reilly, Dr. John, 60
relaxation therapy, 293
relaxing, 115, 116
repetitive strain injury (RSI), 156, 157
reproductive cancers, 28
Rescue Remedy, 228, 260, 262
Rescue Remedy Cream, 228, 262
respect, 179, 182, 183, 184
responsibility, 109, 111, 196, 198
rewards, 109, 111, 138, 181
rhinitis, 37
road safety, 98, 105, 106, 400, 402, 406–7
roman chamomile oil, 246
rubella, 213, 214, 215, 220, 223, 351–52

saccharine, 56, 154
SAD (seasonal affective disorder), 158
safety
    basics, 402
    car, 407–9
    children playing outdoors, 102, 415–16
    cycling, 409–10
    detoxification, 146
    essential oils, 244–45
    flower remedies, 258
    food additives, 152, 153, 154
    herbal medicine, 264, 267
    home, 401–6, 417–22
    homeopathy, 271, 404
    medications, 295
    pact, 416–17
    playgrounds, 102, 405
    road, 98, 105, 106, 400, 406–7
    and sleep deprivation, 137
    sports, 411–12
    tips, 421
    toys/games, 413–14
    vaccinations, 219–21
    water play, 417–18
salmonella, 28
salt, 65
satiety, 61, 62, 69
saturated fats, 11, 12, 15, 38
scaremongering, 399
school
    meals, 63, 86
    phobias, 377–78
    physical education, 63, 100, 101, 102
    start times, 138
    trauma, 374–76
seaweeds, 285
sedentary lifestyle, 60, 63, 91, 100–1
selenium, 24, 284, 437
self-confidence, 172, 176, 178
self-control, 62, 69, 174, 180, 184, 188
self-esteem, 62, 71, 100, 109, 110, 126, 134, 169, 173–76, 180, 189, 197, 399
self-healing, 206
self-image, 62, 65, 173, 174, 178, 197. See also body image
separation anxiety, 133–34, 274
servings, 22–23, 71
Shattock, Paul, 218, 219, 224
shampoos, 143, 243–44
shiatsu, 293

shingles, 378–79
shock, treating, 228, 425–26
shouting (parents), 174, 182, 184, 189
shyness, 172, 379
"sick building syndrome," 158
sick child, care of, 226–28
sickroom, 227
singing, 248, 249
sinusitis, 380
slapping, 189
sleep
    adolescents, 110, 114, 117, 122, 137–39
    associations with, 114, 116, 121, 123, 124, 125–26
    babies, 118, 119–20, 123, 125–26
    crying to, 125, 134
    in dark, 123–24
    deprivation, 115, 116–17, 136, 137
    environment, 117, 123–24. See also bedrooms
    habits, 99, 114–16, 125
    importance of, 116–17
    needs, 115, 117–19
    older children, 121–22
    parental, 134, 136
    problems, 7, 40, 58, 73, 98, 99, 130–39, 380–84
    routines, 116, 119–22
    scheduling, irregular, 139
    sucking to, 126–27
    toddlers, 120–21, 127
    treatments, 132, 378–81
    See also bedtime struggles; bedtimes; falling asleep; naps; waking child
sleep apnea, 117, 383–84
sleepiness, signs, 127–28
sleep-ins, adolescents, 110, 114, 117, 138
sleeptalking, 382
sleep/wake cycle, 127, 128, 138, 155
sleepwalking, 382
Smith, Lendon H., 217
smoking, 5, 209, 283
snacks, 49, 60, 62, 69–70, 71, 412

healthy, 62, 64, 67, 71, 88–89
sodium, 20, 24
sodium nitrate, 74
soft drinks, 6, 21, 55–56
sore throat, 384–85
soy-based (infant) formula, 82
soy milk, 92, 350
soy products, 32, 43
spanking, 188–89
sperm count, 6, 28, 42
spirit, 158, 190, 191–98
spirulina, 285
sports injuries, 99, 411–12
sports, organized, 104, 411
spots, 376
squint, 385
stabilizers (food), 153
stammering, 385–86
star charts, 71, 108, 109, 111, 122, 130, 181, 409
steam inhalations, 243
steroids, 233–34
sticky eye, 386
stings, 426–27
stomach cancer, 31, 65
story tapes, 121, 122, 128, 131, 133
stress, 98, 109, 110, 133, 137, 168, 190, 195, 206, 208, 245, 283–84, 386–88
stroke, 12, 24, 65
strong-willed children, 172
structured (home) environment, 183
styes, 388–89
sudden infant death syndrome (SIDS), 127, 220, 221
sugar, 38–39, 209
sulfites, 74–75
sunburn, 432
sunlight, 93, 158–59
superbugs, 212
supplementation, 22, 66, 67, 72, 92, 93, 282–87

tantrums, 16, 38, 70, 85, 169, 183
tartrazine, 7, 73, 74
tea, 57, 153, 154
teeth, grinding, 354–55

teething, 230, 274, 389
television, 60–61, 63, 99, 100, 101, 104, 105, 106, 116, 121, 122, 133, 163, 192–93
television sets, 155, 157, 163
tetanus, 213, 216, 223
thrush, 389–90
time alone, 189, 194, 195, 196
time-outs, 124, 169, 180
tinctures, 264
tisanes, 264
toddlers
    active, 106
    serving sizes, 23
    sleep, 120–21, 127
tonsillitis, 390–91
toothache, 391–92
tooth decay, 38, 49, 55, 92, 148
toothpaste, 144, 148
touch, 178–79, 276
toxic overload, 30, 73, 86, 141, 152, 206. See also detoxification
toxins, 20, 25, 33, 35, 49, 81, 96, 141, 201–2
toys, 123, 150, 164, 413–14
trans-fats, 12
trauma, 392–93
    at birth, 253
    school, 377–78
travel sickness, 432–33. See also nausea and vomiting
treats, 9–10, 38, 44, 61, 71, 76
trust, 173–74
TSEs, 26–27
tuberculosis, 216–17, 224
tummy aches, 274, 393–94

underweight children, 66–68
unique radiotytric products, 35
unsaturated fats, 12, 66
urinary tract infections (UTIs), 81, 394–96
urticaria (hives), 359

vaccinations, 213–26
vaccines, list, 223–24
vCJD (variant Creitzfeldt-Jakob disease), 25
VDT screens, 155
veganism, 90, 92–93
vegetarians, 67, 91–92

vibrational medicine, 234, 255
video games, 99, 100, 101, 105, 138
visual cues, 186
visualization, 293
vital force, 203–4, 206, 232, 239–40, 267
vitamins, 6, 22, 155, 286, 434, 435–36
    A, 7, 11, 30, 42, 94, 210, 211, 284, 435
    B1, 435
    B2, 30, 435
    B3, 435
    B5, 435
    B6, 435
    B12, 92, 212, 435
    C, 6, 7, 24, 42, 57, 73, 74, 91, 209, 211, 283, 284, 286, 435–36
    D, 11, 92, 93, 436
    E, 7, 11, 74, 211, 284, 436
    folic acid, 435
    K, 436
    P, 286

waking your child, 128. See also sleep/wake cycle
walking, 98, 100, 103, 105, 107–8
warts, 396–97
water, 19–21, 23, 32, 58
water filters, 20–21, 32
weaning, 82–83
white noise, 123
whooping cough, 213, 214, 216, 220, 221, 397–98
winding down, 114, 122, 131, 135
working, part-time (child), 111
worms, 398

yoga, 103, 291–93

zinc, 16, 72, 210, 284, 437